Nursing in Care Homes

Nursing in Care Homes

Second edition

Linda Nazarko
RN, BSc (Hons), MSc, FRCN

Blackwell
Science

© Linda Nazarko, 1995, 2002

Blackwell Science Ltd, a Blackwell Publishing Company
Editorial Offices:
9600 Garsington Road, Oxford OX4 2DQ, UK
  Tel: +44 (0)1865 776868
Blackwell Science, Inc., 350 Main Street, Malden, MA 02148-5020, USA
  Tel: +1 781 388 8250
Iowa State Press, a Blackwell Publishing Company, 2121 State Avenue, Ames, Iowa 50014-8300, USA
  Tel: +1 515 292 0140
Blackwell Publishing Asia Pty Ltd, 550 Swanston Street, Carlton South, Melbourne, Victoria 3053, Australia
  Tel: +61 (0)3 9347 0300
Blackwell Wissenschafts Verlag, Kurfürstendamm 57, 10707 Berlin, Germany
  Tel: +49 (0)30 32 79 060

First edition published as *Nursing in Nursing Homes* 1995 by Blackwell Science Ltd
Reprinted 1996
This edition first published 2002
Reprinted 2003

Library of Congress
Cataloging-in-Publication Data
is available

ISBN 0-632-05226-0

A catalogue record for this title is available from the British Library

Set in 10/12 Souvenir Light
by DP Photosetting, Aylesbury, Bucks
Printed and bound in Great Britain by
MPG Books Ltd, Bodmin, Cornwall

For further information on
Blackwell Publishing, Visit our website:
www.blackwellpublishing.com

Dedication

To Ed, as always, for his help and encouragement and to Rachael and Sam

Contents

Preface

Nursing homes have come a long way in the last 20 years. They have moved from being an often ignored cottage industry to becoming an integral part of government's vision on health care. As you can see from Figure P.1 there are now more beds in the nursing home sector than there are in the NHS[1].

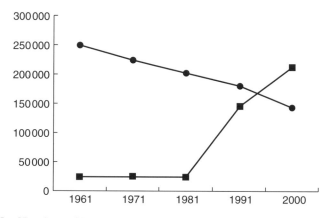

Fig. P.1   Number of beds in the NHS ● and nursing home sector ■.

As I write nursing homes are on the threshold of the greatest changes they have ever experienced, with a series of government initiatives being introduced. In April 2002 the Care Standards Act was introduced; now all homes are known as care homes – the legislation makes no mention of nursing homes. All homes will be regulated by a single body, the National Care Standards Commission. All homes will have to meet national minimum standards.

Older people in differing UK countries are now eligible for different levels of assistance with nursing home care. In England nursing home residents who fund their own care are being paid an allowance towards the care delivered by registered nurses, this allowance is only paid after assessment. In Wales residents receive a non-means tested allowance if they are self-funding. In Scotland nursing home residents are to receive a large contribution towards the costs of nursing and personal care.

In the past, people with continence problems who lived in residential homes had pads supplied by the NHS, but people who lived in nursing homes did not. This situation is now changing and people with nursing needs will be entitled to free incontinence pads.

The Department of Health insist that nursing homes are separate from the NHS but the people who are cared for in homes receive NHS care from General Practitioners (GPs) and other NHS staff either in primary care or within hospitals. Changes to primary care such as Primary Care Trusts will impact on the care nursing home residents receive. New initiatives such as the National Service Framework for Older People outline primary care targets for GPs and identify good practice. GPs will implement this guidance for all of their older patients and targets such as reducing the risk of falls are particularly relevant within nursing homes.

In the 1990s the NHS underwent considerable change – nursing homes quietly developed as nurse led units. Now nursing homes are about to undergo far-reaching change because of new regulation and changes to the way NHS services are delivered.

This second edfition of the book (previously called *Nursing in Nursing Homes*) aims to guide you through the new regulations and to update your knowledge of key issues in the care of older people. It aims to enable you to continue to care for older people in a sensitive and humane way and to offer holistic care. It aims to help you to use research and good practice to provide high quality care.

Nursing in Care Homes has been written so that each chapter is self-contained, giving the information on a particular topic in one place without the reader having to flick between chapters to find all the aspects of the subject. Each chapter also has its own references and further information. Each chapter can thus be used to update your knowledge, or as the basis for further study or teaching sessions. I hope that this approach works for you and I would appreciate comments and feedback.

Nursing remains crucially important to an older person's quality of life. It makes the difference between an older person living life to the full in the remaining months or years of life or feeling as if life is not worth living. It is a real privilege to be able to make a difference and I hope that this book will help you to avoid some of the pitfalls of nursing home nursing and enjoy the rewards.

If you have any suggestions or comments you can send these to linda.nazarko@blueyonder.co.uk

Reference

[1] Department of Health (2000) Shaping the Future NHS: Long Term Planning for Hospitals and Related Services. Consultation Document on the Findings of the National Beds Enquiry. Department of Health, London. This document can be found on the Internet at: http://www.doh.gov.uk/pub/docs/doh/nationalbeds.pdf

Chapter 1

The Legal Framework

Introduction

In April 2002 the legislation that homes in England must meet in order to remain registered changed. The Registered Homes Act of 1984 was repealed and the Care Standards Act 2000 was enacted[1].

This chapter aims to enable you to:

- Understand the main provisions of the Care Standards Act
- Understand how these changes will affect the way homes are regulated
- Be aware of how inspection will change
- Understand the role of the National Care Standards Commission
- Develop an understanding of national minimum standards

The Care Standards Act 2000

The Care Standards Act was introduced in April 2002. It replaced the Registered Homes Act 1984. It aims to end the current fragmented and muddled regulation and the differing standards that health authorities and local authorities use to regulate care. The Care Standards Act does not just apply to nursing and residential homes. It is a massive piece of legislation regulating:

- Children's homes
- Independent hospitals and clinics
- Care homes
- Residential family centres
- Independent medical agencies
- Nurses' agencies
- Voluntary adoption agencies

The Act also:

- Regulates and inspects local authority fostering and adoption agencies
- Establishes a General Social Care Council in England and a Care Council for Wales
- Makes provision for the registration, regulation and training of social care workers
- Establishes a children's commissioner for Wales
- Makes provision for the registration, regulation and training of those providing childminding or day care

- Makes provision for the protection of children and vulnerable adults
- Amends the law about children looked after in schools and colleges

The Act has 123 sections in nine parts and one supplement. The relevant sections are outlined in the rest of this chapter.

Regulation of homes

Under the old system, residential and nursing homes were inspected and regulated separately. Dual registered homes were inspected by two different bodies and expected to comply with different standards. Under the old system local authorities were providers, purchasers and inspectors of residential homes.

National Care Standards Commission

The Care Standards Act establishes the National Care Standards Commission. The Commission takes over from the 95 health authorities and 150 local authorities that currently carry out inspection. This means that one independent body inspects all homes to the same standards. Homes will no longer be inspected by different authorities to different standards. The National Care Standards Commission will inspect to national standards.

How the National Care Standards Commission functions

The National Care Standards Commission (NCSC) is based in Newcastle. It has a chair who works 1–2 days a week. A full time chief executive, Anne Parker (formerly of the Carers National Association), has been appointed. A board consisting of 14 members drives the Care Standards Commission forward. The board consists of lay and non-lay members. Non-lay members are providers or purchasers of health or social care. Lay members have knowledge and/or experience of the sector and of change management and methods of evaluating performance. Box 1.1 outlines the functions of the NCSC.

The work of the NCSC can be divided into four main areas:

(1) Inspection and regulation
(2) Improving the quality of services
(3) Providing information and investigating complaints
(4) Informing and advising government on the range and quality of care services.

Legislative timetable and infrastructure

In April 2002 the Care Standards Act was introduced and old legislation such as the Registered Homes Act 1984 was repealed. Shadow inspection teams developed to the infrastructure for the National Care Standards Commission between April 2001 and April 2002. There are eight area offices. Each area office has a regional director and support services. The NCSC has around 2500 staff. Most have transferred from old inspector

Box 1.1   Functions of the NCSC.

- Advise the secretary of state how to establish offices in specific areas or regions. Inspectors currently work out of 800 offices and the Commission hopes to reduce this.
- Organise staff into divisions. Currently local authority and health authority staff work in separate offices and have their own management structure. The Commission will integrate these structures and establish a new management structure.
- Inform the secretary of state about the availability of provision and the quality of services. The availability of homes varies from area to area. Some areas are well provided for whilst others have an underprovision. The Commission will monitor this, the first time such monitoring has happened. The quality of services varies and the Commission will have a responsibility to monitor quality. It is likely that this will involve introducing a quality audit tool at some time in the near future.
- Encourage improvement of quality and services. This will require the adoption of a nationally recognised quality audit tool.
- Advise the secretary of state on changes required to improve quality. This may involve benchmarking and setting standards.

posts. CCETSW, the Central Council for Education and Training in Social Work, are setting up a post qualification award in inspection, and inspectors will, for the first time, have a relevant qualification.

Regulation of care workers

The Care Standards Act sets up mechanisms to regulate care assistants. They are to be known as 'social care workers'. The Act defines a social care worker as 'a person engaged in the provision of personal care for any person'.

In England social care workers are regulated by the General Social Care Council, and in Wales by the Care Council for Wales. Moves to educate and regulate care assistants are welcome. The precise definitions of a social care worker are:

- Engaged in relevant social work 'social work required in connection with any health, education or social services provided by any person'
- Employed at a children's home, care home or on the premises of an agency
- Supplied by a domiciliary care agency to provide personal care in their own homes for people with a disability, infirmity or illness or who are unable to provide it for themselves.

The following people could also be included in the definition 'social care worker':

- Persons engaged in work for social services
- Persons employed as inspectors of children's homes.

Registration

Social care workers are required to register with either the English or Welsh Council. Each council is required to promote high standards of conduct and practice and promote high standards of training. Each council is required to maintain a register of social care workers. In order to register, social care workers must meet the following conditions:

- Is of good character
- Is physically and mentally fit to perform the work
- Satisfies any rules imposed
- Satisfies training requirements.

Each council will maintain a list of unsuitable persons.

Conduct

Registered Social Care Workers (RSCWS) must abide by a code of conduct. RSCWS will abide by occupational standards – these are to be drawn up by the relevant councils. RSCWS will be required to meet practice standards. RSCWS will meet initial and ongoing training requirements. A person who breaches standards of conduct, practice or the code of conduct will be called to a hearing. If the charges are proven the person may be suspended or removed from the register. There are provisions for restoring people to the register.

The general social care council for England and the care council for Wales will approve courses and make grants and allowances for training. It is not clear if nurses working in homes would be able to access such grants.

Management of homes

Government will require all managers of homes to have relevant management qualifications by 2004. The minimum qualification will be an NVQ level 4 in management or a recognised management qualification. Nurses with relevant expertise and qualifications should be able to use systems such as APL (Acreditation of prior learning) and APEL (Acreditation for prior experiential learning) to help enable them to gain qualifications. This requirement has far reaching implications for homes and nurse managers. For the first time nursing home managers will be required to have a management qualification and experience in working with older people in homes.

These standards will have cost and time implications. Already advertisements for managers are stating that candidates with NVQ level 4 in management are preferred. Who will be expected to fund management qualifications? The introduction of management qualifications will reduce the available pool of managers and increase wage costs – what resources will be made available to meet these increased costs? What will happen if a home is unable to recruit a suitably qualified manager?

Powers of inspection

Homes are required to comply with national minimum standards. These were released in draft form as *Fit for the Future* (1999)[2]. The final standards have now been released. The Minister for Health will have the power to review and amend these standards at any time. Government consider national minimum standards to be a floor below which no home can fall. Government plan to raise standards over a period of time. Many nurses are anxious about what they fear may be a process of continual change.

The Care Standards Act gives regulators a greater range of powers. These powers are:

- Require manager to provide any information concerning the establishment that the inspector requires
- Inspect at any time
- Make any examination into the state of management of the premises and treatment of persons cared for
- Inspect and take copies of records
- Interview manager in private
- Interview person cared for in private if the person consents
- Examine person cared for if the person consents, to ensure the person is receiving proper care; only doctors and nurses may examine the person cared for
- Inspect any medical records
- Seize and remove any document or material thing when there are reasonable grounds to believe that this may be evidence of failure to comply with any condition
- Take such measurements and photographs or recordings as he considers necessary
- Access computer records.

Individual rights

The Act gives inspectors the right to interview any manager, member of staff or resident privately. Managers, staff and residents could feel intimidated by such an interview – the Act does not specify that the person being interviewed has the right to a friend, advocate or supporter.

Offences

The Act specifies offences and lays down penalties for failure to comply with the Act. Offences are:

- Managing an establishment without being registered
- Failure to comply with any condition
- Guilty of an offence under the regulations
- False statements
- Intent to deceive
- Failure to display registration certificate.

Inspectors will have the right to apply conditions to registration, for example they may specify that a particular door is kept locked. The Act lays down penalties for offences. If the manager (or presumably someone who the manager is responsible for) breaches the Act, the manager may be fined up to £5000 or even imprisoned for six months.

National minimum standards

Two years after government released the consultation document *Fit for the Future*, national minimum standards have been released. The responses to *Fit for the Future* have been incorporated into the new National Minimum Standards for Care Homes for Older People.[3] These standards are the *minimum* standards that homes must meet in order to retain registration. The Care Standards Act gives the secretary of state the power to introduce new standards at any time without any further legislation.

Government have announced 38 standards, each with a number of elements. These standards cover seven areas:

(1) Choice of home
(2) Health and personal care
(3) Daily life and social activities
(4) Complaints and protection
(5) Environmental standards
(6) Staffing
(7) Management and administration.

Choice of home

Standards 1 to 6 concern the choice of home. These standards make it clear that the home must justify claims to have the ability to care for a specific client group. If a home claims to care for people with dementia it must clearly state what specific features of care and facilities meet the needs of older people with dementia; for example, if you provide a multisensory room this must be stated in the literature provided to residents. If the manager or other staff have specialist training in dementia care this must be stated. It is not clear what the implications would be of stating that you have a level of expertise and then having key staff leave.

Standard 1
Standard 1 requires homes to produce a statement of purpose setting out the aims, objectives, philosophy of care services and facilities. The home must provide a 'service users guide' written in plain English. The required content of the service users guide is:

- Description of accommodation and services
- Relevant qualifications and experience of the registered manager, provider and staff
- Number of places and special needs or interests cared for
- Copy of most recent inspection report
- Copy of complaints procedure
- Copy of residents' survey
- Information on how to contact the Care Standards Commission, social services and the local authority.

Each home will have to prepare a service users guide. Copies of this could be made available at a central point in the home. The costs of developing and providing such detailed information are substantial. Inspection reports can be 30–40 pages long. It is unclear what the legal position is if you prepare information and some aspect of it becomes outdated.

Standard 2
Standard 2 relates to providing the resident with a contract. The contract must state the room to be occupied, and the resident is issued with details of rights and obligations. The only potential problems relate to moving a resident from one room to another.

Standard 3
Standard 3 requires the home to carry out comprehensive assessment using 13 care categories including falls and continence promotion. Homes must carry out a comprehensive assessment prior to admitting a resident. This is good practice but could prove difficult in certain circumstances. If the person is in Liverpool and wishes to enter a home in London to be near relatives, how will assessments be carried out? What will happen in the case of emergency admissions? The home is (for the first time) legally required to maintain care plans. This has long been good practice but has never been a legal requirement.

Standard 4
Standard 4 requires the home to demonstrate its ability to meet assessed needs and to deliver care that is based on good practice and clinical guidance.

New standards such as *Good Practice in Continence Services*[4] must be adhered to. New standards such as those on prescribing and older people contained in the *National Service Framework for Older People*[5] must be met. Failure to meet such standards could result in loss of registration.

Standard 5
Standard 5 specifies that homes should offer trial visits, and this standard should present few problems. There are provisions for emergency admissions.

Standard 6
Standard 6 relates to intermediate care and is an important standard for homes. The main requirements are:

- Dedicated facilities must be provided for intermediate care
- Rehabiltation facilities must have equipment for therapies and treatment
- Staff have appropriate classifications and training to deliver intermediate care
- Specialist services are provided in sufficient numbers and delivered by competent and skilled professionals
- Intermediate care residents are not admitted to long-term care unless appropriate assessment has taken place.

This standard is significant. Intermediate care (short term care aimed at discharging the individual back to their normal place of residence) is only beginning to come on stream and most contracts are short term and small scale. This standard effectively restricts provision of intermediate care to providers who have the ability to provide dedicated units and specially trained staff. There is a danger that homes will find it impossible to provide such services in the absence of long-term block contracts. Providers may be unwilling to contract with small homes. In such circumstances people could have no option but to move to a corporate home that has a block contract for intermediate care.

Health and personal care

Standards 7 to 11 relate to health and personal care. The aim of these standards is to improve the level of record keeping, assessment and care planning within the home. It is clear that inspectors will use care assessments and care plans to make judgements on the quality of care delivered within the home. These standards make it essential that nurses plan and document care accurately.

Standard 7
Standard 7 duplicates and reiterates standards 3 and 4. Additional requirements are:

- Care plan must detail actions to meet assessed need
- Care plan must meet relevant clinical guidelines
- A risk assessment in relation to prevention of falls must be carried out
- Care plan must be reviewed at least once a month to reflect changing needs
- Care plan must be drawn up in consultation with resident
- Care plan must be accessible to resident
- Care plan must be signed by resident if capable; if not capable must be signed by representative.

This standard is significant. Registered nurses do not generally excel at record keeping. Homes will need to spend significant amounts of time training and supervising staff to ensure that these standards are met. Some residents need their care plans to be updated monthly but others have needs that remain unchanged for years. This standard will increase the time nurses spend completing paperwork and it risks removing them further from the bedside. NHS staff are not required to meet such standards. The issue of preventing falls is becoming more important – this is also emphasised in the National Service Framework for Older People.

Standard 8
Standard 8 is a comprehensive standard relating to maintaining health. The issue of assessing pressure sore risk and prevention and treatment of pressure sores is emphasised. The issue of preventing falls is again emphasised. Homes are required to carry out comprehensive nutritional assessments and to take appropriate action to prevent malnutrition.

These standards are significant in that for the first time homes will be inspected not only on the basis of the facilities they provide but also the quality of care they deliver. Eventually the information held in assessments and care plans will be used to benchmark homes. This means that each home will be measured against others, and its ability to prevent pressure sores, malnutrition, incontinence, falls and other negative care outcomes will be available to the public. This level of scrutiny is unprecedented and provides a real impetus to improve care. Homes that are unable to deliver positive outcomes of care will find it much more difficult to maintain occupancy.

There is a danger though that homes will 'cherry pick' residents to enable them to meet standards. As the number of homes falls, those that remain will find that demand exceeds supply. So homes will be able to choose who to admit. If a person is immobile and has a pressure sore, a home may be reluctant to admit them. If a person is incontinent and has dementia the home may be reluctant to admit them because the presence of dementia makes continence promotion difficult. If a person has Parkinson's disease and a history of falls the home may fear increasing its fall rating by admitting them. When benchmarking is eventually introduced results will have to be interpreted with great sensitivity to prevent such problems.

Standard 9

Standard 9 relates to medication and states that the registered person will ensure that there are suitable procedures for receiving and handling medicines (see Chapter 4).

Standard 10

Standard 10 relates to privacy and dignity when health care and personal care are delivered, and it merely reflects current good practice.

Standard 11

Standard 11 relates to death and dying. It specifically states that the person should be able to die in his or her own room unless there are strong medical reasons to prevent this. It merely reflects current good practice. Residential homes may find it difficult to meet this standard because of staffing implications. There is no mention of providing increased resources if the home has a number of people who are dying. It is possible that regulators will increase staffing requirements in such circumstances, but that homes will lack the resources to meet increased levels of need.

Daily life and social activities

These standards demand that the home comply with good practice in relation to dignity and choice.

Standard 12

Standard 12 requires homes to demonstrate that routines and activities of daily living are flexible and reflect the needs and aspirations of residents. For example, a home that forced residents to rise at 6AM would not meet this standard. A home where staff stated that every resident chose to rise at 6AM would not meet the standard. The only way to demonstrate that you meet this standard is to specifically state the person's preferences on their care plan. The care plan should state, 'Mrs Jones wishes to get up at 7:30AM . . . She prefers to shower rather than bathe. She prefers to shower before breakfast or in the evening'.

Standard 13

Standard 13 requires homes to offer open visiting, which is standard practice. Visitors and friends are to be given written information about the home's policy on maintaining their involvement. This standard will be easily met.

Standard 14

Standard 14 requires homes to enable residents to manage their own affairs, have access to advocates and bring personal possessions to the home. Residents are to have access to their personal records. This means that staff must be careful how they document care and complete daily records. Imagine how you would feel if you read 'Difficult and demanding' in your records. Nurses will have to write carefully and use examples to back up their assertions. For example, 'Mrs Jones appears anxious and needs lots of help to settle into the home. Rang the call bell ten times this afternoon wanting someone to sit with her'.

Standard 15

Standard 15 relates to meals and nutrition. Most of this merely reflects good practice. The items that may require attention are:

- Intervals between meals must be no more than five hours
- The time between the last meal and breakfast should be no more than 12 hours.

If you live in your own home and decide to eat dinner at 7PM, lie in and have breakfast at 10AM the next day, that is fine, but in care homes it is contrary to national minimum standards.

Complaints and protection

Standards 16 and 17 relate to complaints and protection. Most of these merely reflect good practice. The items that may require attention are:

- Complaints procedure should state who deals with the complaint and must give details of how to refer a complaint to the National Care Standards Commission
- Complaints must be responded to within 28 days.

Protection

Standard 18

Standard 18 requires homes to protect residents from abuse and to have policies that state this. A whistle-blowing policy is required. The home must comply with *No Secrets* guidance on prevention and protection of vulnerable adults from abuse. Further details of this are given in Chapter 9.

Environment

Standards 19 to 26 deal with the physical environment of the home.

Standard 19
Standard 19 relates to maintenance and will cause few problems.

Standard 20
Standard 20, the most controversial of the standards, has been considerably diluted in the consultation process. The time-scales have also been extended. The requirements can be summarised as:

- Communal space of $4.1\,m^2$ per resident by 2007 for existing homes
- Total of $14.1\,m^2$ of space provided per resident. If room is larger than $10\,m^2$, communal space can be reduced to 3.7
- Outdoor space accessible to wheelchair users.

Standard 21
Standard 21 details toilet, washing and bathing facilities. From 1 April 2002 all newly-built extensions and first time registrations must have a minimum of an en suite toilet and washbasin. En suite facilities are provided in addition to minimum space requirements in the person's room.

Standard 22
Standard 22 deals with assessment of facilities by suitably qualified persons including an occupational therapist to ensure adaptations are made to enable residents to function to capacity. This specifically refers to adaptations to meet the needs of people with dementia.

In practice few homes employ occupational therapists. There is a national shortage of occupational therapists and community resources are limited. Many NHS community trusts concentrate on using occupational therapists to enable people to remain at home. People living in homes are considered low priority for assessments and services.

Standard 23
Newly-built and adapted rooms must be $12\,m^2$ by April 2002. All single rooms must be at least $10\,m^2$ by April 2007 and by that date 80% of rooms must be single rooms. Single rooms accommodating wheelchair users must have at least $12\,m^2$ of usable floor space. National minimum standards do not define a wheelchair user. This means that we do not know if an immobile person is classified as a wheelchair user. If all people who are immobile are classified as wheelchair users then 78% of new rooms should meet the $12\,m^2$ standard.

Standards 24, 25 and 26
Standards 24, 25 and 26 detail furnishings, heating and hygiene requirements and are not problematic.

Implications of physical standards

The most significant and unclear standard is that wheelchair users must have rooms with $12\,m^2$ of floor space. As the standards do not define what a wheelchair user is it may be left to individual inspectors to try to determine what the standard really means. Hopefully the NCSC will issue guidance to clarify this issue.

The costs of adapting and changing rooms so that each meets new physical standards may be significant and are certain to force the closure of some homes. There is evidence that individual providers are closing homes and providers with more than one home are closing smaller homes. This is because when some homes, especially smaller homes, have been reconfigured, it is no longer possible to run them cost effectively.

Staffing

Standards 27, 28, 29 and 30 deal with staffing matters, the most significant of which are:

- 50% of care assistants to have NVQ level 2 qualifications by 2005
- 50% of agency care assistants to have NVQ level 2 by 2005
- Formal recruitment, references and police checks for volunteers
- Formal recruitment, references and police checks for staff
- Formal six month induction for staff
- Three paid training days a year for all staff.

The implications of these standards are far-reaching. The standards will considerably add to the costs of providing care. Meeting a 50% NVQ target within four years will be difficult for many homes and may prove too expensive for some providers, who will leave the market. Some government assistance with costs of NVQ training has been announced.

Management and administration

Standards 31–38 deal with the management and administration of the home. The only one that may be difficult for most homes is standard 31, the qualifications and competency of the registered manager. The key points are that the manager must:

- Have at least two years experience in senior management in a relevant care setting. This will mean that managers become more sought after and will be able to command higher salaries
- Have an NVQ level 4 or equivalent qualification in management by 2005

- Be a first level nurse if the home is registered for nursing
- Have expertise in caring for older people.

It is unclear what the situation would be if the registered manager left and the home could not find a suitable manager.

Conclusion

Government healthcare policy is changing rapidly. The National Care Standards Commission took over responsibility for regulating care homes on 1 April 2002. On 18 April 2002 the Secretary of State for Health announced plans to merge the National Care Standards Commission, the Audit Commission and the Commission for Health Improvement to form the Commission for Healthcare Audit and Inspection. At the time of writing the date of this merger has not been announced.

The aim of national minimum standards was to provide a clear regulatory framework that ensured that all homes were regulated to the same standards. It now appears that some standards will be applied nationally but others will vary from region to region. The costs of providing care will rise but there are no indications that government intends to provide additional resources to meet these costs. In the short term the introduction of national minimum standards will lead to a reduction in the number of homes.

Further information

The National Care Standards Commission have a useful website: http://www.doh.gov.uk/ncsc/index.htm

References

[1] Care Standards Act 2000. The Stationery Office, London. Copies can be obtained from: The Stationery Office, PO Box 29, Norwich NR3 1GN. Order through the Parliamentary Hotline Lo-call: 0845 7 023474. Fax orders: 0870 600 5533. E-mail: book.orders@theso.co.uk website: http://www.ukstate.com
[2] Department of Health (1999) *Fit for the Future?* Department of Health, London.
[3] Department of Health (2001) *National Minimum Standards for Care Homes for Older People*. The Stationery Office (details above). Also available on the Department of Health website: http://www.doh.gov.uk/ncsc
[4] Department of Health (2000) *Good Practice in Continence Services*. Department of Health, London.
[5] Department of Health (2001) *National Service Framework for Older People*. Department of Health, London.

Chapter 2

Needs Assessment and Funding Care

Introduction

Ten years ago needs assessment had not been invented and funding was fairly straightforward. Now a range of government iniatives and national variations have made everything more complex. Increasingly older people and their families turn to nurses for advice.

This chapter aims to:

- Explain the background to recent policy changes
- Outline current assessment criterion
- Examine new developments
- Update your knowledge of funding
- Explain about national variations in funding

In the 1980s the long stay hospitals that once provided care for older people who required nursing care were closed. The number of places in nursing homes increased dramatically and in 1988 there were for the first time more beds in nursing homes than in NHS geriatric hospitals. Figure 2.1 illustrates

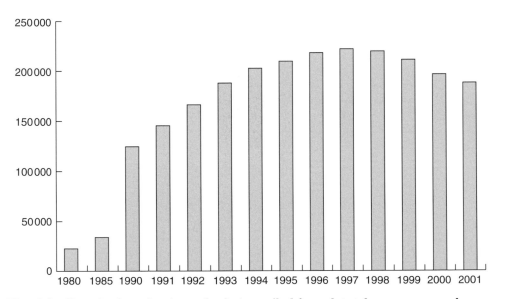

Fig. 2.1 Growth of nursing home beds (compiled from data taken over several years, the most recent being *Care of Older People* (2001) by Laing & Buisson, London).

the growth in nursing home beds. As the number of nursing home beds increased the costs of providing nursing care also rose. The government of the day asked Sir Roy Griffiths to examine the way nursing and residential care was provided. In 1990, as a result of his advice, the NHS and Community Care Act was passed.

The Community Care Act

The Community Care Act was introduced in England, Scotland and Wales in 1993. This gave social services departments in local authorities 'lead responsibility' to assess older people's needs for care. Local authorities were also given budgets to enable them to purchase that care from providers in the independent and voluntary sector. Local authorities had a number of roles:

- Providing care in local authority run homes
- Purchasing from independent sector
- Assessing need for car
- Inspecting residential homes to determine their ability to provide care
- Determining fees for care.

Local authorities were inspectors, assessors of need, providers and purchasers of care. Soon problems developed. Social services departments developed individual assessment criteria to determine whether a person required nursing or residential care. There were concerns that assessment criteria focused more on the person's ability to pay for care rather than the care required[1]. There were also concerns that social services assessment criteria did not meet government standards. Research shown in Figure 2.2 confirmed this[2]. There were also concerns that inadequate assessment and eligibility criteria were preventing older people from receiving the right level of care in the right home[3]. People who required nursing care were being

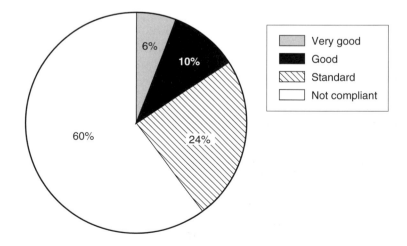

Fig. 2.2   Quality of local authority eligibility criteria. Data from Challis *et al.* 1997[2].

sent to residential homes[4]. People who required complex packages of care were being provided for without reference to district nurses or GPs. An influential report by the Clinical Standards Advisory Group found that 'care packages are financially driven rather than needs led, inappropriate decisions placing people needing nursing care in residential homes rather than nursing homes because it is cheaper[5]'.

The system of community care was discredited and following the 1997 general election the Labour government set up a Royal Commission to examine the funding of long-term care.

The Royal Commission on the funding of long-term care

In the past older people requiring continuing care were cared for in hospital, in long stay geriatric units. The standard of care was often poor and staffing levels were often abysmally low. The standard of accommodation was very poor by today's standards. People were cared for in the old 'Nightingale style' wards. There was little in the way of recreation. But nobody paid. If you needed continuing care you were admitted to a geriatric hospital and the state met your needs. Nursing homes were a very small part of the continuing care sector. Nursing home care was mostly restricted to those who had the means to purchase continuing care. It was a little like private education: you could have it if you wanted to or could afford to but there were always the state schools.

In the 1980s all that changed. Firstly, social security changes made it possible for people of modest means to enter nursing homes. People voted with their feet and nursing homes boomed. The geriatric hospitals were largely closed down and then the problems began. Nursing home care was means tested. If you had more than the income support threshold, you had no option but to pay. That meant spending your life savings and selling your house. Every year 40 000 people were forced to sell their house to pay for nursing or residential home care.

The Royal Commission was asked to examine the options for sustainable funding of long-term care for elderly people, bearing in mind the expectations of older people for dignity and security. Privately, government acknowledged that the current system was a nightmare. Why bother to save for your old age if you would have to spend every penny funding care in your old age? The aim was that the Commission examine ways to fund long-term care.

How the Royal Commission investigated the problem

The Royal Commission held regional meetings throughout the UK to hear the views of the public. The Commission also heard evidence from nurses, and groups such as Age Concern, the Royal College of Nursing and the Alzheimer's Society.

Recommendations of the Royal Commission

Three volumes of commissioned research evidence accompanied the Royal Commission report, which weighed 4 kg[6]. The main recommendations are:

- Free personal care for people living in nursing and residential homes
- Means testing the 'hotel services' element of care
- Increasing the eligibility threshold for means testing to £40 000
- Separating the assessment and purchasing aspects of nursing and residential care
- Establishment of a national care commission to monitor trends including demography and spending and to ensure transparency and accountability; and to set national standards now and in the future
- Enable more people to stay at home
- Increased availability of rehabilitation services
- Allow each individual 12 weeks grace to enable them to recover before a decision is made to place permanently in nursing or residential care.

Minority report
Two members of the Royal Commission disagreed with the report and published a note of dissent that is appended to the report. The dissenters stated that they felt that the NHS should only meet the costs of providing the care delivered by registered nurses and not that delivered by care assistants. They estimated that the registered nurse component of nursing care could be delivered for around £100 a week.

Government response to the Royal Commission
The government response to the Royal Commission report was published a year later[7]. The main points are:

- NHS to pay only for the care delivered by a registered nurse
- Value of person's home disregarded for the first 12 weeks of admission to homes
- Older people no longer forced to sell their homes to pay for care. Loans schemes to enable older people to borrow money from the council and the loan to be paid back when the person dies
- Residential allowance premiums that encouraged placement in independent sector homes abolished in April 2002
- National Commission for Care Standards established.

The importance of assessment

Assessment becomes crucial under national minimum standards. Managers are responsible for ensuring that they can deliver the appropriate level of care to the resident. If the person requires nursing care he or she should not be admitted to a residential bed where this care is not available. If the person requires specialist care because of mental illness it would be inappropriate to admit them to a non-specialist nursing home staffed by nurses who lack qualifications in mental health. The person with dementia may require care in a residential home, a nursing home or a dementia unit but it is rarely possible to determine this merely by talking with family or a social worker.

Many homes now offer both residential and nursing care. Assessment enables you to work out what level of care the person requires and decide which part of the home that care can be delivered in. Assessment enables you to meet the person, find out what specialist equipment and what level of care is required, and decide if you can meet those needs.

Case history

According to the referral letter Mrs Dora Johnston's needs could easily be met in the home and little specialist equipment was required. When Sarah Orem carried out the assessment she found that Mrs Johnston had complex care needs. Mrs Johnston was an overweight lady who had suffered a severe stroke. She was depressed and not able to help nursing staff to move her. She had severe pain that was unresponsive to analgesia. The only way to control the pain was to change Mrs Johnston's position hourly. Mrs Johnston liked to sit out of bed but had fallen out of her chair on many occasions because of poor posture and muscle control following stroke. She had pressure sores to her sacrum and heels that required daily dressings. Mrs Johnston also required supervision while eating because of swallowing difficulties.

In order to meet Mrs Johnston's needs the home needed to supply an electric bed, an alternating pressure mattress replacement, a special chair and additional slings for the hoist. The referral letter gave no indication of these requirements or the relative's expectation that they be supplied. If Sarah had not carried out an assessment, Mrs Johnston could have been admitted without appropriate equipment and without appropriate funding levels having been agreed.

The aim of assessment is to enable nurses to meet the person and to check if the home can meet that person's care needs. Sometimes the home will not be willing or able to meet an individual's care needs and will decline to admit. Older people and their families can choose homes but homes can also choose which residents to admit and which not to admit. In the past, homes have tended to adopt a policy of 'if in doubt admit'. National minimum standards place increased emphasis on the home being able to provide for specific client groups and sometimes homes will have to decline to admit certain individuals because the individual has specialist care requirements. Sometimes homes will decline to admit a person because the person's behaviour could affect the quality of life of other residents living in the home. Sometimes staff within the home do not have the skills to meet that person's care needs.

Nurses sometimes feel upset when they decline to admit a person – they feel inadequate because they feel they ought to be able to care for every person who seeks a place. Sometimes social workers, hospital staff and relatives are angry and rude if you decline to accept a possible resident. It is important to be realistic about the level of care you can offer. Nursing homes are just that; they are not acute general or psychiatric hospitals. Nursing homes normally care for frail older people. Nursing homes are ill equipped to care for acutely ill older people requiring high levels of specialist care and high levels of medical input. Nursing homes are also ill equipped to care for people with acute mental health problems requiring specialist care. Under national minimum standards, the manager will be required to demonstrate staff ability to care for people with specialist care needs.

The single assessment process

At the moment local authorities assess a person's needs for care using local assessment criteria. This means that an older person in Bournemouth may have different access to community care services and to a bed in a care home than an older person in Bolton. Current assessment criteria are inequitable and unfair because they treat people differently depending on where they live. The assessment criteria for social services do not match up with the assessment criteria for continuing care paid for by the NHS, so people can find that they fall between the gaps in services. The Department of Health is now working with professional groups to develop national assessment criteria so that all older people receive coherent assessment that enables them to access care.

Funding care

At present continuing care remains means tested. If an older person meets the local health authority's continuing care criteria she is entitled to have all the costs of care met by the health authority. In the future, Primary Care Trusts will hold 75% of the NHS budget and will be responsible for commissioning all NHS services. Health authorities are to be abolished and 28 strategic health authorities will be created. Primary Care Trusts will take over many of the functions of health authorities in the near future and funding arrangements will change. At the moment, although there are many highly dependent residents in nursing beds who appear to meet continuing care criteria, health authorities fund few of them.

People who have savings above income support levels have to pay for their care. In order to qualify for local authority support in meeting nursing home or residential care costs a person must have capital of £19 000 or below. Capital includes the value of a previously occupied property subject to the following rules.

Disregarded property

Property to be disregarded will include:

- The value of a resident's dwelling if their stay in residential care or nursing home is temporary and they intend to return to the dwelling and the dwelling is still available to them
- Only one dwelling can be disregarded in these circumstances.

Where the resident's stay is regarded as *permanent* their former dwelling can be disregarded for 12 weeks, or totally if it is occupied in whole or part by:

- The resident's former partner (who is not estranged or divorced from the resident)
- A relative of the resident who is aged over 60 or is incapacitated.

The local authority also has the discretion to ignore the property in special circumstances, for example if it is the sole residence of a previous carer of the resident who gave up their home in order to care for the resident. In such circumstances the property will be taken into account if the carer were to die or move out. The benefits agency does not have this discretion for income support purposes.

Jointly owned property

Where a property is jointly owned by the resident and another person whose joint ownership does not enable the property to be disregarded as above, the local authority will take the resident's share into account. However, in doing so it is the value of that interest which is taken into account bearing in mind:

- The resident's ability to re-assign the beneficial interest to somebody else
- There being a market, i.e. the property is saleable.

It may well be construed that because a joint owner has a right to occupy the property it is unlikely that there would be a willing buyer prepared to share in that right to occupy it. The only person who may be interested in purchasing the share would therefore be the joint owner and effectively the 'market value' could be nil. Legal advice should be sought in these circumstances.

The rules for income support purposes are very similar in this respect. Following a Commissioner's decision (CIS/15936/1996) it was held that the valuation of jointly owned property should be based on the actual market value of the claimant's share, and this value may depend on whether there would be a willing buyer of the claimant's interest in the property. If there is a disparity between how the local authority and the benefits agency value the property, which results in the resident not being entitled to the income support element contributing towards their care costs, the amount to be paid by the local authority is that much more. Where the local authority is unsure about the resident's share, or their valuation is disputed by the resident, a professional valuation should be obtained. The name on the deeds of property should establish ownership; however, if ownership is disputed and a resident's interest is alleged to be less than seems apparent from initial information, the local authority will require written evidence on any beneficial interest that the resident or other parties possess.

12-week property disregard

This is effective for all people who enter care homes permanently after 9 April 2001. The local authority will disregard the value of property for 12 weeks and residents will only have to contribute their assessed income less £16.80 personal expenses towards the care home fees. To be eligible for this funding:

- The resident must be assessed as needing *permanent* residential accommodation which can be in either a local authority or an independent care home
- Other capital apart from the value of the property must be below £19 000 and income must be inadequate to meet the full cost of the care.

The 12-week property disregard is mandatory and local authorities are under a statutory obligation to apply it once they are aware of a resident to whom it applies. Delays by local authorities in providing this funding do not affect the resident's entitlement to it and could render them liable to reimburse residents who have consequently paid a higher contribution towards their care costs than they should have during this mandatory disregard period.

NHS nursing care contribution

Residents of nursing homes entitled to a contribution towards their nursing care from the NHS will undergo an assessment for the NHS contribution, which will be paid after the twelve-week property disregard period has expired. During the 12-week disregard period the difference between the local authority's standard rate for the nursing home fees and the resident's assessed charge will be met by the local authority. This is explored in greater detail later in this chapter.

Top-ups for more expensive accommodation

Local authorities would normally pay only their standard rate for accommodation, which is likely to be less than care homes normally charge. In these circumstances residents entitled to the 12-week property disregard will be entitled to top up the local authority contribution from disregarded income, earnings or capital with the proviso that:

- The top-up during the 12-week period must not exceed the lower capital limit, i.e. at the time of writing £11 750 (equivalent to £979.16 per week)
- The level of tariff income assessed (at the time of writing, £1 for each £250 of capital between £11 750 and £19 000) remains the same even though the capital may reduce as a result of topping-up during the 12-week period.

Beyond the 12-week period – the deferred payments agreement

From 1 October 2001 individuals who have not been able to or do not wish to sell their homes to pay for their care may enter into a deferred payments agreement with the local authority. The contribution from the local authority will be secured against the value of their property. This facility is open to those who do not wish to or cannot sell their home and where their other assets are less than the upper capital limits and their income is not sufficient to cover their fees. Local authorities have discretion over whether to operate this scheme, for example they may not wish to enter into an agreement whereby the cost of the chosen care may not be affordable by the individual over the long term.

The possible advantages of an individual accepting a deferred payments agreement are that any growth in the property value will contribute towards the loan, they may be able to let the property and contribute the income towards the fees and the decision to sell the property can be deferred while all options are being considered. However, there are also possible disadvantages, for example:

- The loan is only deferring a liability repayable from the eventual proceeds of the property
- The property will require maintaining and insuring
- Letting property can often be troublesome and rental income is taxable
- The level of local authority funding may restrict the choice of accommodation unless a top-up is affordable over the long term
- Interest will accrue on the loan 56 days after the resident dies
- Councils may ask residents to cover, up front, the costs of land registry searches and any other such legal costs

- If it is intended to sell the property it is probably not to one's advantage to accept a deferred payments agreement if the resident has other capital of below £16 000 and is entitled to an attendance allowance. If the property is *not* on the market it is *not* disregarded for income support purposes. However, if after the 12-week property disregard residents decide to place their property on the market and fund their care independently, they will be entitled to income support with reinstatement of attendance allowance. At the time of writing this is worth an additional contribution of up to £64.65 per week during the period following the 12-week property disregard. Figure 2.3 illustrates this.

(Benefit rates 2002/03)		Local authority deferred loan		No local authority deferred loan Property on the market
		(£)		(£)
Cost of care per week		350.00		350.00
Attendance allowance (not means tested)		(56.25)		(56.25)
Income support (means tested)				
Severe disability premium			42.25	
Pensioner premium (60 and over)	–		44.20	
Personal allowance	–		53.95	
	–		140.40	
Less pension	–		75.75	
Net income support benefits		–		(64.65)
Pension state	75.75		75.75	
Personal expenses allowance	(16.80)		(16.80)	
		(58.95)		(58.95)
Local authority charge against property/shortfall				
First 12 weeks local authority funding		Nil		Nil
Second 14 weeks shortfall		234.80		170.15
Overall cost from capital over 26 weeks		3287.20		2382.10

If it took 26 weeks to sell the property, the current saving by not accepting a deferred payments agreement could therefore be up to £905.10 plus land registry search and legal costs.

Fig. 2.3 Funding options.

Fee plans

Increasing numbers of older people now fund their own care. Around 50% of people in the south-east of England and 30% of people in the remainder of the UK fund their own care. A person with a property to sell could sell the property and purchase an Immediate Need Care Fee Payment Plan liability to pay fees over the long term. Remaining capital can be invested to yield tax-free income and may offer potentially higher capital growth to regenerate the estate.

Top-ups for more expensive accommodation

As with the 12-week property disregard period, individuals who choose more expensive accommodation than the local authority would normally pay for may be entitled to top up their fees from:

- Disregarded income, earnings or capital
- Other capital resources, including the value of the property that is subject to the deferred payments agreement, with the proviso that the resident must be left with total capital resources of no less than the means test lower capital limit, i.e. £11 750. Where the top-up is part of the deferred payments agreement, it is eventually repaid when the property is sold. Local authorities may be reluctant to enter into such agreements if they are not satisfied that the resident contribution including the top-up can be met for the duration of the person's stay in the care home.

The ability for individuals to provide their own top-ups only applies to those benefiting from the 12-week property disregard or the deferred payments scheme. In other circumstances where the local authority is funding the care costs, a top-up may only be paid by a third party who the local authority considers is able to cover the duration of the third party agreement.

NHS nursing care contribution

Residents of nursing homes participating in the deferred payments scheme will, subject to assessment, be entitled to a contribution towards their nursing care from the NHS as if they were normal self-funders. Every case must be considered on its own merits taking into account life expectancy, the property market, the possible loss of benefits, the feasibility of letting against selling and investing in alternative financial products, and the family's wishes to remain independent from state provision.

Before considering whether to be totally independent of the state, there are some important factors residents should bear in mind:

- During any period of interim funding, while the property is on the market the care home fees are likely to be greater than the person's income. How will this shortfall be paid? Can a relative afford it or will the home owner allow it to accrue over the long term if the property does not sell quickly?
- How much will the property sell for and will this provide sufficient money to meet care costs for life? If not, and the capital falls to below £19 000, will the person qualify for help from the local authority (i.e. be assessed as needing the level of care they have chosen at a price the local authority are prepared to pay)?
- Will the home owner agree to keep somebody as a resident in the same accommodation if their capital falls to £19 000 and they can only pay what the local authority offers?

It is sensible to discuss these points with the social services department and the home owner if the resident wishes to follow this course.

Placing a charge on property

Where a resident has a beneficial interest in land that is not disregarded and fails to pay an assessed charge for his accommodation, or chooses to participate in a section 55 deferred payment agreement, from October 2001 the local authority can place a charge on the property to pursue the debt and recover the cost of the accommodation paid on behalf of the resident. In arriving at the value of the property to be treated as capital, the local authority will allow 10% of its value as notional selling costs. The balance of the value will be treated as notional capital and the charge against the property will continue to accrue until such time as that notional capital after deducting the charge is deemed to be below £19 000 and the authority can begin to provide financial support.

Interest can only be charged on the sum due to the local authority under a deferred payment agreement from 56 days after the death of the resident for whom accommodation has been provided.

Property rented

Property rented out will be treated as a capital asset and any rent received will be disregarded as income although it could be paid to the local authority towards the standard charge.

The marital home

For the purpose of the financial assessment, when one member of a couple enters residential accommodation, the value of his or her home is disregarded as long as it is occupied in whole or part by his or her partner. Should the spouse who remains at home decide to sell the property and move into smaller, less expensive accommodation, the resident's 50% share of the proceeds could be taken into account in the charging assessment. However, should the resident wish to make available part of his or her share of the proceeds to the spouse to enable the purchase of the smaller property, the local authority guidance states that it would be reasonable for this amount to be disregarded, leaving only the surplus of the partner's share to be taken into account.

If one member of a couple enters a home the couple should seek professional advice (often obtainable free of charge). Professional advisers should consider whether jointly owned property should be held as a joint tenancy or as tenants in common. The latter would enable a spouse at home to leave their share of the property to an alternative beneficiary rather than to a spouse in a nursing home or residential home who would need to use the value of the property to pay for care costs. Either party can carry out the change in status of ownership without consulting the other.

Seek advice

The financial and legal implications to be considered when paying for care are wide, and require careful planning. Older people or their relatives should seek specialist advice before taking on any commitment that they are unsure of being able to afford. They should seek advice on what their entitlements are from the state, what legal matters they should attend to and how best to use their capital and income to meet ongoing care costs and possible changing care needs.

'Free' Registered Nursing Care

The way that the costs of registered nursing care are met varies across the UK. Older people living in England, Scotland and Wales all have different eligibility criteria because of devolved government. In England government introduced a complex system that it claims meets the costs of registered nursing care in English nursing homes.

The Health and Social Care Act 2001 defines nursing care in a care or nursing home as 'the registered nurse contribution to providing, planning and supervising care in a nursing home setting'. The NHS will pay this component of nursing care when an NHS nurse has carried out an assessment. The NHS will not cover personal or social care costs or the costs of accommodation for residents. However, the NHS will continue to fund the care of residents who meet the criteria for continuing NHS health care where the resident has a primary health need.

Assessing eligibility

In England, Primary Care Trusts have appointed nursing home co-ordinators. In areas where Primary Care Trusts have not yet been established, the health authority will appoint a nursing home co-ordinator. The co-ordinators will be registered nurses. Although some co-ordinators are experienced and well qualified in the care of older people, co-ordinators are not required to have any specific expertise or educational qualifications in the care of older people.

The co-ordinators have received training materials and an assessment tool to enable them to determine the level of nursing need. They also receive one day of training. The tool aims to pay not only for care delivered by a registered nurse but also the time a registered nurse spends teaching, supervising and documenting care[8]. The assessment, a tick-box form, bands care into three categories: high, medium and low[9]. Box 2.1 gives details of the three bands.

Box 2.1   Three bands for registered nursing care (from Health and Social Care Act 2001).

- *Low – £35 per week*   'For those whose care needs can be met with minimal registered nurse input. Assessment indicates that care needs can be met in a setting other than a nursing home, but the person is funding their own care and has chosen to enter a nursing home.'
- *Medium – £70 per week*   'The average amount of care provided (delegated, supervised and planned) by registered nurses in nursing homes.' The person will require RN care on at least a daily basis and may need access to a nurse at any time. Needs are stable and predictable and likely to remain so if existing treatment and care is delivered.
- *High – £110 per week*   This is based on the finding that 'the average amount of care provided for those with complex or enhanced nursing needs is 55% higher than for those with standard needs for care'. This level of funding is for people who have unstable and unpredictable nursing needs. The person will require frequent intervention and assessment by the RN throughout the 24-hour period.

The assessment process takes from 10–45 minutes per person. It is not yet clear how many people will fall into each band. Jacqui Smith, the minister responsible, has indicated that around 10% of people will fall into the lower band and most other residents will fall into the medium band.

Government estimates that the higher level of allowance will pay for ten hours of registered nurse care per week.

Timetable for introduction

People living in nursing homes who are funding their own care were assessed from November 2001 onwards. There are an estimated 42 000 people funding their own care in England so there may be a backlog of assessments. People admitted to nursing homes after 1 October 2001 have their nursing needs assessed if they are self-funding. People who are funded by social services will have their nursing needs assessed from April 2003. This has just been put back a year because of concerns over the number of assessments required.

If the person, or his or her family, is unhappy with the banding for nursing care they are advised to raise their concerns with the home manager. The manager will be responsible for liaising with the nursing home co-ordinator. The person who has been assessed can request a further assessment from the nursing home co-ordinator. The co-ordinator may change the assessment. If the person is still not satisfied then the assessment can be referred to the health authority continuing care panel.

The nursing home co-ordinator will be responsible for making sure that the scheme runs to budget. The system is cash limited – there will be £80 million to spend between October and April 2002. It is unclear what will happen once the budget is allocated. Will people be forced to join waiting lists for registered nursing care? Will people be expected to remain in hospital because the Primary Care Trust is over budget?

Respite care excluded

People who enter nursing homes on a short-term basis are excluded. If a person comes into a nursing home for six weeks or less they will not benefit from free registered nursing care. Older people who live at home with a carer and go into homes for short-term respite care may be eligible for state funding for up to 12 weeks of care. In order to obtain funding the person has to agree to a full financial assessment. Some older people who fund their own care are not aware of the complexities of funding[10].

National variations

In Wales all nursing home residents will receive a flat rate of £100 a week. Nursing home residents will not be assessed individually for nursing care. The Welsh Assembly believes that people who are living in nursing homes are there because they require nursing care. They recognise that £100 a week does not meet the full costs of registered nursing care and hope to be able to increase the allowance each year so that it does at some point meet the full costs of registered nursing care.

In Scotland the Scottish Executive plans to meet the costs of most nursing and personal care for people living in nursing homes[11]. Eligibility will be on the basis of a single holistic needs assessment. The Scottish Parliament hopes by early 2003 to have in place the system to meet these costs. Northern Ireland is expected to follow the English system.

Implications for practice

The nursing home co-ordinator will be working to a limited budget and will have little time to assess the person's need for nursing care. It is vital that your care plans and documentation provide a comprehensive picture of the person. It is useless trying to argue that Mary needs lots of persuasion and that completing her dressing is time consuming, if this is not documented in the care plan and daily record. If Mary has a complex wound that requires time consuming dressings you must document this. You will need to show your wound care assessment and other details. If a person is at risk of falls and requires lots of input and supervision you need to document this. If a person is a brittle, unstable diabetic the funding will not reflect this unless it is documented.

If the person or a relative appeals a banding decision, your documentation will be crucial. If you have not fully documented the care you deliver, then the appeal will fail.

Attendance allowance

Attendance allowance is an allowance that individuals can claim to help them meet the costs of care. It is not means tested. There is little point in people who have fees paid by social services applying for this benefit because if it is awarded other benefits will be adjusted to take account of attendance allowance. Older people who are funding their own care normally claim this benefit. Claim forms can be obtained from the local social security office or the post office. Individuals are not normally considered for this benefit unless disability has persisted for more than six months. Terminally ill individuals are exempt from this ruling. There are two levels of attendance allowance: the higher rate allowance is for individuals who require assistance throughout the day and night and the lower rate is for individuals who only require assistance during the day.

DSS funding and 'preserved rights'

Some older people who enter homes and fund their own care eventually exhaust their capital. They often ask nursing staff to advise them what benefits they are entitled to when their capital reaches £19 000, the level at which they are eligible for help.

When community care was introduced in April 1993, people who had entered homes before that date were allocated 'preserved rights status'. This meant that they continued to claim their fees from the Department of Social Security. In April 2002 preserved rights were abolished and people on preserved rights became the responsibility of the local social services department. It is not yet clear what the implications of this will be. There are fears that social services departments will carry out assessments and decide that people in nursing beds require residential care. If the home only provides nursing care the person could have to move. It appears that people with preserved rights who generally pay lower fees will have their fees met at the higher normal social services rate.

Sources of additional funding

As the gap between the costs of providing care and fee levels paid has grown, it has become very difficult to obtain additional help with home fees. Some charities say that it is not their role to subsidise inadequate state funding. Some organisations have benevolent funds and will consider helping older people with their fees. Many occupations such as the police force have benevolent funds. Individuals who were members of a trade union should contact the union as many have benevolent funds. There are hundreds of charities and benevolent funds that may be able to help. Older people and their families often lack the time and resources to track down possible sources of funding. A number of organisations will help relatives to find additional funding.

Age Concern provides a number of useful fact sheets including information on sources of additional funding:
Age Concern England, Astral House, 1268 London Road, London SW16 4ER. Tel. 020 8765 7200 or 020 8679 8000. website: http://www.ace.org.uk email: infodep@ace.org.uk Tel. 0800 009966 for fact sheets.

Age Concern Scotland, 113 Rose Street, Edinburgh EH2 3DT. Tel. 0131 220 3345.

Age Concern Northern Ireland, 3 Lower Crescent, Belfast BT7 1NR. Tel. 0298 9024 5729.

Age Concern (Cymru), 4th Floor, 1 Cathedral Road, Cardiff CF1 9SD. Tel. 029 2037 1566

Counsel and Care offer information and advice on residential and nursing care: Counsel and Care, Twyman House, 16 Bonny Street, London NW1 9PG. Tel. 0845 300 7585 (10AM–3.30PM) helpline. Tel. 020 7485 1556.

The Nursing Homes Fees Agency offers free advice to all regardless of means. They aim to help people manage their funds well. They produce a number of useful leaflets. Contact NHFA, St Leonards House, Mill Street, Eynsham, Oxford, OX29 4JX Tel. 01865 733000 Fax 01865 733001. website: www.nhfa.co.uk email: enquiries@nhfa.co.uk

Useful address and telephone number

(Use this to enter local information relevant to your work)

Local care managers

Conclusion

The funding of care has become ever more complicated. Often older people and their families are unclear about the level of care required and what assistance they can obtain to pay fees. Research from Counsel and Care found that significant numbers of people who fund their own care are not receiving the benefits they are entitled to because the system is complex and they are unaware of benefits. It is important that nurses are aware of funding systems and can provide information and advice to residents and relatives.

Needs assessment and care funding criteria now differ depending on which country in the UK you work in. It is not yet clear if these changes will prevent older people moving from one country to another to be near family.

References

1 Walker, A. (1994) *Half a century of promises. The failure to realise community care for older people*. Counsel and Care, London.
2 Challis, D., Gill, J., Hughes, J. & Stone, S. (1997) *Eligibility for Social Services for Older People*. A study of local authority criteria for older people. Personal Social Services Research Unit, University of Manchester, Manchester.
3 Millard, P. (1999) *Nursing Home Placements for Older People in England & Wales*. A National Audit 1995–1998. A report commissioned by the Clinical Audit Unit of the National Health Service Department of Geriatric Medicine, St George's Hospital, London.
4 Nazarko, L. (1999) Service Breakdown. *Nursing Times: Nursing Homes supplement*, **1**(2), 24.
5 Clinical Standards Advisory Group (1998) *Community Care for Older People*. A report of the CSAG Committee chaired by Dame Professor June Clark. The Stationery Office, London.
6 Royal Commission on Long Term Care (1999) Chaired by Professor Sir Stewart Sutherland. *With respect to old age: Long Term Care Rights and Responsibilities*. The Stationery Office, London.
7 Department of Health (2000) *The NHS Plan: The Government's Response to the Royal Commission on Long Term Care*. Presented to Parliament July 2000. CM4818–II. Available from: The Stationery Office, PO Box 29, Norwich NR3 1GN. (Mail, telephone and fax orders only) General enquiries 0870 600 5522. website: http://www.nhs.uk/nhsplan
8 A copy of the assessment tool – The Registered Nursing Care Contribution Tool – is available at www.doh.gov.uk/jointunit/freenursingcare
9 Guidance on free registered nursing care can be found on the internet at: www.doh.gov.uk/jointunit/freenursingcare
10 Personal Social Services Research Unit (2002) *Self Funded Admissions to Care Homes*. Personal Social Services Research Unit, University of Kent at Canterbury.
11 Scottish Executive (2001) *Fair Care for Older People*. www.scotland.gov.uk

Chapter 3

Confusion and Dementia

Introduction

The incidence of dementia is growing in line with population ageing and as people live longer it will become one of the major health issues of the twenty-first century. It is the fourth leading cause of death after heart disease, cancer and stroke. In the US almost half of all nursing home residents suffer from Alzheimer's disease. Female Alzheimer's sufferers outnumber men by 2.8:1 but vascular dementia is more common in men[1]. The incidence of dementia increases with age. It affects 1% of 65 year olds, 40% of 85 year olds[2] and around 50% of 95 year olds[3]. Dementia is not a disease[4]; it is a syndrome or a group of concurrent symptoms caused by a number of different illnesses. Individuals whose need for care arises primarily because of mental health needs should be cared for in homes that specialise in caring for people with dementia. They should be cared for in homes that were registered under the old legislation as EMI (elderly mentally infirm) homes and cared for by nurses with mental health qualifications.

However, registered nurses who are general trained often find themselves caring for people with varying degrees of confusion and dementia. Research indicates that large numbers of people living in non-EMI nursing homes and also in residential homes have some degree of confusion. If a person develops dementia when in the home or if the dementia worsens this can pose ethical problems. Is it ethical to transfer a person who develops dementia if the home is not registered to provide dementia care? Is it more humane to care for the person within the home in familiar surroundings? If you decide to attempt to continue providing care within the home, how will this impact on the lives of other residents? If you decide that the person must move, how can you best deal with this and minimise distress?

This chapter is divided into five sections: causes and consequences of confusion, medical treatment of dementia, nursing care of the person with dementia, challenging behaviour, and ethical issues.

Causes and consequences of confusion

The first section aims to enable you to understand the causes of dementia and how this affects treatment.

This section will:

- Examine what dementia is
- Discuss treatable confusional states
- Outline treatment strategies
- Explore the different types of dementia
- Discuss the causes of dementia
- Examine Alzheimer's disease
- Examine Lewy body disease
- Examine vascular dementia
- Explore how dementia affects behaviour

What is dementia?

Dementia is a global term used to describe a group of diseases with common symptoms. It is described as: 'A global impairment of cognitive function that is usually progressive and that interferes with normal social and occupational activities.'

Four main types of dementia account for 90% of all cases of dementia. These are Alzheimer's disease, diffuse Lewy body dementia, frontotemporal dementia and vascular dementia[5]. Before we examine these in detail we will look at treatable causes of confusion.

Treatable confusional states

Dementia is a label that doctors and nurses apply to people. Often they add, 'There's nothing else we can do'. As nurses, when we hear the label 'dementia' we often subtly change our focus to that of palliative care; in most cases that is appropriate. However, dementia is ultimately a progressive untreatable disease and it can be difficult to diagnose, with an estimated 15% of all people labelled demented in fact suffering from treatable illness. Researchers have found that 29% of people diagnosed as suffering from dementia did not have dementia when scanned; some recovered completely following treatment[6]. It is important that we as nurses are aware of the treatable causes of confusion before we accept a diagnosis of dementia.

Older adults are more likely than younger people to develop confusional states because of illness. The cause of confusion may be physical or emotional. It is important to determine the cause(s) of confusion as this enables nurses to offer appropriate care. In many cases, the physical causes of confusion can be successfully treated. Older people are more likely to become confused when they are ill because as we age the body has less reserve capacity. Older adults, because of the effects of ageing on renal, hepatic, cardio-vascular and other systems, find it more difficult to maintain homeostasis. The physical causes of confusion include:

- Infection
- Metabolic causes

- Electrolyte imbalance
- Oxygen lack – (CO_2) narcosis
- Physical trauma
- Sensory problems

Infection

Acute infection can lead to confusion. The commonest sites of infection in the elderly are chest, urinary tract and skin. In older adults, the inflammatory response to illness is often impaired. Many older adults who develop infection fail to become pyrexial. Medication such as steroids, non-steroidal anti-inflammatory drugs and regular analgesia containing paracetamol or aspirin, can mask inflammatory response, including pyrexia, which we tend to view as the cardinal signs of infection[7]. Investigation and treatment of any underlying infection will restore lucidity in such cases.

Nurses can play an important part in reducing the risk of infection. Measures to reduce the rate of infection include:

- Introducing an infection control programme
- Ensuring that the person is as well nourished as possible[8]
- Using risk assessment to prevent the risk of pressure sores[9]
- Encouraging residents who are at risk of developing urinary tract infections to drink cranberry juice.

Metabolic causes

Metabolic causes of confusion can be difficult to identify because changes take place slowly over a period of weeks or months. It can be all too easy to consider these changes part of the disease process. Metabolic causes of confusion include: thyroid disease, renal disease, diabetes and anaemia.

Thyroid disease – The incidence of thyroid disease among older people is not known. However, we do know that the incidence of hypothyroidism increases with age. Features of hypothyroidism include weight gain and slowing of physical and mental function. Thyroid function tests TSH, T3 and T4 detect this problem, which can be effectively treated with thyroxine.

Renal disease – Renal disease can be caused by poorly controlled diabetes (diabetic nephropathy) or hypertension. Renal disease leads to rising levels of urea (uraemia) and confusion. Diuretics can stimulate renal function and postpone the worst effects of uraemia and the associated confusion for as long as possible. It is worth noting that urea and creatinine levels rise naturally with age and older adults can tolerate creatinine levels that would cause confusion in a younger person.

Diabetes – There are between 1 and 1.2 million adults in the UK who have type II diabetes, half remaining undiagnosed. Different races have different incidences of diabetes. In the adult population 4% of white people, 20% of black people, 25% of Asians and 5% of Chinese have diabetes[10]. The incidence of diabetes increases with age and 20% of elderly Caucasians are diabetic[11]. Ageing affects the presentation of diabetes and older people have fewer symptoms than younger people[12,13]. Consider the possibility of undiagnosed diabetes in older people who develop confusion. Older adults who are known diabetics treated with insulin can suffer from transient ischaemic attacks, cerebrovascular accidents and cardiac arrhythmias as a result of hypoglycaemia, and can develop cognitive impairment[14]. Ensuring that diabetics do not run the risks of hypoglycaemia reduces these risks.

Anaemia – Anaemia can be the result of end stage renal disease, carcinoma, blood loss, dietary insufficiency or medication. Medication that can cause anaemia includes phenytoin, which leads to folic acid deficiency and megoblastic anaemia, and non-steroidal anti-inflammatory drugs that can lead to slow blood loss. Anaemia leads to reduced oxygen to the brain (as the ability of red blood cells to transport oxygen is reduced) and confusion. Treatment of anaemia not only resolves confusion but also reduces tiredness and fatigue.

Medication

Older people are more likely to suffer adverse effects of medication because of age related changes. Ageing reduces the efficiency of renal and hepatic systems, which are responsible for breakdown and clearance of drugs from the body, yet older people are more likely to be prescribed a number of medications. As the number of medications rises the risk of adverse reactions increases. Medications which can cause confusion include:

- Hypnotics
- Analgesics
- Tranquillisers
- Antidepressants
- Diuretics
- Digoxin
- Antiparkinsonian drugs

Hypnotics are ineffective after seven days as the body rapidly becomes accustomed to their effects. They suppress the period of REM (rapid eye movement sleep) in which dreams occur and can leave people feeling less refreshed than shorter periods of non-drug induced sleep. Nitrazepam has a half-life of 24 hours and Temazepam 7 hours in healthy young male adults. These half-lives are prolonged in older adults. Using nursing measures and having realistic expectations of how much sleep older adults require, enables older people to avoid the hazards of hypnotics.

Analgesics may cause confusion. These include Co-Proximal, Co-Dydramol, Dihydrocodeine and Temgesic. It is normally possible to offer an analgesic which does not affect the individual's mental state. Perception of pain is linked to anxiety. Consider nursing measures such as massage, touch, diversional therapy, and complementary therapy, which will reduce anxiety and perception of pain and enhance well-being.

Tranquillisers and antidepressants can cause confusion and interact with other prescribed medications. Using measures to reduce anxiety can reduce or eliminate their use.

Diuretics are frequently prescribed for trivial reasons and when they are required, they are often prescribed in larger doses than required. At home many older people 'forget' to take diuretics; GPs think that the diuretic is ineffective and increase the dose. When the older person is admitted to a home nursing staff ensure that the diuretics are given and overdose can occur. Diuretic overdose can lead to hyponatraemia (low sodium levels) and hypokalaemia (low potassium levels), electrolyte imbalance and confusion. Nursing measures include encouraging mobility, elevating limbs, using compression therapy and ensuring adequate fluid intake. Such treatment enables diuretic therapy to be reduced to the smallest possible dose or eliminated.

Digoxin is cleared from the body via the kidneys; impaired renal function (common in older adults) can lead to toxic blood levels. The normal dose of Digoxin in frail elderly people should be 62.5 mcgs daily. If a higher dosage is prescribed, then Digoxin levels should be monitored.

Electrolyte imbalance can be caused by diuretic therapy, vomiting, diarrhoea and metabolic disease. Correcting electrolyte imbalances, and wherever possible the causes, often eliminates confusion.

Hypoxia

Low levels of oxygen and high levels of carbon dioxide are common when older people are suffering from poorly controlled cardiac failure, asthma, chronic bronchitis, acute chest infection and anaemia. Treating the underlying condition whenever possible will improve mental functioning. Other measures include:

- Positioning – to improve oxygen uptake
- Reassurance – which helps improve deep breathing
- Oxygen therapy (nasal oxygen is better tolerated).

Sensory problems

Sensory deprivation is used as a method of torture and can induce complete disintegration of the personality within 48 hours. Many older people suffer from sensory problems.

Visual impairment rises with age – research from the Royal College of Optometrists indicates that 96% of people aged 85 require glasses.

Hearing loss becomes more common with age – research indicates that 25% of people over the age of 85 have moderate to severe hearing loss and would benefit from a hearing aid.

Peripheral neuropathy and neurological problems including cerebrovascular accidents may affect the sense of touch. Older people suffering from a range of neurological diseases may have difficulty in communicating. These problems with seeing, hearing, understanding and making needs understood can all lead to sensory deprivation. Later in this chapter we will consider how nursing practice can also cause or worsen confusion by inadvertently causing sensory deprivation.

Emotional causes

Anxiety, grief perhaps because of the loss of a loved one, and depression can lead to disorientation[15]. In 1961, Lieberman described the disorientation caused by moving the older person from a familiar to an unfamiliar environment as 'Translocation Shock'. Many individuals who enter our nursing homes have been admitted to hospital, transferred from one acute ward to another ward and finally to our homes. Many such individuals are suffering from translocation shock and take some time to familiarise themselves with their new homes and settle in.

Dementia

Diagnosis of dementia is extremely difficult because the only way to conclusively confirm diagnosis is by examining brain tissue either by brain biopsy or more commonly at post mortem. Diagnosis is made by eliminating treatable causes of dementia, assessing mental status, eliminating depression, assessing mental status and ongoing assessment. Brain scans and other investigations combined with ongoing assessment can give an indication of the type of dementia[16].

Alzheimer's disease

This is thought to be the commonest cause of dementia. In 1906, Alzheimer, a German psychiatrist, described microscopic features in the brain of a person who had suffered from dementia. He noted neurofibrillary plaques and tangles in the individual's brain. Alzheimer's colleague Professor Kraepelin described dementia as Alzheimer's disease. However, there is some dispute among doctors about the existence of Alzheimer's disease. Microscopic examination of the brains of older people who have not been suffering from dementia show the same changes as those that Alzheimer (and others) have identified in people suffering from dementia[17]. The brain shrinks with age; memory impairment is a feature of extreme old age. Some doctors argue that lucidity, the forgetfulness that many people develop in old age and Alzheimer's disease lie on a continuum and that what we describe as Alzheimer's is merely one end of that continuum. Although many nursing and medical journals give clear cut definitions of Alzheimer's disease, our knowledge of this disease, its causes and its outcome are far from complete.

Causes of Alzheimer's disease

Early onset Alzheimer's disease occurs between the ages of 35 and 60. This is associated with a number of genetic defects. Chromosome 14 defects are the most common – the responsible gene has been named presenilin-1. It is thought to be responsible for most cases of early onset dementia. Chromosome 1 defects are the next most common – the responsible gene has been named presenilin-2. Chromosome 21 defects in a gene named amyloid precursor protein (APP) have been found in a small number of families worldwide. This fault affects the production of a protein called amyloid. In Alzheimer's there is a build up of amyloid in the brain.

Later onset dementia is linked to a protein called apolipo-protein E (ApoE). There are three types: ApoE2, ApoE3 and ApoE4. A sixth of the population carries ApoE2, the gene least associated with Alzheimer's; 0.5% of the population have two copies of the ApoE2 gene and are at very low risk of Alzheimer's. Around 60% of the popultion have a double dose of the ApoE3 gene and are at medium risk of developing Alzheimer's; about half will develop Alzheimer's in their late eighties. Around 25% of the population have one copy of the ApoE4 gene. This is the gene associated with the highest risk of Alzheimer's. One copy of the ApoE4 gene increases the risk of developing Alzheimer's by four times. Around 2% of the population have a double dose of ApoE4 and this increases the risk of developing Alzheimer's by 16 times, but it is not inevitable that Alzheimer's will develop[18].

Lewy body disease was thought to be a type of Alzheimer's but deterioration is more rapid[19]. It is extremely difficult to diagnose[20]. It can be confused with Alzheimer's and Parkinson's disease because people with Lewy body have clinical features common to Alzheimer's and Parkinson's. Around 88% of people with Lewy body disease are misdiagnosed as having Parkinson's. People with Lewy body disease are more likely to have late onset of symptoms and less likely to have resting tremors[21]. In around 50% of cases people with Lewy body disease have more frequent hallucinations and display symptoms of Parkinson's[22]. In early dementia the incidence of depression, hallucinations and misidentification of people is more marked in Lewy body disease[23]. It is important to diagnose Lewy body disease because many people with this disease react to neuroleptics[24].

Multi-infarct dementia or vascular dementia

This is thought to be the second most common cause of dementia. Vascular dementia is more common in men. It is associated with arterial disease and is of sudden onset. It is caused by small clots causing the death of areas of brain tissue. Vascular dementia can be diagnosed by a brain scan. The scan shows small areas of brain death caused by brain infarctions. There are two types of vascular dementia:

- Acute vascular dementia includes large vessel infarction and lacunar dementia due to small vessel disease including thalamic and caudate strokes.
- Subacute vascular dementia includes Binswanger's disease and cerebral angiopathy. People with vascular dementia often have fluctuating levels of confusion and are more aware than people with Alzheimer's[25].

Treatment of arterial disease and hypertension can prevent or reduce the frequency of further brain infarctions.

Causes of vascular dementia
A mutation on the notch gene on chromosome 19 – cadasil is thought to be one of the causes of vascular dementia[26]. Parkinson's disease can lead to dementia in approximately 30% of sufferers. This dementia normally develops in the later stages of Parkinson's disease. Pick's disease, frontal dementia, and Huntington's chorea are other causes of dementia but onset is usually before the age of 65.

Dementia symptom clusters
The first symptom of dementia is short-term memory loss. It can take some time for this to become apparent and it is estimated that most

people are not diagnosed as suffering from dementia until two years after the onset of the disease. Eventually all aspects of thinking and reasoning are affected. Alzheimer's type dementia causes an individual to suffer four different types of symptom cluster. These have been defined as intellectual losses, personality losses, planning losses and lowered stress threshold.

Intellectual losses lead to loss of memory, initially for recent events. Sense of time is lost and the individual becomes unable to make choices or to problem solve. Judgement is affected and the individual loses the ability to express thoughts. Language abilities decline; the individual has difficulty expressing and understanding others. Intellectual losses may make it difficult for the individual to find their way around the home independently. They may have difficulty recognising their room and may go into other residents' rooms. They may go into the kitchen or leave the taps on and cause a flood.

Personality losses lead to a decreased attention span and the individual with Alzheimer's type dementia (ATD) is easily distracted. Inhibitions are reduced. The individual may take off clothing in public. Emotional liability becomes more marked as the dementia progresses. The individual loses the ability to be tactful, may lose the ability to control temper and delay gratification – wants it now! They withdraw socially – mix and converse less – become increasingly preoccupied with self and uninterested in others. They avoid overwhelming or complex stimuli, and exhibit antisocial behaviour, confabulation and perseveration (recurrent thoughts, ideas or actions).

Planning losses lead to an individual with ATD initially losing the ability to plan the day, then inability to carry out activities which require thought to set goals, organise and complete the task, and functional losses starting with the more complex tasks such as handling money, shopping, etc. As the disease progresses the ability to plan and carry out activities of daily living is lost, usually in the following order:

- Increased fatigue on exertion or mental exertion, loss of energy reserve
- Frustration, refusal to participate, or expression of helplessness
- Bathing, grooming, choosing clothing
- Dressing, walking, using the toilet
- Communicating
- Eating independently.

It is important to note that worry about ability tends to worsen performance.

Progressively lowered stress threshold which is characteristic of individuals with ATD, can lead to catastrophic behaviours, confused or agitated night waking, purposeful wandering, violent, agitated or anxious behaviour, withdrawal and belligerence, noisy behaviour, purposeless behaviour, compulsive repetitive behaviour and other socially unacceptable behaviours. This can lead to individuals becoming unwilling to get up, bathe, dress and use the toilet, and becoming agitated if the carer insists. These symptoms worsen if the ATD sufferer becomes very tired or becomes anxious.

Conclusion

This section has examined the causes and consequences of confusion. Confusion is a symptom. Like all symptoms it should be investigated and treated if possible. Sometimes we as experienced nurses know that there are no cures – no magic pills to make it all better. Dementia is an irreversible terminal disease; the quality of nursing care we offer can enable people to retain ability and to enjoy the best possible quality of life for as long as possible. The next section will examine the medical treatment of people with dementia.

Key points

- The incidence of dementia is growing in line with population ageing
- It is important to distinguish between treatable and non-treatable causes of confusion
- Dementia is not a disease but a syndrome caused by a number of different diseases
- It affects 1% of 65 year olds, 40% of 85 year olds and around 50% of 95 year olds
- Women are more at risk of Alzheimer's
- Men are more at risk of vascular dementia
- Lewy body disease is very difficult to diagnose
- Dementia symptom clusters affect behaviour.

Medical treatment of dementia

Medical treatment currently focuses on finding medication to prevent dementia developing and to treat existing dementia.

The aims of this section are:

- To discuss the latest research on dementia
- To explore current research on preventing dementia
- To discuss the role of medication in preventing dementia
- To explore the role of medication in restoring function and slowing decline
- To discuss treatment of behavioural symptoms

Drug treatment of dementia

Drugs are available to treat five different aspects of dementia. These are:

- Prevention of Alzheimer's type dementia
- Treating specific symptoms, e.g. memory loss
- Restoring function
- Slowing the rate of decline

- Treating behavioural symptoms such as agitation, aggression and hallucinations.

Prevention of Alzheimer's

Research indicates that inflammation plays a major part in the development of dementia[27]. The senile plaques that are the hallmark of Alzheimer's are accompanied by inflammatory changes. These changes lead to raised levels of amyloid beta protein (ABP). These raised levels of ABP are neurotoxic, lead to degeneration of brain function, and the symptoms of dementia develop[28].

Non-steroidal anti-inflammatory drugs (NSAIDS) such as ibuprofen may help treat the inflammation that develops with Alzheimer's. Researchers have found that people who take NSAIDS regularly are less likely to develop Alzheimer's[29].

Oestrogen – Oestrogen regulates aggression, sex drive, impulsive behaviour and hostility. Oestrogen improves cognitive function. When oestrogen levels fall, just before menstruation, many women become clumsy, forgetful and weepy. Oestrogen replacement can be used to prevent and treat Alzheimer's[30].

Benzodiazepines – In a study of 668 older people, carried out over three years, researchers found that people who took benzodiazepines regularly were less likely to develop ATD[31].

Treating symptoms

Most drug treatments are based on the idea that dementia is caused by poor blood flow to the brain. The aim of treatments is to increase cerebral blood flow. At present, there is little evidence that such treatments are effective[32].

Restoring function

Alzheimer's disease causes changes in the basal forebrain cholinergic system (BFCS). Drugs that act to boost function of BFCS, e.g. tacrine and donepezil (Articept), lead to improved ability to reason and function[33]. Tacrine is thought to reverse the dementing process by six months and to maintain the person at that level for 1–2 years. It benefits about 40% of people who are prescribed it. Obviously, people with early or mid stage dementia will benefit most from this. Tacrine is hepatotoxic and there is a high incidence of side effects. Withdrawal can lead to a more rapid decline in ability than if the drug had never been given[34]. Donepezil has a half-life of 104 hours in older adults. Researchers have found it reverses the dementia process by about six months and maintains the person at that level for 1–2 years[35]. Side effects include nausea, vomiting, anorexia and diarrhoea[36]. It can cause outflow obstruction and urinary retention. NICE – the National Institute for Clinical Excellence – which is responsible for determining the effectiveness of drug treatments decided to recommend that tacrine, Articept and donepezil be made available on the NHS. NICE recommends close medical supervision when these drugs are used. They benefit people with mild to moderate dementia.

Nicotine also boosts BFCS function but its action is short-lived. Research using nicotine patches is now being carried out with encouraging results. Side effects include nausea, anorexia, insomnia and a rise in blood pressure.

Nimodopine is an isopropyl calcium channel blocker that can easily cross the blood brain barrier. It is intended to treat ischaemic neurological deficits following subarachnoid haemorrhage. Side effects include hypotension, gastrointestinal problems, headache and nausea. Doctors in the UK and the rest of Europe are using it to treat vascular and Alzheimer's dementia, but there is no convincing evidence that it is a useful treatment for dementia[37].

Ginkgo biloba (available in health food shops) has been found to improve function[38] and no known side effects have been identified[39].

Treating behavioural symptoms

The first response of many GPs when you ask for advice on behavioural problems is to reach for the prescription pad. Drugs may help with some behaviour problems but will be ineffective with others. It is important to determine which behavioural symptoms can be managed by changing practice or the environment. Medication may help in the following cases:

- Hyperactivity
- Agitation
- Psychotic symptoms
- Hallucinations
- Depression

Medication will not help with:

- Wandering
- Stripping off clothes
- Hoarding and hiding objects
- Repetitive questioning

Standard treatment for the symptoms associated with ATD are a group of drugs known as neuroleptics. This group includes drugs such as haloperidol and thioriazine. Nursing home staff face increasing criticism when such drugs are used. Critics seem to ignore the fact that doctors not nurses prescribe these medications. Staff are accused of over medicating individuals to keep them quiet. Paul Flynn, a Labour MP, is at the time of writing attempting to limit the prescription of neuroleptics within nursing homes. He has a point – neuroleptics can, when inappropriately prescribed, adversely affect quality of life. Side effects of neuroleptics include:

- Over sedation and loss of ability
- Drug induced parkinsonism
- Increased risk of infection, incontinence, pressure sores, and contractures.

Recommendations for good practice if using neuroleptics are:

- Neuroleptics should be used as a last resort not a first resort
- Neuroleptics should be given in the smallest possible therapeutic dose
- Neuroleptics should be reviewed regularly (at least every four weeks)
- Nurses should monitor individuals for possible side effects[40].

Conclusion

Our knowledge of dementia has increased enormously in the last few years. Now researchers are predicting that they will have developed effective treatments for dementia within the next five years.

Key points

- Medical treatment of dementia focuses on the use of drugs
- Drugs are used to prevent dementia, restore function and slow the rate of decline
- Current medication merely slows the rate of decline for a short period
- Medication is also used (sometimes inappropriately) to treat behavioural problems.

Nursing care of the person with dementia

The first section of this chapter examined the causes of confusion and how confusion affects individuals. Some of our medical colleagues consider that dementia is a slow but steady march to the grave. En route the individual loses every shred of awareness and dignity and becomes less than human:

'The self has slowly unravelled but caregivers ... assume that there is a person behind the largely unwitting presentation, of the victims, albeit that in reality there is less and less until where once there was a unique individual there is only emptiness'.[41]
'Any real understanding is impossible at the final stages. The patient may be assumed to have no real subjective awareness, no sense of self at all, and to be in this sense mentally dead'.[42]

This section aims to enable you to understand that there is a person behind the dementia and to develop ways of enabling that person to function to capacity.

This section will:

- Discuss how design affects behaviour of people with dementia
- Explore ways to redesign disabling environments
- Explore how nursing practice affects ability
- Discuss ways to improve nursing practice
- Discuss ways to enhance communication skills
- Explore ways to change nursing practice

The nursing perspective

Nurses, possibly because they spend more time with the individuals, have a different perspective on dementia and are developing and introducing research based models of care. The textbooks tell us that people with delirium have fluctuating levels of consciousness but people with dementia do not. However, our experience is that this is not true. The person with dementia can fluctuate not only from day to day but from hour to hour. Why? What are the textbooks missing? My view is that the textbooks see dementia simply in terms of a disease. Real life is seldom so simple. As nurses, we see the person with the disease. The person with dementia, like all of us, reacts and interacts with the environment.

Box 3.1 Conceptual model relating to the well-being of nursing home residents.

Ability is related to the interaction between the competence of the individual and resources within the environment. Individual ability is influenced by:

(1) Biological health
(2) Sensory perceptual capacity
(3) Ego strength.

Resources within the environment are:

(1) Physical and architectural features
(2) Medical regimes for treatment of death and disability
(3) Policy factors
(4) Resident and staff characteristics
(5) Availability of social support.

This section examines the research relating to design of homes and how that enables or disables the person with dementia, then examines the effects of nursing practice on individuals.

Nursing home design

Unit size

Small is beautiful – research demonstrates that people with dementia respond better when nursed in small units. The optimum size of a unit is 8–10 people. Small units have fewer staff, so the individual has fewer people to relate to. Staff have the opportunity to get to know residents really well as people. This leads to appropriate, organised, individualised care. The amount of bustle and noise is reduced and this helps reduce anxiety levels and the risks of catastrophic reactions.

Our nursing homes are becoming larger. In 1984 the average nursing home had 20 beds; in 2002 it has 40 beds and nursing homes with 20 beds or less are barely viable. There are fears that new national minimum standards will sound the death knell for smaller homes, yet research reveals that nurses feel more comfortable with them and consider that they can provide more personal, higher quality care within small units. Some, but not all, of the corporates break down their homes into smaller units. Takare, now part of BUPA, have 30 bed houses that act as virtually self-contained units and are staffed separately. Bettacare break their homes into 20 bed units. Some nurses work in large or extended homes on several floors; these homes are not physically separated into smaller units. So how can we meet the needs of the demented person for smallness within our large units?

Lounges and dining areas

A number of small lounges and dining areas are better than one large area. If you have only one large lounge, do everything within your power to change this. In large lounges we end up arranging the furniture around the edges simply to enable people to move around freely. Noise levels rise in large rooms and staff are constantly bustling around. Small lounges make a big difference. Noise levels are reduced. People with dementia have great difficulty in interpreting and processing information; reducing the noise level, bustle, and frequency and volume of stimuli reduces anxiety and problem behaviours significantly.

Primary nursing

Primary nursing, also known as a key worker scheme, enhances the quality of care. Allocating a primary nurse and a limited number of care assistants (normally no more than three) to provide care has a number of effects:

- The individual with dementia only has to relate to a limited number of people. This is less stressful for resident and carer.
- Staff get to know the individual well. They feel responsible for their residents and develop a sense of ownership and pride in their work.
- Staff who see residents as individuals are less likely to burnout and I am convinced that the possibility of abuse is greatly reduced.

Primary nursing is something that many units claim to practice but do not in reality. There is more to primary nursing than being responsible for a care plan. When primary nursing is really practised nurses are not moved around every eight weeks and matron does not make all the decisions or take all the responsibility. Roles change with primary nursing. Staff have more control over the care they deliver, and the matron/manager's role changes from a directive one to a supportive and educational role.

Designing to dement

The ideal unit in which to nurse people with dementia is on one floor, without stairs and long corridors. It is specifically designed to reduce background noise. Reducing excess background noise (the clatter of dishes, the drone of the Hoover, staff chattering) and distractions (visitors, deliveries, bells ringing) and minimising staff movement enables people with dementia to concentrate, and it improves ability[43]. Our nursing homes are not like that – they have long disorientating corridors, stairs, high noise levels and busy staff. What can we do to change the environment so that it enables, rather than disables, people with dementia?

Redesigning disabling environments

Corridors

People with dementia (and people who are not demented) find long corridors with identical signs disorientating. So individuals mistake the clinical room for their bedroom or matron's office for the toilet. Disguising doors that we do not wish residents to enter so that they blend with the background, is extremely effective. These doors can either be painted or papered. Highlighting doors that we wish residents to notice helps them to find their way around. A simple way is to colour code doors. One nursing home in Northern Ireland painted all bedroom doors peach and all toilet doors pink. Other nursing homes have found that painting all toilet doors red (a colour easily seen even by the visually impaired) and all bedroom doors yellow is effective. This use of colour enables not only people with dementia but other residents and visitors to associate door colours with use.

The problem then is how to help an individual find their bedroom. In many nursing homes, the doors have discrete labels. Consider using a large A4 size piece of brightly coloured card to produce a sign combining a picture, the resident's name, and details of her carers. The use of pictures enables residents who can no longer read or understand writing to identify their rooms. Pictures are selected, wherever possible, by the resident or by the resident's family. Pictures can either be computer clipart or can be cut from magazines. The important points are that the picture means something to the resident and that it is big enough to see.

Being visible
People with dementia are less confused and anxious when they can see a member of staff at all times. This can be difficult but small changes, such as encouraging staff to write reports, fill in forms and complete paperwork within sight of residents, increase resident ability.

Familiar decor
Confusion and anxiety levels are reduced when individuals are surrounded by familiar decor and appliances. As nurses, we can easily help provide such an environment. Relatives are usually only too happy to bring in old familiar items of furniture, pictures, the 'wireless', and photographs.

Bedroom. Making the resident's bedroom look like her bedroom at home, instead of a tasteful but sterile carbon copy of the room next door, enables the person to function better.
Lounges too can be made to look and feel like home. Replace the CD player with a radiogram or record player bought from a car boot sale. Encourage those residents who do not require specialist seating to bring in their old battered armchair from home. It is very difficult for an individual to pick out their chair when all the chairs are the same!
Lighting plays an important but little recognised role in mood. Fluorescent energy-saving lights are now becoming very popular. Research though has shown that by providing soft low lighting in the evening, anxiety, confusion and behavioural problems are reduced. Researchers found that switching off the fluorescents, putting on wall lights and playing soothing music resulted in residents becoming less distracted, eating more and taking less time to eat[44]. If you think about it this makes sense; restaurants have been doing it for a long time and the only people who expect us to eat under fluorescent light are fast food outlets who also expect us to eat with our fingers.
Decor can increase or decrease confusion and mobility levels. Wallpaper

with complicated patterns can set people on edge. Many units now use pastel colours with pictures to provide splashes of colour. Carpet and floor covering can affect mobility. People with dementia have great difficulty processing information. They may perceive floor coverings with strong patterns as changes of level. They may also perceive dramatic colour and pattern contrasts between floor coverings as changes of level[45]. Using the same colour of floor covering and avoiding strong patterns can enable people to remain mobile and prevent falls.

All the suggestions given in this section are simple and do not cost a lot, but they can enable us as nurses to negate some of the effects of the poorly designed environments that we work in. It would, of course, be much simpler if those who design nursing homes asked those of us who work in them to assist them in designing non-disabling environments.

Nursing practice

Nursing practice can enable or disable people in our care. If your opinion is that the person is incapable, they will very soon live down to your expectations. If you or your staff tend to do things for the person because 'it is quicker', then sooner than you think you will have no choice but to do those things because the person will have become totally dependent. When older people consider that nothing they do is right, that they continually fail to meet your expectations, they give up trying and develop 'learned helplessness'[46]. This sets up the vicious circle where staff do not expect the person to be able to communicate or to be able to do anything. Low expectations and high dependency follow, and staff feel that they were 'right' because what they predicted – the person 'going downhill' – has come to pass. Nursing practice can reinforce behaviour that encourages the person to do as much as possible or it can reinforce dependent behaviour. Communication is one of the most important features that helps us to nurse people as individuals and to enable rather than disable them.

Communication
Many nursing home residents can be thought of as having been sentenced to solitary confinement. Their only chance of communicating is through the efforts of staff who try to remove as many barriers to communication as possible. If people are not encouraged to use speech and are not stimulated, they will deteriorate quickly and unnecessarily[47]. In dementia language breaks down in stages:

- In the early stages, speech becomes empty and vague, sentences are not completed
- Then word finding becomes a problem – the person has increasing difficulty naming things
- Speech becomes increasingly repetitive
- Speech and conversation are related only to the individual
- Mutism may follow[48].

This inability to communicate can irritate and sometimes overwhelm staff.

Enabling the person to communicate

- Ensure aids such as hearing aids and spectacles are used at all times
- Make sure the environment is right – eliminate distractions such as television, radio and other people chattering or working in the room; if necessary, take the person to a quiet place
- Mean what you say. People with dementia (because they have difficulty in processing verbal communication) appear to be extremely sensitive to body language. Make sure that your facial expression and posture are relaxed. Use open postures. Sit at the same level. Make eye contact. Use the person's name.
- Use touch and gestures to reinforce your presence and what you are saying.
- Speak simply and slowly. Use short sentences, ideally seven words. Introduce only one idea in each sentence.
- Allow the person time to answer you. The person with moderate dementia takes five times longer than the older person without dementia, to process information.
- Listen. Learn to pick up cues and prompts.
- Listen for the meaning beneath the surface. People with dementia often use metaphors to communicate.
- Don't assume that lack of response means lack of understanding. The person may be thinking or may not wish to respond.
- Illustrate what you are saying. Use objects, gestures and body language.
- Don't be confusing. Don't twiddle your earrings and talk about teeth!
- Even if thought process or words get mixed up you may still be able to understand what is being said. One resident asked me to get 'a packet of ball-points'. When I asked him what he would do with them, he replied 'Shave of course'. He used Bic disposable razors and Bic, as we all know, also make ball-points. Another resident asked for 'Kippers no ... Kiplings'; what she wanted was Mr Kipling's Cherry Bakewells.
- Check that you have understood what has been said: 'So you want me to get you some of those yellow Bic razors to shave with?'
- Don't laugh at their attempts to communicate with you. The person is trying very hard. Do not denigrate their efforts or strip them of their dignity.
- Be prepared for a display of emotion – many people are grateful for the opportunity to communicate.
- Do not avoid communication because you feel it may upset the person. You are actually helping and enabling the person to express their thoughts and fears.
- Ensure that you are calm.
- Don't appear rushed – even if you are.
- Concentrate
- Let the person know that you are aware of the effort she has made to communicate with you and that you appreciate the effort made.

Sensory integration therapy
Consider the way some of our residents spend their days:

- Sitting in the same place in the same chair – their view of the world is restricted
- Sitting on a vinyl chair
- Feeling the textures of cotton, polyester cotton and nylon
- Hearing a blaring TV programme or the noise and bustle of other residents and staff
- Smelling only air freshener, furniture polish and soap
- Being touched only when care is required
- Being cared for in a constant temperature
- Having no idea of the weather outside or the passing of the seasons
- Rarely getting the opportunity to go out.

Routine is important to people with dementia. It helps them to make sense of their world and their lives. However, consider making small changes to the person's routine to increase stimulus and enrich and enhance quality of life. Consider introducing sensory integration therapy.

Staff education and development
Staff attitude and behaviour is of crucial importance if we are to enable rather than disable the individual with dementia. Staff though can only offer enabling care if they are taught to do so. All staff – registered nurses, care assistants, and domestic staff – require education and training if we are to enable people within our homes to function to the highest possible level.

Creating an environment open to change
Education though is not enough. You read, you attend seminars and you go back to your unit full of enthusiasm and keen to change things. Some of you will succeed, others will achieve nothing. You may even become frustrated because of this. Why? As nurses, we need to learn how to manage change, how to introduce change without it appearing to threaten and devalue all that has gone before. We also need to create environments that welcome ideas and are willing to try new things. Some of the things we try will not work. We need to create environments where staff are not crucified when things fail – supportive environments where people learn from their failures and have the support and the courage to try again. Building up a support network will also help you to cope with managing change. Ultimately the difference between providing quality care is not just about having enough staff and enough training, it is also about passion, commitment and courage.

Conclusion

Nursing people with dementia makes many demands on staff. If we are to believe the medical model, we are nursing empty shells that once contained unique individuals. The medical model is comforting and safe because we are all vulnerable. It allows us to put some distance between ourselves and the questions that nursing people with dementia raises. Frailty, madness, dying and death and frightening. The medical model enables us to keep our distance and to stay safe.

   There are dangers though in adopting the medical model. The medical model encourages us to believe that there is no one at home – we are merely nursing breathing corpses – the intellect, and presumably, the spirit have died. Then we cease to nurse people and merely perform a series of tasks for the 'living dead'. Seeing human beings as 'less than human' encourages us to see them merely in terms of work to be done – as fast as possible – never mind the quality – does it really matter? The nursing model of working to make contact with the person is less safe but ultimately more life affirming, and the nurse gains as much if not more than the person with dementia.

Key points

- Signage and visual clues affect ability
- Familiar décor lowers confusion and anxiety levels
- It is possible to enhance communication skills
- Staff education and development is crucial to providing quality care
- Introduce change without devaluing that which went before.

Challenging behaviour

The type of resident cared for in nursing homes has changed dramatically in recent years. Now, higher dependency levels and staffing shortages can mean that nurses are run off their feet. At one time, the average nursing home had one or two residents with behavioural problems; now nurses often find a third of residents have challenging behaviour.

This section aims to discuss the reasons why challenging behaviour occurs and then to offer some solutions.

This section will:

- Discuss the person we are caring for
- Explain the ABC technique
- Look at the reasons why challenging behaviour occurs
- Explore the reasons why a person wanders
- Explore the risk factors for aggression
- Discuss the reasons for shouting and screaming

Who are we caring for?

Dementia leads to profound difficulties in communicating. Often it is difficult for us to find out about the person. It is impossible to offer individualised care if we do not know who the person is. Doris may be spitting out her beef casserole because she hates beef, does not like gravy, or detests onions. Doris may attempt to rip off her red blouse because she hates red. Doris may spend hours rubbing her arms because she cannot bear the Yardley's lavender you have thoughtfully sprayed on. Doris may yell 'Peter' all day, but how can you respond when you do not know who Peter is? Life history books enable you to offer care that is as individual as Doris[49]. These books are designed to record important details about the person's life and can include pictures and other papers[50]. These books point out that life is a movie, not a snapshot. Our view of the resident is limited. We see only an old man or woman. The child, the young adult, the parent, the worker, and all other aspects escape us. Encouraging relatives and friends to help the resident prepare a collage can help us to see the whole person. The individual or others can use the collage as a talking point. Using a life history book or collage helps staff learn about the person and enables them to tailor care to the person's needs. You can easily draw up your own life history books and encourage family and friends to complete them.

The ABC technique

Challenging behaviour can be very disruptive and stressful. Often nurses are so involved in day to day care that it is difficult to step back and work out what is happening. The ABC technique aims to help you work out what is happening and how to sort things out:

Antecedent or activating event. What set this off? Perhaps you tried to persuade Mary to have an extra spoonful of pudding.
Behaviour. What happened? What did Mary do in response to this trigger? Perhaps she threw the spoonful of food at you, or spat it out and pulled the tablecloth and all the dishes off the table.
Consequences. What happened next? How did you respond?

The most important question to ask is, 'Is she trying to tell me something?'. Perhaps the metal of the spoon touched a sensitive tooth. Perhaps she's had enough pudding and she's fed up with you force feeding her.

Why does challenging behaviour occur?

There is usually a reason for the challenging behaviour. Our challenge is to identify the reason. The next paragraphs look at specific behaviour and ways of dealing with it.

Wandering
Wandering is: 'Moving about with any definite purpose or destination'. We think of wanderers as poor lost souls moving around without any purpose but we are mistaken. Wandering is rarely aimless; wanderers wander with a purpose[51]. One researcher mapped the journeys of wanderers and found that 93% of journeys led to a logical destination. Most (59%) were to a person or a group of people and 29% to a window with an outside view. When a person wanders, you should ask the following questions:

- Is this a problem? When people who wander are cared for in settings that are not designed for them, wandering can cause enormous problems[52]. Is the person's wandering a problem or is it the environment? Many homes have introduced wandering walkways with seats and interesting things to do along the way. Others have introduced safe enclosed gardens with interesting features such as wind chimes and bubble fountains.
- Is this person wandering alone or with a friend?

- Does the wandering appear aimless? Is the person looking for someone or something?
- Is the person distressed, perhaps looking for a child?
- Is the person happy?
- Is the wandering constant or does it occur only at certain times?

Use the ABC technique to help you identify causes and work out solutions.

Case history

George's wandering was driving everyone in the nursing home mad. At around 6AM he would collect pieces of paper, write on them, and then go around the bedrooms putting the papers under the doors. A life history revealed that George was a former postman. George was delivering everyone's post. Staff decided to ask George to sort out the post and deliver it to residents. The post came at 7.30 so George waited by the door for it to arrive. Often he chatted with the postman. Then George sorted out the post, very accurately, and delivered it to residents. Now George's behaviour was no longer a problem.

Case history

Elsie was always wandering around the home looking for something. She would go into residents' rooms and turn out their wardrobes and chests muttering, 'it is here somewhere, I know it is''. Eventually staff found that Elsie was looking for her handbag. They provided a handbag, complete with purse, compact and tissues, and Elsie's wandering stopped.

Aggression

'Violence is the voice of the unheard' – Martin Luther-King. Aggression and violence can cause staff to fear and dislike residents. However there is always a reason for aggression and violence[53]. Use the ABC technique to help you identify causes. Possible causes include:

- Misunderstanding care as an assault
- Having some insight and trying to cope or hide the condition
- Being unable to perform a task and becoming frustrated
- Sensory deprivation, e.g. poor eyesight, hearing, etc.
- Staff may be perceived as aggressive and trigger a defensive reaction
- Understimulation
- Poor environment – disabling, causing frustration and aggression
- Being thought of as dependent and not being given the chance to do things for self
- Being ignored or not consulted
- Too many carers
- Different approaches and expectations from different staff
- Noise or disturbance disrupting sleep patterns.

Shouting and screaming

'Help, help help.'
'Peter, Peter, Peter.'
'Nurse, nurse, nurse.'
Often the person who shouts, screams or repeats the same thing over and over again is ignored. The more she yells the less we hear. We say to

concerned visitors 'Don't worry – she's always saying that. She's okay.' The problem is that she is not okay and we don't feel too good either. Use the ABC technique to identify problems. Sometimes shouting and screaming is caused by overstimulation. Sometimes it is a response to understimulation, a response to sensory deprivation[54]. Sensory integration therapy often helps. Sometimes the person is calling for someone and having access to the person's life history will help.

Case history

Ruby shouted 'Peter' from morning till night. The nurses were baffled. According to the social worker Ruby had no family or close friends. Then a neighbour visited. Peter was Ruby's budgie and was staying with the neighbour. Peter came to stay with Ruby and sang most of the day. Ruby no longer called for Peter.

Seeking help

If you are unable to manage a person's behaviour remember that none of us can be experts at every type of care – call in an expert. Your local mental health team can advise you how to manage behavour and can give you support and advice.

Key points

- Life histories enable you to offer individualised care
- It is important to work out the causes of challenging behaviour
- Wandering is not a purposeless activity – the challenge is to find out the purpose
- Aggressive episodes can be reduced using the ABC technique
- Drug treatment has its limitations and should be used with care and constant monitoring.

Further reading

Allan, K.M. (1994) (ed.) *Wandering*. Dementia Services Development Centre, Stirling University, Stirling, Scotland.

Fox, J. (1995). *Understanding the Behavioural Problems in Early Onset Dementia*. Julia Fox.

Harvey, M. (1990) *Who's confused?* Prepar Publications. Birmingham.

Roberts, C. (1997). *The Management of Wandering in Older People with Dementia*. The Foundation of Nursing Studies, London.

Stokes G. (1988) *Screaming and Shouting*. Winslow Press, Bicester.

Ethical issues

The aim of this section is to explore ethical issues concerning the care of people with dementia. As nurses, we are bound by a professional code of conduct. Increasingly nursing literature is critical of what is termed 'medical or nursing paternalism'. Nurses are urged to respect the individual, to nurse the whole person, to respect the person's wishes, values and rights. Enabling the individual to live their own life even when their goals and values are different from our own, is now considered good practice. However, not all people are capable of making decisions.

People with dementia are human beings; we must work to preserve their choices and rights. But the individual's capacity may change according to the environment, the people caring for her, the time of day, prescribed medication and physiological state. People with dementia are vulnerable and in need of protection and support. As nurses, we have a great deal of power over our residents' lives. How do we protect the individual without dominating? How do we help without taking over, rendering them powerless and fostering learned helplessness?

Ethical principles

The basic principle of ethics is 'beneficence'. That means that the nurse acts in the individual's best interests. The nurse chooses 'goodness over badness'. Sometimes, in the real world things are not black and white only shades of grey. Look at the following cases, which involve some ethical issues, and consider how you would deal with them.

Case history – The issue of choice

Mr Peters has dementia. He is sitting in the lounge and you suspect that he has defecated in his pants. You take him to his room and your suspicions are confirmed. He refuses to remove his clothes or let you help him bath and change. What would you do?

Case history – Personal freedom versus safety

Mrs Leeds has a very poor short-term memory. You are aware that if she leaves the home unaccompanied she may get lost, forget where she lives or get run over on the busy main road. Snow has been falling steadily all day and the pavements are like polished glass. You meet Mrs Leeds in the hall. She is wearing her hat and coat and tells you, 'Nice of you to visit dear. I'm just off to collect my children from school and do some shopping before my husband comes home. Do let yourself out when you've finished.' She is adamant that she is going. What do you do?

Case history – Can you justify dishonesty?

Neighbours call the police because they are worried about two elderly sisters, Doris and Ethel, who live alone. The police break into the house and find both sisters are cold, undernourished and ill. They are both taken to hospital. Doris dies. You are caring for Ethel and she asks you how Doris is. You cannot pass the buck to the doctors because, say, they are all away at a conference. What would you do?

Case history – Informed consent

Mrs Jones is 89 years old. She is hallucinating and is extremely confused and agitated. She screams constantly and complains that her hair is on fire, rats are eating her toes and you have stolen her baby. Her GP prescribes Stelazine 5 mg daily. Mrs Jones settles down and although she remains confused, she appears happy and contented. Her family are relieved. Things are just settling down when you receive an unannounced inspection. The registration officer accuses you of breaching your professional code of conduct by giving medication without consent. She points out that Mrs Jones is unable to understand the effects of Stelazine and give her consent to taking it. How do you explain that your actions are ethical?

Case history – Medical treatment

Mrs Anderson has lived at the nursing home for eight years. She has end stage dementia. She is mute, immobile, doubly incontinent and depends on nursing staff to give her puréed diet and fluids. She is now refusing all diet and fluids. Her family are aware that without artificial methods of hydration she will soon die. They state that it will be 'a happy release' and that she has had a good life. Her GP visits and asks you to help him insert a fine bore nasogastric tube to enable rehydration. Matron and her deputy are away at a nursing homes conference and you have no way of contacting them. What would you do?

Conclusion

Often with ethical issues, there is no easy answer. The 'right' answer in one situation will be 'wrong' in another. The principle that we are acting in the resident's best interests and making every effort to ascertain their view is all that we have.

Further reading and information

BMA & RCN (1995) *The Older Person: Consent and Care*. BMA, London.
Counsel & Care (1992) *What If They Hurt Themselves*. Counsel & Care, London.
Alzheimer's Disease Society, Gordon House, 10 Greencoat Place, London SW1 1PH, Tel. 020 7306 0606. Fax 020 7306 0808.
email: enquiries@alzheimers.org.uk This charity produces a number of useful factsheets on all aspects of Alzheimer's disease, including *Dementia: drugs used for behavioural problems*, a useful handout for relatives. The website: www.alzheimers.org.uk has lots of interesting and downloadable information and fact sheets. Order enquiries for publications can be made by telephoning 020 7306 0606. Fax 020 7306 0808.

References

[1] Forsyth, E. & Ritzline, P.D. (1998) An overview of the aetiology, diagnosis and treatment of Alzheimer's Disease. *Physical Therapy*, **78**(12), 1325–1331.
[2] Bolla, L.R., Filley, C.M. & Palmer, R.M. (2000) Dementia DDx. Office diagnosis of the four major types of dementia. *Geriatrics*, **55**(1), 34–37.
[3] Fratigilioni, L., De Ronchi, D. & Aguero-Torres, H. (1999) Worldwide prevalence and incidence of dementia. *Drugs, Aging*, **15**(5), 355–375.
[4] Goldsmith, Malcolm (1996) *Hearing the voices of people with dementia. Obstacles and opportunities*. Jessica Kingsley, London.
[5] Bolla, L.R., Filley, C.M. & Palmer, R.M. (2000) Dementia DDx. Office diagnosis of the four major types of dementia. *Geriatrics*, **55**(1), 34–37.
[6] Farina, E., Pomati, S. & Mariani, C. (1999) Observations on dementias with possibly reversible symptoms. *Aging* (Milano) **11**(5), 323–328.
[7] Roy, R. (1984) *Immunology and infection in the elderly*. Churchill Livingstone, Edinburgh.
[8] De Week, A. (1992) Immune Response in Ageing, constitutive and environment aspects. In: Munro, H. & Schlief, G. (eds) *Nutrition of the Elderly*. Raven Press, New York.

[9] Young, J.B. & Dobrzanski, S. (1992) Pressure sores epidemiology and current management concepts. *Age & Ageing*, **2**(1), 42–57.

[10] British Diabetic Association (1996) *Diabetes in the United Kingdom*. A report by the British Diabetic Association. BDA, London.

[11] Meneilly, G.S. & Tessier, D. (1995) Diabetes in the elderly. *Diabetic Medicine*, **12**, 949–960.

[12] Sinclair, A.J. (1994) Diabetes care in the aged: time for a reappraisal? *Practical Diabetes*, **11**(2), 60–62.

[13] Gale, E. & Tattersall, R. (1990) *Diabetes Clinical Management*. Churchill Livingstone, Edinburgh.

[14] Langan, S. *et al.* (1989) Recurrent hypoglaecemia causes cumulative cognitive impairment in patients with type 1 (insulin dependent) diabetes. *Diabetic Medicine*, **6**(2) 7a (supplement).

[15] Chester, R. & Smith, J. (1995) *Older People's Sadness*. Counsel & Care, London.

[16] Alzheimer's Disease Society (1997) *Diagnosis and assessment*. Fact sheet. Alzheimer's Disease Society, London.

[17] O'Brien, J.T. & Levy, R. (1992) Age associated memory impairment. *British Medical Journal*, **304**(6818), 5–6.

[18] Alzheimer's Disease Society (1997) *Genetics and Alzheimer's disease*. Fact sheet. Alzheimer's Disease Society, London.

[19] Cox, S.M. & McLennan, J.M. (1994) *A Guide to Early Onset Dementia*. Stirling Dementia Services Centre.

[20] Papka, M., Rubio, A., Schiffer, R.B. & Cox, C. (1998) Lewy body disease: can we diagnose it? *Journal Neuropsychiatry Clinical Neuroscience*, **10**(4), 405–412.

[21] Louis, E.D., Klatka, L.A., Lui, Y. & Fahn, S. (1997) Comparison of extrapyramidal features in 31 pathologically confirmed cases of diffuse Lewy body disease and 34 pathologically confirmed cases of Parkinson's disease. *Neurology*, **48**(2), 376–380.

[22] Ala, T.A., Yang, K.H., Sung, J.H. & Frey, W.H. (1997) Hallucinations and signs of Parkinsonism help distinguish patients with dementia and cortical Lewy bodies from patients with Alzheimer's disease at presentation: a clinicopathological study. *Neurology, Neurosurgery Psychiatry*, **62**(1), 16–21.

[23] Ballard, C., Holmes, C., McKeith, J., Neill, D., O'Brien, J., Cairns, N., Lantos, P., Perry, E., Ince, P. & Perry, R. (1999) Psychiatric morbidity in Lewy Bodies: a prospective clinical and neuropathological comparative study with Alzheimer's disease. *American Journal Psychiatry*, **156**(7), 1039–1045.

[24] Papka, M., Rubio, A., Schiffer, R.B. & Cox, C. (1998) Lewy Body Disease: can we diagnose it? *Journal of Neuropsychiatry Clinical Neuroscience*, **10**(4), 405–412.

[25] Kunlik, M.E., Huffman, J.C., Bharani, N., Hillman, S.L., Molinari, V.A. & Orengo, C.A. (2000) Behavioural disturbance in geropsychiatric inpatients across dementia types. *Journal Geriatrics, Psychiatry and Neurology*, **13**(1), 49–52.

[26] Roman, C.G. (1999) Vascular dementia today. *Rev Neurol*, **155**, supplement 4, S64–72.

[27] Leblhuber, F., Walli, J., Tilz, G.P., Wachter, H. & Fuchs, D. (1998) Systemic changes of the immune system with Alzheimer's Dementia. *Dtch Med Wochenschr*, **123**(25–26), 787–791.

[28] Verbeek, M.M., Otte-Holler, I., Ruiter, D.J. & de Waal, R.M. (1997) Inflammatory mechanisms in the pathogenesis of Alzheimer's disease. *Tijdschur Gerontol Geriatric*, **25**(5), 213–218.

[29] Prince, M., Rabe-Hesketh, S. & Brennan, P. (1998) Do anti-arthritic drugs

decrease the risk for cognitive decline? An analysis based on data from the MRC treatment trial of hypertension in older adults. *Neurology*, **50**(2), 374–379.

30 Rodriguez, M.M. & Grossberg, G.T. (1998) Estrogen as a psychotherapeutic agent. *Clinics Geriatric Medicine*, **14**(1), 177–189.

31 Fastbom, J., Forsell, Y. & Winblad, B. (1998) Benzodiazepines may have protective effects against Alzheimer's disease. *Alzheimer's Disease Associated Disorders*, **12**(1), 14–15.

32 Schnieder, L.S. & Tariot, D.N. (1994) Emerging drugs for Alzheimer's disease. Mechanisms of action and prospects for cognitive enhancing medication. *Medical Clinics of North America*, **78**(4), 911–934.

33 Lawrence, A.D. & Sahakia, B.J. (1998) The cognitive psychopharmacology of Alzheimer's Disease: focus on cholinergic systems. *Neurochem. Res.*, **23**(5), 787–794.

34 Norman, I. (1998) Treating dementia. *Elderly Care*, **10**(1), 14–15.

35 Shintani, E.Y. & Uchida, K.M. (1997) Donepezil: an anticholinesterase inhibitor for Alzheimer's disease. *American Journal Health Systems Pharmacology*, **54**(24), 2805–2810.

36 Packer, T. (1999) Rationing memory. *Elderly Care*, **10**(1), 16–17.

37 Lopez-Arrieta, J.M. & Birks, J. (2000) Nimodipine for primary degenerative, mixed and vascular dementia. *Cochrane database review*: HD:2: CD000147 2000.

38 Maurer, K., Ihl, R., Dierks, T. & Frolich, L. (1997) Clinical efficacy of Ginkgo biloba special extract EGB761 in dementia of the Alzheimer type. *Journal Psychiatric Residents*, **31**(6), 645–655.

39 Stevermer, J.J. & Lindbloom, E.J. (1998) Ginkgo biloba for dementia. *Journal Family Practice*, **46**(1), 20.

40 Tarriot, P., Gaile, S.E., Castelli, N.A. & Porsteinsson, A.P. (1997) Treatment of agitation in dementia. *New Directory of Mental Health Services*, **79**, 109–123.

41 Fontana & Smith (1989) Alzheimer's Disease victims, the unbecoming of self and the normalisation of competence. *Sociological Perspectives*, **32**(1), 43–45.

42 Jacques, Alan (1992) Understanding Dementia. Churchill Livingstone, Edinburgh.

43 Kelly, M. (1993) *Designing for People with Dementia in the Context of the Building Standards*. University of Stirling, Dementia services Development Centre, Stirling, Scotland.

44 Ford, Fox and Fitch (1986) Light in the darkness. *Nursing Times*, 7 January.

45 Social Services Inspectorate (1993) Inspecting for Quality: Standards for the Residential Care of Elderly People with Dementia. The Stationery Office, London.

46 Lubinski, I. (1991) Dementia and Communication. Decker, London.

47 Jones, Gemma (1992) A communication model for dementia. In: *Care Giving and Dementia Research and Application*. Tavistock Routledge, London.

48 Griffiths, H. (1991) The psychiatry of old age: the effects of dementia on communication. In: Gravell, R. & Frances, J. (eds) *Speech and Communication Problems in Psychiatry*. Chapman Hall, London.

49 Midwinter, Eric (1996) *Getting to Know Me*. Third Age Press, London.

50 Irving, E. (1996) *The Landscapes of a Lifetime*. Third Age Press, London.

51 McGregor, I. & Bell, J. (1994) Buzzing with life, energy and drive. *Journal of Dementia Care*, **2**(6), 20–21.

52 Allan, Kate (1994) Dementia in acute units: wandering. *Nursing Standard*, **9**(8).

53 Holden, U. (1994) Dementia in acute units: aggression. *Nursing Standard*, **37**(9), 11–14.

54 Stokes, G. (1996) *Screaming and Shouting*. Winslow Press, Cheshire.

Chapter 4

Medication Management

Introduction

The registered nurse's role in relation to medication is changing as the role of nursing homes changes. The nurse has a number of roles:

- To order, store and audit medication
- To dispense medication
- To enable residents to take medication
- To observe residents for signs of adverse effects to medication
- To work with medical staff and the pharmacist to minimise medication and avoid polypharmacy
- To ensure that residents on medication are reviewed
- To dispense homely remedies
- To prescribe medication if a nurse prescriber.

Some of the roles a registered nurse undertakes within a home are alien to nurses who work in hospital settings where pharmacists are employed.

This chapter aims to:

- Make you aware of good practice
- Enable you to order, store and record medications
- Enable you to provide an audit trail for medications
- Enable you to fulfil legislative requirements
- Provide practical help in implementing good practice in your workplace

---

Ordering medication

Medication is ordered on an individual basis for individuals in nursing homes. Stock medication cannot be ordered and stock bottles cannot be kept. If ten individuals are prescribed digoxin 62.5 mcg then ten individual prescriptions must be issued. Each prescription issued by a GP must have the individual's name and address on it. No more than seven items can be ordered on one prescription form (FP10). Prescription items are normally ordered every 28 or 30 days for all individuals in a home. Items such as a course of antibiotics are ordered when prescribed and for a set number of days.

When a GP has supplied a prescription, the nurse completes the back of it on the individual's behalf. She indicates, by ticking a box, that the individual is over retirement age (and thus entitled to free prescriptions) and stamps and signs the prescription. Details of all prescriptions ordered should be recorded. This can either be a computer record or entered in a bound book kept specially for this purpose. The record or book should have details of date ordered, name of resident, drug ordered, dose, and amount of medication ordered. The home should keep a book of medication received. This book should have details of date of delivery and space for two nurses to sign when the medication is received. This book provides a record of all medication received into the home. Individuals who enter the home from hospital or the community should have any medication that they bring in with them entered in this book. Failure to do this can cause problems when auditing medication.

Controlled drugs

It is good practice to record any controlled drugs ordered in red and to write the amount ordered in words and figures. Controlled drugs must be entered in a controlled drugs book.

Choosing a pharmacist

Nurses who have been appointed to work in a new home will be approached by a number of retail pharmacists who are anxious to supply the home with a pharmacy service. Older people living in nursing homes receive medical care from GPs who prescribe medication by writing a prescription on a form FP10. Normally prescriptions are left with the home, which obtains the medication from a retail pharmacist.

Retail pharmacists are paid for each prescription item they dispense and nursing home business is extremely lucrative so they compete with each other to supply nursing homes. Nurses are often unaware of this and arrange for the first pharmacist to approach them, or the nearest pharmacist, to supply the home. It is advisable for nurses to ask pharmacists what services they will supply before appointing. It is important that an out-of-hours service is available so that nurses can obtain emergency prescriptions 24 hours a day, 365 days a year, if required. This service should be available as standard and not given as a favour or grudgingly. A delivery service should be provided for regular and emergency items. It is important to enquire if the pharmacist has a computerised system. Pharmacists with computer systems, or another method, can provide monthly or four weekly printouts of resident prescriptions, which can be used when auditing medication. They will also be able to supply records of a person's usage of a particular medication going back months, if required for auditing purposes. Pharmacists should be willing to take part in drug audits and assist and advise nurses in implementing good practice. Pharmacists can make an enormous contribution to quality of care. One study showed that pharmacist review of medications within nursing homes led to fewer drugs being prescribed and lower death rates[1].

Medication in nursing homes is prescribed to individuals. Enquire how the pharmacist proposes to deliver a monthly supply of medication. The pharmacist who delivers it jumbled up in a couple of cardboard boxes is wasting your time and does not deserve your business. Choose the pharmacist who will deliver every individual's medication in an individually labelled bag. This will save nursing time when checking medication received and will make it easy to store medication and find it in the stock cupboard when it is required.

If you find a number of pharmacists who can meet your requirements, ask them which nursing homes they currently supply. The staff of another home will normally be pleased to tell you the pharmacist's good and bad points. A little time taken choosing a pharmacist will save so much time and trouble that it really is worth choosing your pharmacist with care. There is no reason why nurses should feel compelled to choose the nearest pharmacist, if a better service is available from a pharmacist some distance away and delivery arrangements are satisfactory.

Getting the best from an existing pharmacist

Many nurses inherit a pharmacist when they go to work in a home. A good pharmacist plays an important role in ensuring that a first class pharmacy service is delivered to a home. Sadly there are some pharmacists who do little more than dispense medication. Some nurses are expected to collect and deliver prescriptions and medication to their homes and are expected to use emergency pharmacists for out-of-hours services. Nurses who find themselves in such situations should meet with the pharmacist and negotiate a service such as that outlined in the section above. Most pharmacists who are aware of nurses' needs and expectations will be eager to change and tailor their service to the home's requirements, as they would not wish to risk losing the business.

Homely remedies

The use of homely remedies in nursing homes is increasing. In some areas the GP and the home manager agree a written list of non-prescription medicines which nursing staff may give without a prescription. These items normally include paracetamol and cough medicines. The agreement stipulates the length of time these may be given, usually between two and four days. This is verified or agreed by the district pharmacist.

If homely remedies are given, the home needs to have a supply of stock items such as paracetamol and simple linctus. These must be purchased from a pharmacist and dispensed as agreed. Nurses need to be alert when giving homely remedies. Mrs Jones may simply have a headache that will respond to paracetamol, but it might be something more serious.

Nurse prescribing

The first courses in nurse prescribing for nurses who are not working as district nurses are now in place. The courses have a taught element and a period of supervised practice. Nurse prescribing has the potential to make a huge difference to care within homes. Nurses will have the ability not only to prescribe but also to review medications and to discontinue those that are no longer required.

Storing medication

As all medication is prescribed and dispensed on an individual basis, storage of medication can be difficult. Homes should have a drugs trolley (or trolleys) with a drawer for each individual. All medication in current use for the individual should be stored in the drawer. Additional bottles and packs of medication can be stored in bags with the individual's name on the bag, in a locked cupboard, preferably in the treatment room. Some medication, such as eye drops, may require refrigeration. It is not good practice to store such medication in a refrigerator in the kitchen; the treatment room should be equipped with a small fridge where medication can be stored. Fridge temperatures should be checked daily and recorded.

Medication for external use such as lotions and creams, should not be stored with medicines for internal use, such as tablets and syrups. They are usually stored in a cupboard in the treatment room. The storage of controlled drugs is governed by the Misuse of Drugs (Safe Custody) Regulations 1973. Controlled drugs must be stored in a specially purchased metal cupboard designed for their storage.

Administration of drugs

Homes should have written policies regarding the administration of drugs. Written policies safeguard individual residents and nurses and reduce the possibility of errors. At one time most hospitals insisted that two nurses carried out drug rounds, one dispensing medication while the other checked it and administered it. It is now common practice in many hospitals for one nurse to administer medication. This increases the possibility of error and in a nursing home environment, where many individuals require help to take their medication, makes administration much slower.

Nurses within homes should discuss and decide policy on medication administration; it will depend on the size of the home and the numbers of trained staff on duty at any one time. Some homes have policies that state that whenever possible medication should be administered by two registered nurses, but when staffing levels or workload make this impractical, one registered nurse may dispense medication. You may ask a care assistant to give medication (other than controlled drugs) that you dispense. This means that you dispense the medication and watch the care assistant give the medication.

Unacceptable practices

Nurses in many settings will encounter registered nurses who dispense medications into medicine pots and place the individual's name on the pot. Several individual's medications are dispensed at once and all are placed on a tray. The nurse then carries the tray around and gives out the medication. This practice is known as secondary dispensing and is in contravention of UKCC guidelines. It is extremely dangerous – the possibilities of medication error are enormous – and is totally unacceptable. Written drug policies for the home should make it absolutely clear that this is forbidden.

Some nurses dispense medication and then sign for all medication on the unit after the drug round. This is totally unacceptable. How can the nurse possibly remember who is prescribed medication at this time and who has required PRN medications? If medications have been changed since the nurse last looked at the chart she may give drugs in error or omit prescribed drugs.

Nurses should not alter labels. Wrongly labelled medication should be returned to the pharmacy. Nurses should not transfer medication from one container to another.

Identifying residents

People admitted to hospitals are given wristbands showing their name and hospital number. In nursing homes the emphasis is on providing nursing care in a homely domestic environment and the use of name bands for identification purposes is rare. Usually the residents are well known to staff working at the home but occasionally newly appointed staff, agency or bank staff who are unfamiliar with all the residents, are required to give out medication. The use of a photograph fixed to the drug chart enables nurses to identify individuals without resorting to institutional devices such as name bands.

Drug charts

Nurses are required to keep a record of all medication given. Normally medication is written up on a drug chart. In many homes nurses transcribe on to the chart the prescription written on an FP10 prescription by the individual's GP, and the doctor signs this chart. It is possible to buy ready-printed medication charts but nurses can have their own charts printed especially for their home (or group of homes) for little more than the cost of buying preprinted charts. Many preprinted charts run for 90 day cycles without requiring rewriting. This discourages regular medication reviews by doctors. It is good practice to use charts that require rewriting every 28–30 days. A sample chart is shown in Fig. 4.1.

Medication charts should have space in which to record drugs not given, the reasons for their omission, time, and the signature of the nurse. They should also have a separate section for 'as required' prescriptions; this should have sufficient space for nurses to indicate the time of administration and, if appropriate, the dose given. The chart should also have a section for 'once only' medications such as vaccinations. The sample chart (Fig. 4.1) also has a space labelled pharmacy. This space is used by nurses to record the date on which a new bottle of medication is commenced and how many tablets were in the bottle when it was opened. This is explained in detail in the drug auditing section later in this chapter.

Recording medication

It is essential that nurses maintain records of medication given. Medicine charts and resident records should be maintained for eight years after resi-

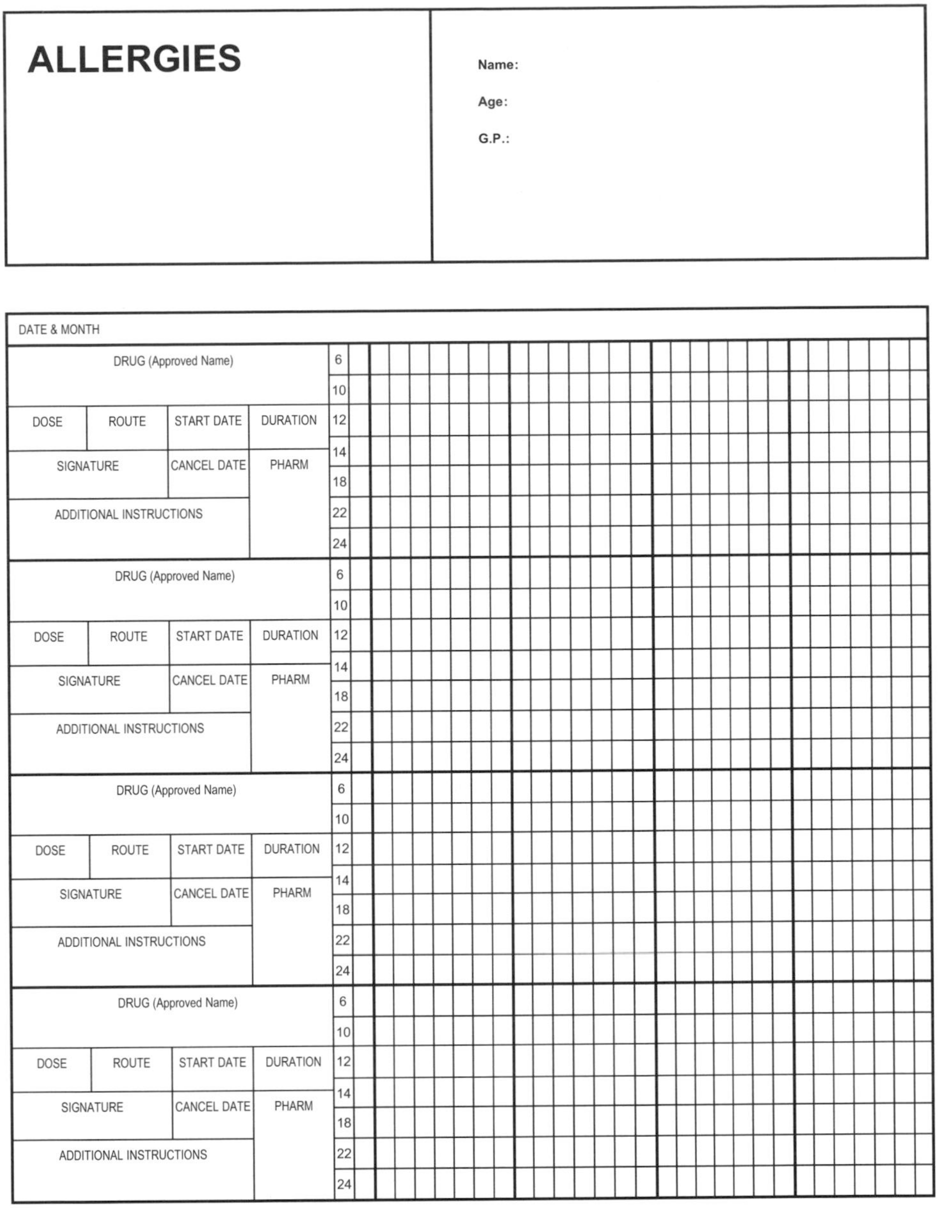

Fig. 4.1 Sample medication chart.

dent discharge or death. Medications are prescribed on a regular or 'as required' basis. Nurses should never give medication with which they are unfamiliar; they should look up the drug in an up-to-date version of the British National Formulary (BNF) or another reference book. Retail pharmacists are usually happy to supply complementary copies of the most up-to-date versions of these books to nursing homes they supply with drugs.

The nurse has a duty to withhold prescribed medication if she feels it is unsafe or unwise to administer it. A nurse who encounters a higher than normal dose of medication, or a chart and bottle showing different dosages, should withhold medication. The nurse who suspects that an individual is suffering an adverse drug reaction should withhold medication. In these circumstances the nurse should inform the person's GP. She should record her reasons for withholding medication on the medication chart in the 'drugs not given section' and also in the nursing records. The nursing records should include details of any action she has taken such as returning medication to this pharmacy or requesting that a doctor alter an incorrectly completed medication chart.

Controlled drugs

Controlled drugs should be recorded not only on the medication chart but also in the controlled drugs register. Controlled drugs registers can usually be purchased from the district pharmacist's office, which is usually based at the local hospital. They can also be purchased from the Stationery Office – your local telephone directory will provide details. A separate page is required for each medication. Two nurses should sign that they have checked and administered the prescribed medication. In small homes where only one registered nurse is on duty on a shift, it is often possible for drug administration times of regular medications to coincide with handovers so that two nurses are available. If this is not possible, perhaps because medication is being given on an 'as required' basis, the registered nurse should ask a care assistant to check and sign that she has witnessed the registered nurse administering the medication to the resident. This is not a legal requirement but such practice protects both the resident and the nurse.

Drug audits

Nurses should audit medication every 28 to 30 days. The interval will depend on the prescription cycle in use by doctors who are providing medical care to older people within the home. In many homes one doctor cares for the majority of residents but in others there are a number of doctors. It is much easier if all doctors use the same prescription cycle and this can usually be arranged.

Auditing at first appears to involve a lot of hard work and the first reaction of some nurses is to think that it is creating work for work's sake. Auditing has two main functions. It enables nurses to monitor the usage of drugs and to ensure that they are being given correctly. It also ensures that each resident has sufficient drugs to carry them through a prescription cycle. This saves a lot of time and effort and with efficient auditing systems drugs do not run out, nurses do not have to constantly re-order drugs, and pharmacists do not have to keep rushing up and down to the home with prescription items. Auditing systems quickly repay the time and effort involved in setting them up.

When nurses have worked out the prescription cycle they will use they need to draw up a table of audit dates, medication order dates and delivery dates. The interval between the order date and delivery date should be discussed with the pharmacist. It is sensible to allow a week or ten days between order and delivery dates.

Pharmacists should be involved in drug audits whenever possible. In some circumstances the pharmacist cannot take part in every audit but should be involved in as many as possible. The pharmacist supplies a printout or typed list which gives details of each individual in the home and the name, dosage and frequency of each medication including details of 'as required' medication. The nurse and pharmacist check that the list and medication charts are identical and that there have been no recent changes that are not included on the pharmacist's list. Each regular medicine is counted and nurse and pharmacist ensure that there is sufficient medication until the next delivery date.

A note of the amount of medication required for the next prescription interval is put on the printout. This will usually be the same amount but it can vary. In some cases the amount of tablets prescribed has been reduced and a lesser amount can be ordered for the next prescription cycle. This eliminates waste. In other cases an individual has been admitted to hospital during a prescription cycle and so all medication prescribed has not been used and the hospital have usually provided a further two weeks' supply of medication on discharge. Medication prescribed on an 'as required' basis can either be counted or estimated depending on usage. This skill is rapidly acquired. Individuals admitted during a prescription cycle have their medication counted and sufficient is ordered to bring them in line with the prescription cycle.

Auditing enables pharmacist and nurse to compile a prescription list that is accurate and reflects the amount of medication required during the cycle. This is then entered on computer so that the pharmacist can keep accurate records of each individual's drug usage. A copy of the list, or the relevant sections relating to the individuals on a doctor's list, is sent to the doctor. The nurse and pharmacist retain a copy of the list, which can be posted, faxed or delivered to the home by the pharmacist. A copy of all prescriptions required can be either recorded on computer or written into the drug ordering book by the nurse and checked by another nurse to ensure accuracy. The doctor(s) then issue individual prescriptions which are sent to the nursing home where they are checked for accuracy, stamped and collected by the pharmacist. This system has a number of checks that minimise the possibility of error.

The process of auditing sounds daunting and time consuming but once the system is in place the nurse and pharmacist can complete an audit on an average 39 bed nursing home in under two hours and it saves countless time over the prescribing period.

Avoiding auditing pitfalls

Changes of medication or dosage during a prescription cycle can cause problems with auditing. If a medication is prescribed during a prescription cycle, the amount of medication required to last until the next delivery date should be calculated. The doctor is then asked to prescribe this amount. The normal amount for the cycle is then ordered on the ordering date. When medication is increased the additional amount required until the next delivery cycle must be calculated and ordered. Short courses of medication such as antibiotics can be ordered as a complete course regardless of prescription cycle as they will not cause auditing problems. It is acceptable to order variable dose medications, such as warfarin or steroids, which are being reduced in amounts greater than the cycle, as the additional medication enables doctors to prescribe as clinically indicated without necessitating frequent calls to the pharmacy. The drug audit will enable the nurse and pharmacist to check that the individual's stock levels of variable dose medication are sufficient.

Effective auditing is dependent on the nurse and pharmacist working together. It is essential that the nurse is able to rely on a cooperative professional pharmacist if the system is to function effectively.

Keeping records of medication entering the home

Details of all medication ordered and received should be kept in a bound book, giving details of the date of order, name of resident, drug, dosage and amount ordered. When medication is received this should be checked, either by the pharmacist and the nurse or two nurses, against the order; any discrepancies or shortfalls should be noted and both should sign. This book should contain details of any medication brought from hospital or home by individuals or supplied by doctors in an emergency situation. Failure to record all sources of medication will make auditing impossible. In some areas it may be acceptable to keep these records on computer – check with your district pharmacist if in doubt.

Dealing with medication no longer required

Using a drug auditing system reduces excess stock within homes, but there are occasions when the nurse is left with medication that is no longer required. Discontinued medication should be returned to pharmacy. The medication of deceased residents should also be returned to pharmacy. It is recommended that nurses should remove medication for deceased residents from the medicine trolley, place it all in a container with a note stating the date of death, and lock this in a medicine cupboard. It should not be returned to pharmacy until seven days after the individual's death, in case the coroner wishes to have the medication examined. A record of all medication returned to pharmacy should be kept. This should be a bound book that should state the date, individual's name, name of medication, dose, amount returned and reason for returning to pharmacy. The nurse returning medication and the pharmacist receiving the medication should check these details together and should both sign the register of returned medications. There is no legal requirement to do this but it is good practice and ensures that every item of medication entering and leaving the home can be accounted for.

Medication review

More than 90% of people aged 75 and over are prescribed regular medications[2]. Older people receive 43% of all prescribed medicines and are the largest consumers of medicines[3]. The average old person living at home takes 3.5 prescribed medications[4] and the average person living in a nursing home takes six medications.

All medications have adverse effects and for every benefit a drug offers there is also the risk of adverse reactions. These can have a profound effect on an older person's quality of life. It is policy on some elderly care units for doctors to discontinue all medication, monitor resident condition carefully and prescribe only when absolutely necessary. Some older adults, though, move through the health care system acquiring more medications as doctors treat them symptomatically. Older people are more likely to suffer from adverse reactions from medication because their renal and hepatic systems are less efficient and drugs remain in the system for longer.

Medical staff have responsibilities under the National Service Framework for Older People to carry out medication reviews and to document these reviews. Nurses can help by reminding doctors to review medications regularly to ensure that older people are not prescribed medications which they no longer require. Nurses are the people in the best position to monitor residents for adverse effects of medication because they spend so much time with residents. If you suspect that a resident is suffering adverse effects from a medication you must withhold the medication and seek medical advice.

It is important that medications are monitored. If a person is prescribed Lithium, blood levels must be checked at least six monthly. If a person is prescribed thyroxin, thyroid tests should be carried out at least once a year. It is important to work with the doctors who care for residents in the home to develop systems to ensure that regular checks are carried out. In a small home these could be written in the diary and the resident's care plan. In larger homes more formal systems may be required.

Nursing practice can have an important influence on the type of medication prescribed and the amount used. The aims of quality care are to avoid polypharmacy and the use of sedatives and hypnotics and to promote an environment where drug use is minimised and quality of life maximised[5]. Box 4.1 outlines good practice in prescribing[6].

Each chapter in this book that relates to a clinical condition will examine drug treatment and explore drug interactions in depth. This section aims to flag up types of medication to which you should pay particular attention.

Hypnotics

The use of hypnotics in nursing homes is falling as medical and nursing staff become more aware of the dangers of night sedation. Hypnotics decrease the level of awareness and increase the risk of daytime drowsiness and nocturia. Reduced ability to metabolise drugs rapidly can prolong drug half-lives and the older person may be less alert during the day. Reduced levels of alertness can increase the risk of falls, reduce mobility and muscle strength and reduce diet and fluid intake, causing the older person to become weaker.

Box 4.1   Good practice in prescribing.

Minimise drug treatments
- Ensure that the drug is still necessary
- Consider risks and benefits
- Review all medicines

Optimise compliance
- Avoid complex drug regimes
- Simplify dosage use one daily regime if possible
- Use appropriate dosages to minimise side effects
- Ensure person can swallow tablets otherwise prescribe medicine in another form

Consider polypharmacy when prescribing
- Consider non drug treatments
- Pay attention to [possible adverse reactions

These changes increase the risks of developing infection and pressure sores. The use of hypnotics is now discouraged and they are no longer recommended for long term use. If a person is admitted to the home on hypnotics and there are clinical indications for these to be discontinued they will have to be reduced gradually as dependency can occur with long term use.

Many older people find it difficult to sleep when admitted to a home. The person is in a strange place, sleeping in a strange bed and surrounded by strangers. It is important to offer the person high levels of support on admission. Nursing measures such as providing a hot drink, helping the person to get comfortable and dimming lights can enable older people to sleep well.

Some older people want to go to bed very early. In winter some residents request to be put back to bed at around 4.30 PM when it gets dark. This is a difficult issue. If you help the resident back to bed she will be asleep by suppertime and wide awake at midnight. In some units older people are assisted to bed by staff at around 7 PM. This discourages evening visits from friends and family. The need for sleep diminishes with age and it is quite normal for an older person to require only six or seven hours of sleep. An older person who is asleep by 7 PM can be wide awake at 1 AM and nursing staff can report that insomnia is a problem and hypnotics can be prescribed. The real problem of course is nursing practice! Nurses need to understand that old people tire easily and need one or more naps a day to help recharge batteries. This, combined with a reasonable night's sleep, allows the person to be refreshed.

Having realistic expectations about how much sleep an adult requires is the first step. Encouraging friends and relatives to visit even for a few minutes can help an older person go to bed happy and relaxed and more likely to have a good night's sleep. Encouraging older people to stay up later, perhaps watching a video, playing cards or reading a book, will ensure that they go to bed when ready to sleep and not simply out of boredom. Bedrooms should be warm and comfortable. Offering hot milky drinks and ensuring night staff make minimal noise when moving around the home all help older people to sleep. Nurses who use their skills to help ensure older people are given a comfortable environment will find that they can virtually eliminate the use of hypnotics within the nursing home.

Diuretics

Nursing home residents are often prescribed diuretics; in one study 48% were on diuretic therapy, often for swollen ankles. Diuretic therapy can lead to urgency, frequency and urinary incontinence. Urinary incontinence can be greatly reduced in nursing home residents if nursing staff treat postural oedema by encouraging exercise wherever possible, elevation of legs and the use of support stockings and tights. Diuretic therapy can, because of the fear of incontinence, cause elderly people to become less mobile, and loss of mobility increases the risk of falls, leads to a reduction in muscle strength and increases the risk of the individual developing infection.

The inappropriate use of diuretics can cause older people to become caught on a downward spiral of depression and loss of physical strength. Nursing intervention can successfully reduce or eliminate oedema and enable the use of diuretics to be greatly reduced.

Psychotropic drugs

Large numbers of people living in homes are prescribed psychotropic drugs[7,8]. These reduce the level of alertness and individuals prescribed psychotropic drugs are at great risk of falling. The national Service framework (NSF) for older people identifies falls as one area where doctors should examine specific risk factors including the use of medication. The implementation of the NSF may lead to a reduction in the use of psychotropic medications. Diet and fluid intake can be reduced due to drowsiness. Reduced alertness can also lead to incontinence. Nurses should encourage doctors to prescribe psychotropic drugs on an 'as required' basis and should give them only as a last resort. The nurse can help older people who are unhappy and depressed by promoting an atmosphere within the home that enables people to maximise their remaining abilities rather than focusing on disabilities; more information is given in Chapter 12.

The nurse can help an older person more by listening and spending time discovering what is bothering them, rather than dispensing psychoactive drugs. Good nursing practice can significantly reduce the use of psychotropic medication within the nursing home.

Summary

Older people are more likely to be prescribed a number of drugs than younger people and are at greater risk of suffering from adverse reactions to them than younger people. GPs are busy and do not always have time to review the need for medications. Nurses can influence the amount of drugs used within a nursing home and by working in partnership with the older person and by using their nursing skills, they can ensure that residents are not prescribed medication unnecessarily.

Dealing with drug errors

Any nurse who makes or discovers a drug error has a duty to report that error. The home should have a written policy that outlines action to be taken in such circumstances. It is important for the manager to discover the reasons for the error and wherever possible to change practice to avoid such errors in the future. The UKCC has expressed concern that nurses who have made mistakes under pressure of work and have reported such errors are subject to disciplinary action.

The use of disciplinary action in such circumstances may discourage nurses from reporting drug errors. It is important that the home's policy is just and fair and that the manager carefully considers the circumstances, and advises, counsels, identifies training needs and changes practice within the home if necessary. Disciplinary action will not rectify problems associated with busy periods of the day when nursing staff feel pressurised to complete the medication round as quickly as possible; but rearranging work patterns will help avoid future errors.

Conclusion

The nurse should be aware of the effects of medication and should inform the person's doctor if an individual is suffering from side effects from medication. The nurse can remind doctors to review medication regularly and can advise on its effectiveness. The use of a drug audit enables the nurse to check all medication that is brought to the home and detect errors in administration. Written policies on drug ordering, administration, disposal and the procedure to be followed if an error occurs, protect resident and nurse.

References

[1] Furniss, L. Burns A. Craig, S.K. *et al.* (2000) Effects of a pharmacist's medication review in nursing homes. *British Journal of Psychiatry*, **176**, 563–7.

[2] Harris, C.M. & Darjdar, R. (1996) The Scope of repeat prescribing. *British Journal of General Practice*, **46**(412), 649–653.

[3] Audit Commission (1994) *A Prescription for Improvement. Towards more Rational Prescribing in General Practice.* The Stationery Office, London.

[4] Purves, I. Kennedy, J. (1994) *The Quality of General Practice Repeat Prescribing.* Department of Primary Health Care, University of Newcastle upon Tyne, Newcastle upon Tyne.

[5] Broderick, E. (1997) Prescribing patterns for nursing home residents in the US. The reality and the vision. *Drugs, Aging*, **11**(4), 255–260.

[6] Shepherd, M. (1998) The Risks of Polypharmacy. *Nursing Times*, **94**(32), 60–62.

[7] Hatton, P. (1990) Primum non nocere – an analysis of drugs prescribed to elderly patients in private nursing homes registered with Harrogate Health Authority. *Care of the Elderly*, April, (2), 4.

[8] Schneider, Justine (ed.) (1997) *Quality of Care: testing some measures in homes for elderly people*. Report of a study funded through Northern and Yorkshire NHS Executive under the Department of Health Research and mental health initiative. Discussion paper 1245, Personal Services Research Unit, University of Kent at Canterbury.

Chapter 5

Infection Control

Introduction

Older people are more vulnerable to infection than younger people. People living in nursing and residential homes are the frailest of their generation and are most at risk of infection. High quality care can reduce the risk of infection, enable older people to experience the best possible quality of life and reduce nursing workload.

This chapter is divided into six sections. This chapter aims to enable you to minimise infection within the home.

This section aims to enable you to:

- Understand how the body defends itself against infection
- Understand how ageing and illness increase the risks of infection
- Understand how ageing affects the body's ability to combat infection
- Understand how infection affects older adults.

Causes and effects of infection

Infection rates

In UK hospitals the infection rate is rising. One survey found that 6% of hospital patients acquired an infection[1] and later figures indicated that this had risen to 11%[2]. The rates of infection within hospitals are highest in elderly care wards. Medical and orthopaedic wards have the next highest rates of infection. People cared for in medical and orthopaedic wards are often elderly. Infection rates in UK hospitals are now surveyed; however no surveys are carried out on infection rates within nursing homes. There is little published information about infection rates within UK nursing homes. In North America researchers have been publishing work on infection rates since the 1960s. North American research indicates that the infection rate within nursing homes varies between 10 and 16%. Clearly older people are more susceptible to infection than younger people. Older adults living in nursing homes are the most disabled of their generation. They are more likely to suffer from chronic illness. They are often prescribed a number of medications. They are more vulnerable to infection than people of the same age who are in good health and able to live at home. This section examines how the body defends itself against infection and how ageing and illness affect those defences.

External and internal defences

The body has two lines of defence against invaders – external and internal defences. External defences are to prevent micro-organisms gaining entry to the body. If there is a breach in the wall of the body's external defences the internal defences are activated. People who have indwelling urinary catheters, intravenous catheters, nasogastric tubes and other external devices are at greater risk of contracting an infection; the device breaches the body's external defences and provides a 'portal of entry' for micro-organisms.

Table 5.1   External defences against micro-organisms.

Defence mechanism	How ageing affects this
Eyes are protected by lysozome, an enzyme with a bactericidal action found in tears	Tear production reduces with age
The mouth is protected by lysozome in saliva	Saliva production decreases with age
The respiratory tract is protected by cilia which waft micro-organisms out	This process becomes less efficient with age
The gastrointestinal tract is protected by the acidity of the stomach	Reduced stomach acidity and increase in achlorhydria
The bladder is protected by flushing of acid urine. This prevents bacteria adhering to the genito-urinary tract	The bladder muscle empties less efficiently. Residual urine increases. Bacteria can breed in this stagnant pool of urine.
The prostate gland produces a bactericide	Ageing leads to decreased production of prostatic bactericide. Prostatic enlargement leads to increased residual urine.
Vaginal secretions ensure that the vagina is acid. These acid secretions inhibit the growth of bacteria and fungi	Vaginal secretions are reduced, become alkaline and are less effective at inhibiting fungi and bacteria
Skin – sebaceous and sweat secretions produce lactic acid. This 'acid mantle' of pH 5.5 kills bacteria.	Reduced secretions, increased dryness, and loss of collagen and subcutaneous fat all reduce the ability of the skin to protect against infection

Internal defences

When micro-organisms breach the body's defence systems and enter the body, inflammation takes place. Inflammation is a non-specific immune response. It has two functions:

- To destroy micro-organisms as quickly as possible
- To prevent invading micro-organisms from spreading.

There are three stages of inflammatory response:

(1) *Histamine* is released from the mast cells. This causes blood vessels to dilate, blood flow to the area is increased, the area becomes hot and red.

(2) *Prostaglandins* increase the permeability of blood vessels. Plasma and white blood cells migrate into tissues, and the area becomes swollen.

(3) *Swollen tissue* increases the pressure on nerve endings and the area becomes painful.

How ageing affects inflammatory response

The immune system becomes less effective with age[3] and the inflammatory response is less efficient. Older adults have greater difficulty in destroying invading micro-organisms and limiting their spread. Other factors associated with impaired inflammatory response include:

- *Malnutrition* – this is very common in older people. Malnourished people can be obese, of normal weight or thin. Vitamin and mineral deficiencies impair immune response and make the older person more susceptible to infection. Medication can impair absorption of vitamins and minerals. Low levels of vitamins and minerals can reduce the ability of the immune system to fight infection.[4]
- *Medication* can impair the inflammatory response and reduce the ability of the body to contain and fight off infection. Antihistamines block the release of histamine from the mast cells. Non-steroidal anti-inflammatory drugs and steroids reduce the level of inflammatory response and increase the risk of infection.

Phagocytes and their role in combating infection

Invading micro-organisms and damaged tissue triggers the inflammatory response. When the blood flow to the area has increased, special white blood cells called phagocytes appear. There are two types of phagocytes:

(1) Polymorphonuclear neutrophil leucoytes (neutrophils)
(2) Mononuclear macrophages.

These phagocytes recognise, seek and destroy invading micro-organisms by engulfing them. This process is more efficient if the foreign cells have been marked by antibodies or proteins. The process of marking is called oponisation. It is carried out by the complement system.

The complement system
The complement system is a system of proteins or enzymes. They circulate in the blood in a dormant state and are activated by invading micro-organisms. They act by:

- Attracting neutrophils
- Enhancing phagocytosis
- Punching holes in the membrane of invading cells so that phagocytes can destroy them.

Specific immune response

Phagocytes are unable to kill all invading micro-organisms. Some micro-organisms can survive and multiply inside phagocyte cells. Lymphocytes are second line of defence against invading micro-organisms. Lymphocytes are round cells. They vary in size. All have a large round nucleus and a small edge of cytoplasm. Our knowledge about the types of lymphocytes and their specific function is still incomplete. We are aware of two types of lympho-cytes:

- *Short-lived lymphocytes* are produced in the bone marrow and live for a few days.
- *Long-lived lymphocytes* are produced in the thymus and lymph tissue and may live for months or years.

There are two types of long-lived lymphocytes:

- *T-lymphocytes* originate in the bone marrow but have to be processed by the thymus gland to gain the ability to perform their immune func-tions. They circulate in and out of the thymus gland. They recognise the antigen produced by an invading micro-organism. T-lymphocytes destroy abnormal cells such as tumour cells. They also destroy cells (including phagocytes) infected with viruses and micro-organisms. Two thirds of all circulating lymphocytes are T-lymphocytes.
- *B-lymphocytes* originate in the bone marrow. They produce antibodies against specific invading micro-organisms. Both T and B-lymphocytes work together and interact with phagocytes and the complement system.

The thymus gland

The thymus gland lies in the front of the neck and upper part of thorax. It increases in size up to the age of 16 and then becomes smaller. Our knowledge of its functions is not complete. We know that it is a source of lymphocytes before birth. It is a source of long-lived lymphocytes. It pro-cesses and matures T-lymphocytes.

How ageing affects specific immune response

The thymus is thought to become less efficient at processing and maturing T cell lymphocytes. The number of T cells declines with age. Remaining T cells are less able to respond to infection. When T cell function declines, this affects B cell function.

Researchers took thymus and bone marrow cells from new-born mice. They irradiated the cells to prevent rejection and transplanted the cells into old mice. They found that the immune system of the old mice became more effective.

How infection affects older adults

Many older people die as the result of infection. Others suffer long-term effects because of infection. An infection can, for many older people, mark the beginning of a downward spiral. Infection leads to the loss of ability. This loss of function causes the older person to become at risk of a number of further potentially life threatening conditions.

The downward spiral of infection

Infection often leads to the older person becoming less mobile. The first sign of a chest infection is often 'going of the legs'. People with urinary tract infections are more likely to develop continence problems. They become less mobile because of the fear of wetting and because of depression. People with infected leg ulcers often become less mobile because of the pain associated with the inflammatory response. People with pressure sores are often encouraged to rest or remain in bed to encourage healing. Immobility rapidly leads to muscle wasting. The immobile person is at high risk of developing continence problems. Immobility predisposes the person to urinary tract infections. Immobility reduces the appetite and increases the risk of malnutrition. Malnutrition increases the risk of infection. It also leads to loss of respiratory muscle and increases the risks of chest infection. Immobility increases the risks of constipation. Constipation can lead to urinary retention and increased risk of urinary tract infection. Immobility leads to reduced blood flow and increases the risk of venous incompetence. This can lead to leg ulceration in some residents. Immobility increases the risk of developing pressure sores.

The older person who acquires one or more of these problems can become depressed and miserable. She may begin to feel that life is not worth living. Nursing workload increases enormously. Nurses rush around responding to one crisis after another. There is no time to think or to plan ways of getting out of this downward spiral. Assessing each individual's risk status and taking measures to reduce the rate of infection enables nurses to work proactively and not reactively. The next section examines ways to assess risk.

Key points

- Infection rates in UK hospitals have almost doubled in a decade
- There are no national surveys on infection rates in UK nursing homes
- Age related changes reduce the body's external defences
- The immune system becomes less effective in old age.
- Chronic illness, poor nutrition and some prescribed medication impair immune response
- Infection can lead to irreversible loss of function and mortality rates are high
- Infection increases nursing workload.

Infection risks in nursing homes

Nursing homes now care for people who are more frail and vulnerable than ever before. Increased frailty and changing practice increase infection risks.

This section aims to:

- Improve your understanding of the types of infection common in nursing homes
- Inform you about infection risks
- Enable you to understand the significance of infection rates
- Develop an awareness of how antibiotic use contributes to antibiotic resistance
- Enable you to explore your role in preventing infection

Why do we need to assess infection risks?

Until the mid 1980s acutely ill, chronically ill and dying older people, the very people who are at greatest risk of developing infection, were cared for in NHS hospitals and continuing care units. Now over 200 000 vulnerable older people live in our nursing homes[5]. In hospital settings nurses caring for older people could easily contact the hospital-based infection control nurse. Although older people requiring continuing care have moved from hospitals to nursing homes, there are few community-based nurse specialists. Infection control within nursing homes is an issue that has received little attention. At present there is little published guidance regarding infection control in nursing homes. The rate of infection within UK nursing homes is not known. We have no information relating to the percentage of residents receiving antibiotic therapy at any one time. We do not know if antibiotic resistance is widespread within UK nursing homes. Only by examining North American research, much of it at least ten years old, can we begin to discover who is at risk of developing infections and why.

Types of infection prevalent within nursing homes

Research indicates that the commonest infections within nursing homes are:

- *Urinary tract infection* – one survey found that 50% of all nursing home infections were urinary tract infections. Residents most at risk were those with indwelling catheters. Further research indicated that 50% of non-catheterised nursing home residents had bacteria in their urine.
- *Chest infections* accounted for 23% of all infections.
- *Wound infections* accounted for a further 23% of infections.

Infection rate within nursing homes

North American research indicates that infection rates within nursing homes are high. The reported rate varies from 10% to 16%. Research indicates that the rate of infection is related to the size of the nursing home. One team of researchers investigating antibiotic resistance in nursing home residents admitted to hospital found that large nursing homes had three times the rate of infection of smaller nursing homes. The reasons for the increased infection rate in larger nursing homes were unclear. Individuals cared for in larger US nursing homes may have been more susceptible to infection than those cared for in smaller homes. A host of other factors could have been responsible for this finding and clearly further research into this area of infection control is required.

Antibiotic use within nursing homes

Research indicates that the number of antibiotics prescribed by GPs has doubled since 1990. Prescribing patterns indicate that GPs are prescribing newly introduced antibiotics that are being heavily promoted by manufacturers. New generation antibiotics, such as aminopenicillins, cephalosporins, macrolides and quinololes, are being prescribed in ever increasing numbers by GPs. Researchers suggest that the reason for the increasing number of prescriptions and the link between prescription levels and the growing level of antibiotic resistance, are investigated.[6]

No records of antibiotic use within nursing homes are maintained in the UK. Medical care for nursing home residents is provided by GPs. In some nursing homes one GP cares for most of the residents. However homes may have a number of different GPs who care for their patients within the nursing home. A research study discovered that 15 GPs were providing medical care within one nursing home. When a number of GPs are providing medical care none will have enough information about infection within the home and care can easily become fragmented. However when one GP provides medical care for all residents this too can cause problems. Researchers discovered that more than half of GPs who cared for 50 or more residents within a single nursing home found their workload 'unmanageable'.[7]

Researchers have found that the rate of antibiotic prescription within nursing homes is high and many residents are prescribed several courses of antibiotics within a year. Some GPs, unlike their colleagues in hospitals, tend to prescribe antibiotics without sending off specimens for culture and sensitivity. This strategy may be effective for patients living in the community but is it effective for nursing home residents? Prescribing antibiotics without checking for culture and sensitivity assumes that antibiotic resistance is not a widespread problem within nursing homes. Is it safe to make this assumption? Let's examine the research relating to antibiotic resistance within long-term care.

Antibiotic resistance within nursing homes

Antibiotic resistance is a growing problem. In US hospitals 13 300 patients died in 1992 from infections resistant to antibiotics[8]. Research carried out in seven nursing homes over a period of a year discovered horrifying levels of antibiotic resistance:

- Ampicillin resistance was 66%
- Cephalothin resistance was 66%
- Trimethoprim resistance was 52%
- Gentamicin resistance was 21%.

Later research found high levels of aminoglycoside resistant enterococcus in nursing home residents.

Aminoglycosides

Aminoglycosides are active against many Gram-negative aerobic and some Gram-positive bacteria. They are not absorbed from the gut and must be given parenterally. Aminoglycosides can damage renal function and hearing if blood levels are not closely monitored. Commonly used aminoglycosides are gentamicin, tobramycin, amikacin, neomycin and streptomycin.

Epidemics caused by antibiotic resistant bacteria

Antibiotic resistant strains of bacteria have caused epidemics within nursing homes[9]. There are published reports of epidemics caused by:

- methicillin-resistant *Staphylococcus aureus* (MRSA)
- Salmonella species
- Ceftazidimine-resistant Klebsiella pneumonia
- Aeronomas hydorphilia.

Clearly, antibiotic resistance is a major problem within North American nursing homes. We have no reason to believe that residents in North American nursing homes are any different from those in the UK. If the incidence of antibiotic resistance within UK nursing homes is similar, then current GP prescribing practices within nursing homes will contribute to growing antibiotic resistance. Inappropriate antibiotic prescription encourages the development of resistant strains of bacteria. Non-resistant bacteria are killed by the antibiotic and resistant bacteria have more space and a greater food supply. This enables them to multiply and grow[10]. People admitted to hospital from nursing homes are three times more likely to die because of infection than older people admitted from home. Developing infection control programmes can reduce the rate of infection within nursing homes. This will enable older people to retain the highest possible level of function and retain independence. It will also reduce nursing workload.

Assessing infection risk in nursing homes

Researchers have identified factors that increase the individual's susceptibility to infection.

Ageing increases the risk of infection. The immune system becomes less effective in old age and the body is less able to combat infection. Older people take longer to recover from infection. Interestingly 25% of older people have an immune system that can combat infection as *effectively* as young adults[11].

Immobile nursing home residents are three times more likely to develop infections than mobile residents are. Immobility leads to a reduction in muscle strength, reduces appetite, increases the risk of incontinence, increases the risk of constipation and increases the risk of developing pressure sores.

Malnutrition inhibits mobility and delays recovery[12]. Older people are at risk of becoming malnourished and the risk increases with age[13]. Research indicates that many healthy older people living at home suffer from vitamin deficiencies. Older people are most likely to suffer from deficiencies of iron, zinc and vitamin C. Vitamin supplements that correct these deficiencies lead to a reduced rate of infection[14]. Many older people are admitted to hospital malnourished; unfortunately many become even more malnourished in hospital[15]. Weight loss leads to muscle loss, which affects respiratory muscles and leads to reduced respiratory function. This makes it more difficult for individuals to cough and expectorate and increases the risk of chest infection.

Medication can directly or indirectly increase the individual's risk of developing infection. Non-steroidal anti-inflammatory drugs can cause gastro-intestinal bleeding and lead to iron deficiency anaemia. Anticonvulsant drugs such as phenytoin reduce the absorption of folic acid. This increases the risk of anaemia. Anaemia increases the risk of infection. Anticonvulsants also impair vitamin D absorption, leading to reduced bone density, osteoporosis and increased risk of fracture. Medication can often cause nausea, anorexia and constipation, all of which can impair appetite and increase the risk of infection. Psychotropic medications increase the risk of infection, possibly because of their effect on appetite, mobility and other aspects of the individual's lifestyle.

Dementia increases the risks of developing an infection. This may be because of medication given to control behavioural symptoms, because of immobility, because of malnutrition or because of incontinence.

Congestive cardiac failure increases the risk of infection because poor circulation impairs the body's ability to fight off infection. Effective medical treatment of cardiac failure reduces the infection risk. Nursing treatment, including enabling the person to remain mobile and continent, also reduces infection risks.

Hospital admission increases the risk of infection. Older people who have been discharged from hospital within four weeks are four times more likely to develop an infection than those who have remained in the nursing home.

Antibiotic therapy is associated with an increased risk of infection. Inappropriate antibiotic therapy enables resistant bacteria to multiply and cause infection.

Preventing infection

Older people living in nursing homes have a wide range of abilities. Some will be extremely vulnerable to infection. Assessing each individual to determine risk factors will enable nurses to prevent infection and deliver high quality care. An example of a risk assessment form is given at the end of this chapter.

Putting research into practice

Using research enables you to identify residents who are vulnerable to infection and to plan care to minimise infection risks. If an older person with a pressure sore is sharing a room, ensuring that they do not share with a catheterised resident will reduce infection risks.

Adopting a problem-solving approach enables you to reduce each individual resident's risk of developing infection. If the person is immobile, is it possible to enable them to regain mobility? If the person is malnourished, how can you improve nutritional status? If the person is incontinent, can you help her to regain continence? If the person has an indwelling urinary catheter, find out why it has been inserted; if there are no sound indications (such as urinary retention) consider removing it.

Conclusion

Assessing infection control risks enables nurses to plan care and improve the older person's quality of life. Infection leads to a loss of ability. Often abilities that are lost are never fully recovered. The older person's quality of life is reduced and the nursing workload is increased. Assessment and planning enable nurses to work proactively instead of reacting to infection and its consequences. When infection does occur, nurses will have time to minimise the loss of ability which can occur.

Key points

- Nursing homes now care for the people most at risk of infection
- Nursing home staff rarely have easy access to infection control and microbiology staff
- North American research indicates that infection rates within nursing homes are high
- GP prescribing rates have doubled in a decade. This can contribute to antibiotic resistance
- Antibiotic resistance in US nursing homes is high and has led to epidemics
- Assessing infection risks enables us to work proactively, reduce our workload and improve residents' quality of life.

Urinary tract infection

Urinary tract infections are very common in frail older people. Research suggests that many urinary tract infections remain undiagnosed; many of those diagnosed are treated ineffectively.

This section aims to:

- Enable you to understand how ageing increases the risk of urinary tract infection
- Enable you to understand how illness and disability increase the risk of urinary tract infections
- Examine the other factors that increase the risk of infection
- Understand how to minimise infection risks

How ageing affects the urinary system

The kidneys become smaller and lighter with age; the weight of the average kidney decreases from 250 grams to 200 grams between the ages of 20 and

80. The majority of cells lost are in the renal cortex, which contains the largest number of functioning glomeruli. It is estimated that the decrease in functioning glomeruli is between 30% and 50% in extreme old age. These changes do not normally cause problems in older adults unless diseases cause further stress. The surface area of the remaining glomeruli is reduced and there is thickening of the glomerular basement membrane. These structural changes affect the blood flow through the nephrons and decrease the ability to concentrate urine and to maintain PH balance.

The bloodflow to the kidneys is affected by arteriosclerotic changes. Research has demonstrated that renal blood flow decreases from 600 ml per minute at the age of 40 to 300 ml per minute at the age of 80. It has been suggested that this reduction is caused partly by decreased cardiac output and the decreased renal vascular bed[16].

Glomular filtration rates (GFR) have been shown to decline significantly with age. One study of healthy men living in the community demonstrated a decline of 30% to 50% in GFR in two thirds of the men studied, but a third showed no decline in GFR with age. The age related decline in GFR is of great significance to nurses caring for older adults. Many older adults are less able to excrete drugs normally excreted rapidly from younger more efficient kidneys. Older adults are more at risk of the toxic effects of many drugs such as digoxin, cimetidine and cephalosporins that are excreted from the kidney and are affected by changes in GFR. Illness can further lower GFR and can lead to elevated levels of phosphate, uric acid and potassium and lower levels of bicarbonate.

The kidneys are less able to concentrate urine. There are several theories to explain this. There is not thought to be any change in the levels of anti-diuretic hormone (ADH) produced in old age but it is thought that kidney response to ADH diminishes with age. Rennin activity is diminished with age and this leads to a reduction in aldosterone. This can lessen the kidney's ability to reabsorb sodium, potassium and water in the distal tubule. Older adults are as a result of these changes more at risk of electrolyte imbalance. This risk can be increased by the use of diuretic therapy that is currently widespread among the elderly population. The use of potassium sparing diuretics and of potassium supplementation with diuretics such as frusemide is not without its hazards. One study found that 73% of cases of hyponatraemia in elderly people were caused by diuretic therapy. Older adults are less able to dispose of large fluid loads and run the risk of cardiac failure resulting from increased blood volume if too much fluid is given too rapidly. Intravenous fluids must be given with particular care because of this risk.

How ageing affects bladder function

The bladder muscle – the detrusor – is smooth muscle which expands and contracts in all directions. The detrusor is primarily under parasympathetic control. Parasympathetic stimulation releases acetylcholine, causing detrusor contraction and assisting bladder emptying. Sympathetic control is via the beta-adrenergic receptors, which are situated in the body and fundus of the detrusor. Stimulation of these receptors assists in bladder relaxation and filling. The main age related bladder changes are all intrinsically linked. The afferent sensors in the bladder become less sensitive with age.[17] The main effect of this change is that older adults are not aware of the desire to void until their bladders are 90% full; younger adults are aware of the desire to void when their bladders are 50% full. This means that older people have less time to find a toilet and when combined with disabilities which impair mobility, it can lead to incontinence. There is a reduction in the contractility of the bladder muscle; it no longer stretches and contracts as efficiently as before, the amount of fibrotic tissue in the bladder increases and this further decreases bladder capacity.

How ageing affects the urethra

There are also age-related changes to the urethra, which can affect an older adult's ability to maintain continence. The female urethra may become de-oestrogenated with age and this can lead to decreased urethral closing pressures and in some cases to stress incontinence. It must be emphasised that many women are able to produce sufficient oestrogen to maintain adequate urethral closing pressures throughout their lives. The pudendal nerve is responsible for inhibiting micturition and is under voluntary control.

How ageing affects the prostate

Older men have larger prostate glands than younger men do, as the prostate gland enlarges with age. This change is not pathological in many men but if prostatic growth is into the bladder neck (this is common in prostatic malignancy) this can lead to decreased sphincter control. Benign prostatic enlargement can lead to an increased amount of residual urine because of urethral obstruction. This residual urine if in excess of 350 ml can cause back-flow to the kidneys, renal damage and infection. Older men are much more at risk of urinary tract infections because as they age the prostate produces less prostatic bactericide, which prevents urinary infections.

How illness and disability increase infection risks

Research[18] indicates that over 70% of nursing home residents suffer from neurological disease, 24% have 'mental disorders' and 29% have ortho-paedic problems (some residents had more than one diagnosis). Neuro-logical diseases such as MS, dementia, Parkinson's disease and strokes increase infection risks because they can lead to incomplete bladder emptying. A pool of stagnant urine in the bladder is the ideal breeding ground for bacteria[19].

Almost a third of our residents are admitted because they fail to regain mobility following a fracture. Immobile residents are thirteen times more likely to develop a urinary tract infection than mobile residents are. There are several reasons for this. Immobile residents do not walk and the airflow to the genital region is reduced. Immobile residents may cut down on fluids in an effort to cut down on urine output and avoid 'bothering the nurses'. Immobile residents are more likely to develop postural oedema of the legs and are more likely to be prescribed diuretics to reduce oedema. Diuretics can lead to dehydration and dehydration increases the risk of infection.

Other factors

Nursing practice can contribute to urinary tract infections developing. It is important to wash the genital area from front to back. This avoids transferring *E. coli* commensals from the anal region to the urethral area where they can easily ascend and cause urine infections. It is important to stamp out 'magic gloves syndrome'. Magic gloves are usually worn by care assistants though some registered nurses also use them. These gloves are put on at the beginning of a shift and remain on for hours. They move unwashed from resident to resident transferring *E. coli* and other bacteria from resident to resident.

Nursing practice can reduce mobility: 'it's quicker to wheel her', 'don't get up – you might fall', 'don't walk on your own, wait for a nurse', 'don't put her frame next to her, it's in the way', 'let's put the frames in the corner out of the way, we don't want anyone to fall over them'.

Nursing practice can contribute to poor fluid intake. Does everyone have a glass and a water jug? Are drinks placed where residents can reach them in the lounge? Do you offer second cups of tea?

Nursing practice can contribute to dehydration: if Mrs Brown's legs are becoming swollen, do you take her for walks, elevate her legs, or ask the GP to prescribe medication?

Minimising risk of infection

Minimising the risk of infection is simple but not easy:

- Ensure hand washing has the highest possible priority
- Train and educate your staff to the highest possible level
- Ensure domestic and laundry staff also receive training in infection control
- Use risk assessment so that you do not place two highly vulnerable residents in the same room
- Constantly reinforce the need for infection control measures
- Enable residents to retain abilities for as long as possible – don't allow a dependency culture to take hold.

Catheterised residents

Infection is inevitable in people with long-term catheters, within 12 days of catheterisation[20]. The infecting organisms are often the person's own commensals such as *E. coli*. The person is vulnerable to other bacteria, fungi and yeasts because the catheter acts as a portal of entry. Infection can occur because the drainage bag is left on the floor. Infection can be transferred on the unwashed hands or magic gloves of staff. Infection can be transferred if the bag becomes contaminated with faeces. In all these cases infection travels along the outside of the bag and catheter and into the urethra and bladder. Bacteria can also migrate from inside the drainage bag up the internal lumen of the tubing and catheter and into the bladder. We now know that a biofilm develops within urine drainage bags and catheters. Bacteria move from the bag to the bladder and are not deterred by the 'non return valve'[21].

Preventing infection in catheterised residents

In hospitals people who have been catheterised suffer more complications and have longer stays than similar patients who have not been catheterised. Avoid catheterisation when possible. If catheterisation is unavoidable:

- Ensure adequate drainage, use straps to support leg bags, use night drainage bags on stands at night. Ensure that the tubing is not kinked. Inadequate drainage leads to a pool of stagnant urine in the bladder. If more than 350 ml collects there is the danger that urine will backflow into the ureters and cause renal infection.
- Ensure the person has an adequate fluid intake – this dilutes bacteria and flushes the bladder, reducing the risk of infection.
- Change leg bags twice weekly; dating them allows you to monitor this.
- Change leg bags if they become visibly contaminated.
- Wash hands before and after emptying catheter bags.

Night drainage bags

In the community people are advised to wash out night drainage bags in warm soapy water and to hang them up to dry. These bags are then reused for about a week. Some continence advisers recommend that nursing home staff do this. However there have been several cases where nursing home residents developed Gram-negative bacteraemia due to inadequate disinfection of night drainage bags. The mortality rate of Gram-negative bacteraemia is 40%. Single use night drainage bags solve the problem of inadequate disinfection and they are much cheaper than night bags designed to be reused.

Catheter valves

The bladder normally fills and is emptied. Catheterisation causes the bladder to shrink. Catheter valves eliminate the need for urine drainage bags and reduce the risk of infection. The valve is used to empty the bladder at two to four hourly intervals. They reduce the risk of urethral trauma caused by overfull urine bags. Consider using catheter valves for selected individuals. Mobile male residents catheterised because an enlarged prostate has caused voiding difficulties, often find valves ideal. Residents catheterised because of retention do well. Immobile residents with small unstable bladders are usually unsuitable.

Catheter hygiene

Research indicates that cleansing the meatal area with antiseptics is ineffective in preventing infection[22] and can lead to infection with multi-resistant organisms[23]. Normal washing is all that is required. It is important to ensure that dependent male catheterised residents have the foreskin retracted and the glans cleaned at least daily. Poor hygiene can lead to infection, phimosis and urethral strictures. Confusion about bathing and showering is common.

One researcher asked patients with catheters to bathe in water full of fluoresce dye but found no evidence of dye in their bladders.

Urinary sheaths and infection

Wearing a urinary sheath increases the risk of developing a urinary tract infection. One study found that 87% of older men who wore urinary sheaths developed infection over a five month period[24]. You can prevent complications by taking the following action:

- Ensure that you assess the person's suitability for a sheath.
- A man who has a large residual urine (over 150 ml) may be suffering from outflow obstruction and a urinary sheath would be inadvisable
- People with compromised immune status are at high risk of developing infection
- People with allergies may react to adhesive or material – test by cutting a piece of sheath off and strapping to inner aspect of arm for 48 hours, then inspect
- Men who are circumcised are more at risk of tissue damage because urine comes in direct contact with the tip of the penis.

Cranberry juice

Cranberry juice has been used since 1932 to prevent and treat urinary tract infections. It acts by preventing bacteria and yeasts adhering to mucosal cells. It inhibits the growth of bacteria and yeasts. Cranberry juice reduces and usually eliminates the odour of catheterised urine. Individuals should drink 400 ml each day to prevent infection[25].

Conclusion

Nurses have more influence than any other professional on infection control practice. Infection within nursing homes is not inevitable. Nursing practice can reduce infection rates, increase resident quality of life and reduce nursing workload.

Key points

- Older people are more vulnerable to urinary tract infections
- Neurological disease, common in nursing home residents, increases vulnerability
- Immobility, inadequate fluid intake and poor practice increase infection risks
- Enabling practice of infection control procedures can reduce risks and enhance resident quality of life.

Preventing wound infection

This section will focus on how you can prevent wound infection and enable wounds to heal.

This section aims to:

- Update your knowledge of wound healing
- Discuss how chronic wounds are susceptible to infection
- Update your knowledge of research-based practice
- Discuss when and how to cleanse wounds
- Update you on larval therapy
- Enable you to choose appropriate dressings
- Discuss how to set up good infection control practices

Structure of healthy skin

The skin is the largest organ in the body. It is the barrier between the body and the environment. The skin consists of three layers of cell:

(1) The epidermis
(2) The dermis
(3) Subcutaneous tissue

The epidermis

The epidermis is the outer layer of the skin. The cells of the epidermis are dead and constantly being shed and replaced by cells from the deep layers. The epidermis contains no blood cells.

The dermis

The dermis is the middle layer of the skin. It supports and attaches firmly to the epidermis. Complex protein fibres called collagen in the dermis provide strength and elasticity. The skin's blood vessels, nerve endings, hair follicles, sweat glands and lymphatic drainage vessels are situated in the dermis. The blood vessels carry blood that contains the nutrients required to keep the skin healthy. The blood vessels also regulate heat – dilating to increase blood flow and allowing heat loss, constricting to reduce blood flow and to conserve body heat. The dermis cannot regenerate if it is destroyed. It heals by formation of granulation tissue that is replaced by scar tissue.

The subcutaneous layer

The subcutaneous or fatty layer carries the larger blood vessels that supply the skin. Its thickness varies enormously depending on the area of the body and the individual. It acts as a thermal barrier and energy store for fats and water in the body and disperses localised pressure, protecting the superficial skin from the effects of sharp internal boney prominences.

The functions of the skin

The skin has five main functions: protection, sensation, heat regulation, storage and absorption.

Protection – The skin provides a barrier to prevent harmful bacteria from entering the body. It protects the internal organs from damage. It prevents the leakage of vital chemicals and fluids.

Sensation – The sensory nerve endings in the skin warn the body of changes in stimuli including temperature, touch, pain and pressure.

Heat regulation – The skin plays an important part in regulating body temperature. The diameter of the blood vessels alters depending on environmental conditions. Sweat glands also regulate body temperature.

Storage – Water and fat stores in the subcutaneous tissues act as a protective layer protecting muscle and bone against mechanical forces as well as providing insulation and nutritional stores.

Absorption – Absorption of ultraviolet light aids the body in manufacturing vitamin D.

Damage to the skin can interfere with all of these vital functions. A healthy blood supply is vital to them all. The skin receives up to a third of the body's circulating blood.

Wound healing

Wounds heal in two distinct ways. Surgical wounds and wounds where both edges of the wound are pulled together either by sutures or steristrips heal by primary intention. The body only needs to produce a small amount of tissue to promote wound healing. Primary healing is completed within days.

Secondary healing

A wound extending into the dermis or deeper tissues results in a greater loss of tissue. That tissue must be replaced with new tissue and finally covered with epithelium. Secondary healing takes weeks or months, depending on the site and size of the wound (intrinsic factors) and the nutritional status, health status and age of the individual (extrinsic factors).

Preventing infection in chronic wounds

The commonest chronic wounds in nursing homes are pressure sores and leg ulcers. Chronic wounds heal by secondary intention. There are four main ways that can reduce the incidence of wound infection:

(1) Introducing and *maintaining* good infection control practices
(2) Introduce routine surveillance to detect and deal with outbreaks of infection
(3) Use research-based practice to enable rapid wound healing to take place
(4) Prevent the occurrence of wounds.

The process of healing

Wound healing consists of four phases that overlap:

(1) Inflammatory phase – lasting 1–3 days
(2) Destructive phase – lasting 3–5 days
(3) Proliferation phase – lasting 5–24 days
(4) Maturation phase – lasting from 24 days to up to a year.

Inflammation

The first response to tissue damage is inflammation. It is a normal phase of wound healing. It is a protective mechanism causing increased capillary permeability and oedema and the stimulation of pain fibres. The five signs of inflammation are:

(1) Heat
(2) Redness
(3) Pain
(4) Swelling
(5) Loss of function

The inflammatory phase of healing can be prolonged in large wounds. If inflammation is prolonged then infection or wound damage caused by wound cleansing agents or dressings should be investigated. The inflammatory response is essential for healing. It can be depressed in the frail elderly. Those with diabetes or taking steroids or non-steroidal anti-inflammatory drugs have a depressed and prolonged anti-inflammatory response.

Destructive phase

During the destructive phase polymorphs and macrophages remove dead tissue and stimulate the multiplication of fibroblasts.

Proliferation

During this phase fibroblasts begin to produce fibres of collagen. New capillary loops grow into the collagen and form granulation tissue.

Maturation

During this phase more collagen fibres are produced and reorganised, strengthening the scar. Finally epithelial tissue covers the wound.

Why are chronic wounds susceptible to infection?

Chronic wounds have a large exposed surface area. They take weeks or months to heal. Until the wound is completely healed it is vulnerable to infection. Some wounds are particularly susceptible to infection. Individuals who are doubly incontinent are more likely to develop pressure sores, especially on the sacrum. Sacral pressure sores are at risk of faecal contamination and infection.

Nursing practice

Nursing practice should be research-based and aim to enable rapid wound healing to take place. This includes not only treating the wound but also the person with the wound. Whenever possible treat any underlying problem that will affect wound healing. A modified aseptic technique – the clean technique – is recommended for chronic wounds[26]. Box 5.1 gives details.

Box 5.1   Modified aseptic technique.

Aim
To avoid the introduction of potential pathogens to the wound
To prevent the transfer of pathogens to residents and staff

Indications
- Dressing of wounds healing by secondary intention
- Removal of sutures
- Removal of intravenous lines
- Removal of drains
- Endotracheal suction
- Dressing tracheostomy sites

Principles
(1) Ensure that all equipment is ready and that a clean area is available to place it on
(2) Explain the procedure, obtain consent and position resident
(3) Wash hands – disinfect with alcohol handrub
(4) If direct contact with blood or body fluids is anticipated wear clean gloves and a plastic apron
(5) Soak off dressing – this can either have been done in bath or shower or using sterile saline
(6) Clean wound with either water or sterile saline only if necessary[27]
(7) Apply sterile dressing
(8) On completion of procedure, dispose of any gloves, apron and dressing
(9) Wash hands.

Wound healing and bacteria

Chronic wounds, which heal by second intention, become colonised by bacteria. Researchers have discovered that, in most cases, bacterial colonisation does not delay wound healing. Necrotic tissue encourages bacteria to multiply, increases the risk of infection and delays healing[28].

Necrotic wounds covered in black hard dry eschar need to be rehydrated so that autolysis (the breakdown of dead tissue) can take place and healing begin. Hydrogels such as Intrasite or Granugel covered with a film dressing are suitable. Hydrogels should be changed *every* day if infection is present but otherwise can be left for up to three days. Hydrocolloids such as Granuflex and Comfeel prevent water loss from the dry wound bed and this enables the wound to rehydrate and heal. Hydrocolloids should be left in place for no more than seven days. Rehydrating necrotic wounds as rapidly as possible reduces the risk of infection.

Wound cleansing – promoting healing

Cleaning wounds reduces their temperature below body temperature. Healing is slowed until the wound regains temperature. Cleaning wounds reduces the rate of cellular repair[29].

Wound antiseptics are less commonly used than before. Researchers have tested the effects of wound cleansers on the ears of rabbits. This research normally involves checking blood flow before and after cleansing with a variety of cleansers. Other research involves checking the effects of wound cleaners on living human and animal cells in a laboratory.

Many cleansing agents have been proven to damage granulating wounds; these include Eusol, which kills granulating tissues. Chlorhexidine and cetrimide damage granulating tissue and also have been proven to reduce blood flow to the wound bed. Providone iodine has been proven to close off capillary blood flow to granulating wounds for five days. However specialists are now reconsidering the role of iodine in wound healing[30]. Cadexomer iodine, i.e. iodine ointment and iodine impregnated dressings, deliver a low level of iodine to the wound – 0.00225%. This level of iodine appears to be non toxic and appears to stimulate antioxidant activity and fibroblast proliferation[31]. One study investigated the effect of iodine on ulcers colonised with *Pseudomonas aeruginosa*. Pseudomonas produces an entoxin that is thought to delay wound healing. Iodine killed the pseudomonas but 12 weeks later when the iodine was discontinued the pseudomonas returned. This was a small study involving only four patients[32]. Using gauze to clean wounds can damage fragile new granulation tissue and impede healing.

Larval therapy

The use of larvae or maggots to cleanse wounds is becoming increasingly popular. Sterile larvae are obtained from the biosurgical research unit in Wales. The larvae are the size of pinheads on arrival. The wound is prepared by using an occlusive dressing around the wound so that the wound itself is exposed. Saline is added to the larvae pot and the larvae and saline placed on the wound. A fine nylon mesh is taped over the wound and a secondary dressing applied. The larvae liquefy and ingest slough and necrotic tissue[33]. The secondary dressing can be changed daily if required. The larval secretions kill *Streptococcus* and *Staphylococcus* bacteria[34]. Most hydrogels kill larvae so it is important to irrigate wounds well if you were using a hydrogel to debride the wound before applying larvae[35]. Larvae are now being used in hospitals to treat wounds infected with multi-resistant strains of bacteria[36]. Larval therapy is cost effective, safe and simple. It is now being used throughout the world to treat wounds and prevent or treat infection[37].

Larvae are extremely effective in debriding wounds and you will notice a reduction in exudate and smell within 24 hours. The larvae look like pieces of cotton within 24 to 48 hours of application. When they are ready for removal they look like earthworms.

Many nurses fear applying larvae. Nurses fear that larvae will become lost in cavities – this does not happen. They fear that they will turn into flies but the larvae need somewhere dry in order to pupate and wounds are not suitable environments for this. Generally, once nurses have used them they become enthusiastic. People treated with larvae sometimes report a tickling sensation, but generally this treatment is well accepted.

Recommendations for good practice

It is now recommended that wounds are not routinely cleansed at each dressing change but only when clinically necessary. Reasons for cleansing might include removal of debris or excess exudate. Chronic wounds can be washed with clean warm water when the resident is showering, cleaned in a bucket of warm tap water or cleaned with saline. Irrigation is preferable to using cotton wool or gauze swabs as this avoids damage to the fragile granulating tissue at the wound bed.

Minimise dressing changes. If all seems well do not take a dressing down 'to have a look'. Gardeners do not dig up their seeds to see if they are rooting!

Do not use harsh disinfecting agents to clean wounds. Do not clean wounds unnecessarily. Do not traumatise wounds when changing dressings – soak dressings off. Use a dressing, which is appropriate to the stage of wound healing. Clean and dry equipment between dealing with each resident.

Wound dressing

It is important that dressings encourage healing. Moist wound healing using occlusive dressings encourages healing and reduces the risk of infection.

Preventing wounds occurring

The most effective way to prevent wound infection is to prevent wounds developing. Proactive nursing practice that anticipates and prevents the occurrence of problems is the most effective but least visible part of nursing. Use scoring systems to determine who is at risk of pressure sores and do everything in your power to prevent them. Use compression stockings and encourage residents with a history of venous problems to continue walking. Handle residents with great care to prevent knocks that can easily turn into leg ulcers. Use padding on frames and furniture if necessary.

Introducing and maintaining good infection control practices

Hand washing is the most important aspect of infection control. It is now considered good practice to soak off dressings and often this is done in the bath or shower. Often a care assistant will be responsible for bathing a particular individual. If care assistants are not trained in infection control procedures they can easily spread infection from resident to resident during their shift.

- The person who removes a dressing should ensure it is disposed of immediately according to the home's procedure.
- Dressings should not be left lying about in bathrooms or showers.
- Hands should be washed after removing or handling a used dressing.
- Baths should be washed out with hot water and detergent after each person. A rinse is not sufficient if a dressing has been removed.
- Ideally the individual with a wound should be bathed last. The bath can then be thoroughly washed and dried after use.
- If a basin or bucket is used to soak off a leg dressing, each individual should ideally have his or her own bowl or bucket. If this is not possible the bowl or bucket should be washed with hot water and detergent and dried between each person. Drying is important as Pseudomonas can thrive in damp containers. The container should be lined with a bin liner that is disposed of after each use.

- If barrier creams and emollients are used these should be labelled with the individual's name and should not be shared, as the bacteria can be shared around. It is important to explain the reasons for this to care assistants or they may fail to comply.
- Research indicates that infection control practices 'slip' and everyone becomes more careless after a while. Infection control nurses recommend using notices and posters to keep infection control on everyone's mind. These are most effective if they are rotated, e.g. infection control tip of the week. If the same posters are always up no one notices them after a while.

Introducing routine surveillance to detect infection

Introducing infection control programmes will enable you to monitor infection within the home. If cross infection occurs you can detect this quickly, investigate and tackle the breakdown in your infection control procedures. Hospital-based researchers have found that infection control monitoring has two main effects. Firstly it sends out the message that you are serious about infection control. This tends to make staff more conscious of basic infection control procedures. Secondly, hospital-based research demonstrates that monitoring can reduce infection rates by 40%. Secondary infection is detected and treated early, reducing the risk of cross infection. When cross infection does occur it can be dealt with promptly.

Enabling rapid wound healing

Research-based practice enables nurses to help heal wounds as rapidly as possible. The sooner a wound is healed, the sooner infection risks are eliminated.

Conclusion

In infection control as in all things prevention is better than cure. Preventing wound infection is a team effort, which involves not only registered nurses but also care assistants and domestic staff. Explaining, teaching and constantly reinforcing infection control measures is essential. Routine surveillance will enable you to monitor your success and to pinpoint problems. Be generous with your praise when you are successful.

Key points

- Prevention of infection is of crucial importance
- Hand washing is the most important aspect of infection control
- Good infection control practices must be constantly reinforced
- Introduce routine surveillance to monitor infection
- Research-based practice enables rapid wound healing to take place and reduces infection risks
- Do everything possible to prevent wounds occurring.

Preventing infection

Introducing policies and practices to reduce risks

All staff employed in homes have an important role to play in preventing infection. Bacteria thrive in dirty and dusty conditions, and high standards of cleanliness prevent infection. Domestic staff are important members of the team and the nurses should ensure that they are valued and feel that their role is appreciated. Staff who feel that their work is important and valued are motivated and their work is of a higher standard than the work of those who feel they are 'just the cleaner'.

Disposal of waste

Safe disposal of waste plays an important part in preventing infection. It is easier to ensure that waste is disposed of properly if written policies exist which inform staff how to dispose of waste. Nurses have a duty to ensure correct disposal of waste under the Environmental Protection Act 1990. Different types of waste should be stored in colour-coded bags and dealt with in different ways.

Domestic waste

Domestic waste can be stored in black plastic bags. These are normally emptied into domestic dustbins in smaller homes, and in larger homes into large bins designed for commercial waste, such as Paladin bins which are normally supplied by the local council. Domestic waste is normally collected by the local council and arrangements can be made to have waste collected weekly, or daily on weekdays. Nursing homes are classified as businesses and the council charges a fee for each bin emptied. Many homes have large amounts of waste and having it collected can be expensive. Some homes purchase compacters which compact waste and reduce the number of collections required.

Glass, broken crockery and aerosols

Glass, broken crockery and aerosols should be stored in a cardboard box and placed in a separate bin (usually a domestic dustbin) which has 'Glass' painted on it.

Clinical waste

Clinical waste should be collected and stored in yellow plastic bags. Clinical waste includes incontinence pads, and many homes have large amounts. Clinical waste is not collected with domestic waste, but in a separate vehicle. Many councils run a clinical waste collection service and arrange to have the waste collected once or twice a week, with a nominal charge of 50p or £1 per sack. Many nursing homes have great problems in storing volumes of clinical waste, and council clinical waste services were often designed as a service for local doctors' and dentists' surgeries and were not designed to cope with the large volumes of incontinence pads which some homes can generate.

If local council services cannot cope, nurses can organise alternative means of disposal. Private companies offer special bins and clinical waste collection services, but these are expensive. The costs of collecting clinical waste from a typical 39 bed nursing home with an incontinence rate of 60% would be around £400 to £500 per month.

Pads can be incinerated but the Environment Protection Act 1990 specifies that the incinerator must reach extremely high temperatures and must satisfy stringent emission controls. The local council must also grant a licence before any incinerator can be used. Incinerators which meet such standards normally cost more than £10 000 and are beyond the means of most homes.

Pads can be broken up into a pulp in a macerator and pumped into the drains. A macerator offers a practical solution for many homes and the cost, usually around £2000, is quickly recovered. Homes must have a licence from the waste treatment and sewage department of the local water authority, which allows them to discharge macerator waste into the local sewage system. This licence normally costs a nominal amount, around £15 to £20, and is renewed annually. Soiled dressings, latex gloves, colostomy bags and disposable items such as catheters and catheter bags cannot be disposed of in macerators. Macerator blades get fouled up on such items.

The use of a macerator significantly reduces the amount of clinical waste, and council services or private contractors can be used to dispose of any remaining clinical waste. This is normally reduced to one or two bags per week. This clinical waste should be stored in yellow bags in dirty areas such as sluices. It should never be stored in clinical areas, resident areas or clean areas.

Sharps

Sharps such as lancets, syringes, needles, stitch cutters and any other item likely to pierce the skin cannot be placed in a yellow bag. They should be stored in a sharps bin, which should be placed in treatment rooms. In some cases a sharps bin can be stored in an individual's room. If a diabetic individual is receiving regular insulin injections and blood glucose monitoring, the risk of needlestick injuries can, in some cases, be reduced by placing a sharps box in the room. Nurses will have to balance this against the risk of the individual or other residents injuring themselves by investigating the sharps box.

It is possible to contract with private companies who will supply sharps bins and replace them at monthly, bi-monthly or quarterly intervals. The costs of this service normally depend on frequency of collection. All companies supply spares so that bins do not become overfull, and they will change bins on request.

Dealing with linen

Many homes have their own laundries and employ staff to launder bedding, towels and residents' clothing. It is important to set out clear, written policies for storage of and cleaning linen.

All used linen should be stored in either clear plastic bags or white bags which are used specially for laundry. Soiled linen should be placed in red bags. It is possible to buy special bags with an alginate strip. These bags are placed in washing machines on a special sluice cycle, the alginate strip dissolves on contact with water, and the bag opens. The sluice cycle removes soiling and at the end of the cycle the alginate bag is disposed of and the linen is washed in the machine. The use of alginate bags ensures that soiled linen is handled only once and this reduces the risk of infection. Staff handling soiled linen should wear an apron and gloves. Hands should be washed after the gloves and apron have been removed.

Items such as tablecloths should be washed separately from bed linen or clothing. Ensuring that the home is kept clean, that waste is disposed of appropriately and that linen is stored appropriately and laundered correctly, ensures that environmental hazards are reduced and basic safeguards are in place. Nurses can then go on to introduce specific measures to reduce infection within nursing homes.

Universal precautions

The single most important action staff can take to prevent infection is to wash their hands before and after attending to each resident. Bacteria are normally transferred from resident to resident on the unwashed hands of care givers. The importance of handwashing and its role in preventing cross infection cannot be overemphasised.

Homes should provide facilities to ensure correct handwashing techniques. Handwashing facilities should be provided in treatment rooms, sluices, toilets, bathrooms and other areas. Wash-basins should have taps which can be operated using wrists or elbows. Disposable paper towels should be used to dry hands. A foot-operated bin should be provided for disposal of used towels. Liquid soap in wall-mounted dispensers should be used; perfumed soaps and soaps containing lanolin should be avoided as these can cause allergies and dermatitis in some individuals.

When staff should wash their hands

- At the beginning of each shift
- Before serving meals
- Before giving out medications
- After handling laundry and making beds, before physical contact with a resident, after physical contact with a resident, and after removing aprons and gloves
- Before, during, and after performing aseptic techniques
- At the end of each shift.

Methicillin-resistant *Staphylococcus aureus* (MRSA)

In the 1980s many nurses working in hospitals and homes worried about methicillin-resistant *Staphylococcus aureus* (MRSA). Now it seems that we take MRSA for granted and do little to prevent its spread. MRSA can be relatively harmless but it can also lead to life threatening illness.

This section aims to:

- Update your knowledge on bacteriology
- Discuss the consequences of staphylococcal infections
- Discuss how *Staphylococcus aureus* has developed antibiotic resistance
- Discuss current treatment of MRSA
- Update you on transmission of MRSA
- Enable you to differentiate between colonisation and infection
- Enable you to set up strategies to prevent the spread of infection

MRSA has caused outbreaks of infection in UK hospitals since the 1980s. There is evidence to suggest that the prevalence of MRSA has been increasing in southern England since 1986[38]. Older adults are particularly at risk of contracting MRSA infection. The incidence of MRSA infection within nursing homes is not known. Nurses throughout the UK report that increasing numbers of older people with MRSA are being referred to nursing homes. In the early 1990s, nursing home staff feared that if they accepted older adults with MRSA they would be placing their residents at risk[39]. Some social services departments have informed nurses that they will refuse to place any individuals in homes where there is a known case of MRSA. In the past, nurses in homes had no firm guidance about the risks that MRSA poses in nursing homes. Many are unsure of their role in preventing the spread of MRSA while enabling the older adults colonised or infected with MRSA to lead normal lives.

Epidemiology/What is MRSA?

Staphylococcus aureus is a common bacteria. It consists of non-spore forming Gram-positive cocci that appear as golden tinged clusters when seen under a microscope. It commonly colonises normal skin. It thrives in warmer parts of the body such as the axilla, groins, perineum and nose. *Staphylococcus aureus* causes superficial skin infections such as boils, abscesses, septic spots and impetigo. It can also cause life-threatening illness such as septicaemia and pneumonia. Some strains produce a toxin that is responsible for 'toxic shock syndrome'. Some strains can cause acute gastroenteritis if ingested. Staphylococcus is responsible for approximately a third of all wound infections in hospitals. MRSA is a methicillin-resistant strain of *Staphylococcus aureus*. Resistant strains of *Staphylococcus aureus* developed shortly after the introduction of antibiotics in 1941[40]. This is illustrated in Table 5.2[41].

Strains of MRSA

Currently 17 strains of MRSA have been identified. They can be considered as four main groups:

(1) Penicillin sensitive strains
(2) Penicillin resistant; sensitive to methicillin and cephalosporins
(3) 'Borderline' resistant strains sensitive to methicillin

Table 5.2 MRSA and antibiotic resistance.

Antibiotic	Introduced	Resistance identified
Penicillin	1941	1940s
Streptomycin	1944	mid 1940s
Tetracycline	1948	1950s
Erythromycin	1952	1950s
Methicillin	1959	Late 1960s
Gentamycin	1964	mid 1970s
Cephalosporins	1980s	1986 epidemic strains reported in London
Mupirocin	1980s	1990
Vancomycin	1980s	1998

(4) MRSA resistant to methicillin and cephalosporins. Most strains of MRSA are also resistant to erythromycin, clindamycin, tetracycline and aminoglycosides[42,43].

Treatment of MRSA

Currently most strains of MRSA resistant to other antibiotics too are sensitive to vancomycin. Resistance to vancomycin is new and as yet there is little information about its prevalence. Vancomycin is given intravenously. The normal dose is either 500 mg every six hours or 1 g every 12 hours. It is given by slow intravenous injection over an hour. Vancomycin is extremely toxic and can damage hearing and renal function. Blood levels are carefully monitored (usually daily) to avoid toxicity. Older people are normally given reduced doses. Vancomycin is usually given for life-threatening infections. Residents requiring treatment with vancomycin are cared for in hospitals.

Mupirocin (Bactroban) ointment is often applied to skin lesions infected with MRSA. Some strains of MRSA have already developed resistance to mupirocin[44].

Tea tree oil is being used to treat mupirocin and vancomycin-resistant MRSA in some clinical settings.

Transmission of MRSA

MRSA is rarely spread by airborne transmission. There is little evidence to suggest that nasal carriers of MRSA transmit disease[45]. Despite this there have been attempts to eradicate MRSA in nasal carriers. Attempts to eradicate MRSA in colonised individuals have been found not only unnecessary and ineffective but also 'potentially hazardous' because MRSA strains isolated after attempted eradication had acquired resistance to even more antibiotics[46]. MRSA is normally spread from resident to resident on the hands of nursing and medical staff. The time it remains on the hands varies from minutes to hours. MRSA can be removed by washing hands thoroughly with soap and water.

Colonisation or infection?

Many individuals are colonised with *Staphylococcus aureus*. Research indicates that 40% of adults demonstrate nasal carriage of methicillin-sensitive *Staphylococcus aureus*[47]. Many individuals are colonised with *Staphylococcus aureus* but have no evidence of disease. Nursing home residents in common with the general population are colonised with a number of bacteria including *Staphylococcus aureus*[48]. It is important that the nurse ascertains if an individual is colonised or infected with MRSA as this will affect the infection control measures required.

Infection	*Colonisation*
Bacteria present	Bacteria present
Pyrexia	Apyrexial
Signs of infection, e.g. wound, urine, chest	No signs of infection
Appears unwell	Appears well

Who is at risk of contracting MRSA infection?

MRSA is not a danger for healthy individuals. Staff caring for residents are not at risk. They will not carry the infection home and put their families and children at risk. Visitors, including pregnant women, babies and young children, are not at risk. In nursing homes only residents who have urethral or supra-pubic catheters, nasogastric or gastrostomy tubes, tracheostomy, leg ulcers, pressure sores or are extremely frail, are at risk. MRSA can only enter the body if the person is very debilitated or there is a portal of entry.

Preventing the spread of MRSA in nursing homes

The numbers of individuals with MRSA in UK nursing homes is unknown. It has been suggested that many individuals in UK nursing homes suffer from undetected MRSA infection and that their readmission to hospitals perpetuates a cycle of infection[49]. North American research indicates high levels of MRSA in nursing homes and the spread of MRSA within these homes is attributed to inadequate knowledge of infection control strategies and poor nursing practice. The introduction of an infection control programme will enable nursing staff to determine which bacteria are causing infection within their nursing home and to use appropriate strategies to prevent cross infection[50].

Handwashing

The most important aspect of preventing the spread of MRSA is hand washing. Each time a member of the nursing staff attends to a resident she should wash her hands with soap and water and dry them with a paper towel. Research shows that the average nurse spends 20 seconds washing her hands. Although most infection control nurses recommend a one-minute handwash, even a ten-second handwash removes micro-organisms effectively. Drying the hands with a paper towel or using a hot air dryer removes bacteria. Cloth towels act as a breeding ground for bacteria and can undo the effects of handwashing[51]. Some practitioners advocate the use of chlorhexidine hand disinfectant followed by a chlorhexidine alcohol hand rub but further research is required into the necessity and cost effectiveness of this policy. The routine use of hand disinfectants and alcohol rubs can cause hands to become very dry and crack; dry cracked skin is at risk of becoming infected with MRSA so such strategies may well lead to further outbreaks of MRSA.

Unfortunately many nurses fail to wash their hands at all even after 'dirty' procedures when their hands are visibly contaminated[52]. One research study found that nurses only washed their hands 28% of the time. Only half of all nurses washed their hands when they were visibly contaminated. This study found that nursing workload and the availability of soap, towels and washbasins affected handwashing. Most nurses used gloves when these were available. The authors commented that gloves were often not available[53]. Staff are less likely to wash their hands when facilities are poor.

Gloves

Some practitioners recommend the use of latex gloves when touching colonised or infected patients. This practice could upset and alarm older adults. The use of latex gloves is not a substitute for hand washing. Gloves can give nurses a false sense of security and they may omit hand washing because they are using gloves. Gloves can endanger nurse and patient. Now 10% of nurses have some form of latex allergy – allergies may be caused by either the powder or proteins in the gloves. There have been several reports of nurses having asthma attacks triggered by powdered latex gloves. The incidence of latex allergy in patients is also growing. Gloves split and leak. Gloves will not protect residents within the home from the risks of cross infection. Unless hands are washed after removing gloves, hands contaminated with MRSA during glove removal can spread MRSA. Published recommendations on caring for patients with MRSA state clearly that wearing latex gloves is not necessary[54]. A summary of these guidelines is given in Box 5.2. Latex gloves should be used when handling body secretions from individuals who are MRSA infected. Cuts or areas of broken skin on a nurse's hands should be covered with an occlusive waterproof dressing.

Caring for people with MRSA infected wounds

Wounds infected with MRSA should be covered with an occlusive waterproof dressing that effectively contains exudate. A strict aseptic technique

---

Box 5.2   Guidance on caring for people with MRSA – recommendations from combined working party on MRSA.

- MRSA carriage should not normally prevent discharge to a nursing home.
- Carriers are not a hazard to residents, staff or visitors if simple hygienic measures are followed.
- Basic principles of infection control are the same as those in hospitals. The single most important one is good handwashing.
- There should be an infection control policy with written procedures and a designated person responsible for infection control. This person should have access to training.
- Effective communication between doctors, infection control staff and nursing home staff must be established.
- Hospitals must facilitate the re-admission of the MRSA carrier if clinical condition deteriorates.

should be used. The nurse should wear latex gloves and a disposable plastic apron, which should be discarded after the dressing is completed. Ideally the nurse dressing this wound should not dress other residents' wounds. If this is not possible the MRSA infected wound should be dressed after all other dressings have been completed.

Can MRSA infected individuals share a room?

It is preferable to nurse MRSA infected individuals in single rooms. Some nursing homes still have shared rooms and individuals may be sharing with a spouse, sibling or a friend. It is possible to nurse MRSA infected individuals in shared rooms provided they meet the criteria in the next paragraph and strict infection control procedures are adhered to. One study found that there was a greater incidence of MRSA spread from individuals in single rooms than in shared rooms. The study, however, gives no details of infection control procedures within the nursing homes concerned[55]. The message from this and other studies is that the spread of infection cannot be contained by ritual barrier nursing. Nurses need to have a basic knowledge of infection control policies.

Box 5.3   Criteria for containment of MRSA.

MRSA in wound
An occlusive dressing effectively contains exudate.

MRSA in sputum
The individual uses tissue or sputum pot to contain sputum.

MRSA in urine
The individual is continent and uses toilet
The individual has a catheter, which is patent, and there is no spillage of urine.

MRSA in faeces
The individual is continent of faeces
The individual has a stoma and stoma appliances effectively contain faeces without leakage.

The resident needs to be alert and able and willing to assist nursing staff in preventing MRSA spread. The resident's room-mate must not have a wound, pressure sore, catheter, nasogastric, gastrostomy tube or tracheostomy. MRSA infected or colonised residents should not share a room with any individual who has a skin lesion, an indwelling catheter, nasogastric or gastrostomy tube or a tracheostomy or is very frail, as such individuals are at risk of contracting MRSA infection.

An MRSA infected individual who fulfils the criteria for room sharing can lead an unrestricted life both inside and outside the nursing home. She can take part in normal social activities and join others for meals in the dining room; there is no need to use disposable crockery or cutlery. She can go out to the shops or to visit her family. If nursing staff experience difficulty in containing infected sputum, wound exudate, urine or faeces they should contact the local infection control nurse for further advice.

Communication

An individual who is MRSA positive should have this recorded on her care plan. Infection control measures, actions, intentions and evaluation of care should be recorded. If a visit to a hospital, perhaps for an outpatient appointment, is planned, hospital staff should be notified of the individual's MRSA status before the appointment. Ambulance staff should also be notified if she is travelling by ambulance. Ambulance staff do not require protective clothing, gloves and masks. The ambulance does not need to be fumigated after use. If the individual is attending an Accident and Emergency unit, staff should be informed of the MRSA status so that they can use appropriate infection control measures. Communication between hospital and nursing home is essential if the spread of MRSA is to be minimised. Hospital staff also have an important role to play in informing nursing home staff of residents' MRSA status.

Conclusion

The guidance on MRSA in nursing homes helps clarify infection control measures required in nursing homes. Unfortunately it assumes that all MRSA infection is in wounds. It is possible to have MRSA in a number of sites, including the chest, urine and sputum. Introducing effective infection control policies within nursing homes can contain the spread of MRSA and other more potentially hazardous bacteria. MRSA infected individuals can be safely cared for in nursing homes and can enjoy quality of life without compromising the safety of others if infection control measures and strategies for containment are applied. Further research is required to determine the extent of MRSA infection within nursing homes. As antibiotic resistance becomes more prevalent it is essential that nursing home staff develop policies to prevent infection occurring.

Setting up an infection control programme

This section aims to discuss practical aspects of setting up an infection control programme within a nursing home. It is based on my experience of setting up such a programme in my workplace.

This section aims to:

- Enable you to assess infection risk
- Discuss how to set up an infection control programme
- Discuss how you can audit infection in your home
- Discuss practical ways to reduce infection rates

Why set up an infection control programme?

Older people are particularly vulnerable to the effects of infection, and older people in nursing homes are more vulnerable than healthy older people living at home. Setting up an infection control programme will help you to:

- Enable older adults to enjoy the highest possible quality of life and function to capacity
- Reduce high nursing workload associated with infections and their complications
- Monitor rates of infection within the home
- Reduce infection rates
- Reduce unnecessary antibiotic prescriptions
- Ensure that antibiotics prescribed are appropriate
- Cut GP prescribing costs.

Work hard to get nursing staff involved in planning the infection control programme. Listen to their ideas and suggestions.

Baseline audit

Before you can decide where you want to go you need to discover where you are at the moment. Carrying out an audit of antibiotic use over the last year indicates infection rates (or suspected infection rates). Auditing antibiotic use is fairly straightforward. Check medication charts over the last year. Make a note of how many courses of antibiotics were prescribed. Pay particular attention to cases where an antibiotic prescription was followed by another within a short period, e.g. 6–8 weeks.

Auditing over a shorter period will not give you accurate data. If you audit over winter months (when chest infections are more common) you will not get an accurate picture of the incidence of chest infections. The information you obtain from your audit will help you to gain the co-operation of GPs.

Discussing protocols with medical staff

One of the greatest barriers to setting up an infection control programme is securing the co-operation of medical staff. Involve medical staff in the programme when you have completed your baseline audit. You will have to work hard to 'sell' the infection control programme to them. If you are successful they may eventually think it was their idea!

The easiest way of getting the medical staff to consider the infection control programme is to give them a copy of your data on antibiotic use within the home over the last 12 months. If you have an efficient pharmacist with a computer system he can present you with a print-out detailing the costs of that treatment. GPs are conscious of prescribing costs. The idea of enhancing quality of care and reducing prescribing costs will appeal to many GPs. Outline the benefits of establishing protocols as part of the infection control strategy for the home:

- Reducing rates of infection
- Determining if infection is present using protocols
- Reducing the number of unnecessary antibiotic prescriptions
- Ensuring that appropriate antibiotic is prescribed – and treatment is effective
- Reduction in GP prescribing costs
- Reduction in unnecessary calls to GP
- Enhanced quality of life for residents.

Discuss protocols that you consider most important. The most worthwhile protocols are those involving suspected urinary tract, wound and chest infection. Examples of protocols for these are given at the end of this chapter.

Involving the infection control nurse and consultant microbiologist

Your protocols will involve nursing staff taking the decision to send off urine for culture and sensitivity, and send wound swabs and sputum specimens when these are clinically indicated. You will need to have results sent directly to the nursing home if you are to follow through infection control procedures. If they are sent directly to GPs there may be a delay in treating those who require treatment. If you have more than one GP visiting the home there is a risk that none will have an overview of infection control. If all results are returned to the home then vital pieces of the infection control jigsaw are not filed in individual patients' notes in different surgeries. Visit the infection control nurse and if possible the consultant microbiologist. Show them your draft protocols and explain your aims. Explain that you intend to send urine, sputum and wound swabs according to your protocols. Explain that the request forms will be marked with the relevant GP's name but that the return address will be that of the nursing home. The microbiology laboratory can then enter this information on their computer system. If you fail to do this all results may be automatically sent to the GP. Begin to build up a relationship with the infection control team.

Finally agree final protocols with the GP(s). These protocols should be signed by the GP(s) and copies retained by the GP(s) and the home.

Implementing protocols

Before implementing protocols you need to make sure that staff are clear about their use. Ideally staff will have been involved in drawing these up.

Staff education

Implementing protocols will ensure that antibiotics are used appropriately. Other general infection control measures will reduce infection control rates further. All staff within the home – domestics, catering, laundry, care assistants and registered nurses – have a part to play in reducing infection rates. You must ensure that every member of the team knows how important his or her contribution is. Many staff are willing to help but do not know how. Educating staff through one-to-one and formal teaching sessions is important. The most important aspects are:

- Ensuring that the home is clean.
- Ensuring that spills are cleared up promptly.
- Make sure that handwashing is a priority. Signs above each wash basin, in toilets, sluices, bathrooms and the kitchen all improve handwashing rates.
- Examine your wound care practice. Are you still using topical antibiotics and iodine-based ointments and dressings? These can sensitise skin and delay wound healing. They should be used rarely and after a great deal of thought.

- Examine your wound-cleansing agents. Few (if any) wounds require cleansing with agents other than saline.
- Work to prevent wounds occurring. Prevent pressure sores and 'knocks' that can easily develop into ulcers.
- Work to prevent urinary tract infections:
  Encourage fluids
  Ensure good perineal hygiene – teach staff and residents to wash from front to back to prevent bacterial infection.
  Ensure residents do not become constipated – this increases the risk of urinary tract infections (UTIs)
  Encourage residents to walk – this reduces the risk of UTIs
  Consider cranberry juice if the person suffers from recurrent UTIs
  Ensure that catheter hygiene is maintained.
- Work to prevent chest infections:
  Encourage mobility, however limited
  Ensure hydration is adequate
  Ensure nutrition is as good as possible.

Monitoring infections

Monitoring, the final part of infection control, is the most important. Monitoring will enable you to measure your success. It will allow you to monitor infection rates within the home, and antibiotic usage. Monitoring enables you to detect bacteria that could potentially cause problems – for example haemolytic streptococci, *Clostridium difficile* and methicillin-resistant *Staphylococcus aureus* – and to take action to head off problems before they occur.

Conclusion

Introducing an infection control programme involves some planning and additional work in the short term. It is worth the effort involved because of the long-term benefits to older adults within the home and nursing staff. Introducing infection control programmes can result in an overall reduction of 40% in antibiotic usage. Our greatest success has been in eliminating unnecessary antibiotic prescriptions when wound infection was suspected. We also successfully reduced antibiotic usage relating to urinary tract infections. Now, because we send off specimens for culture and sensitivity routinely, residents are rarely prescribed serial antibiotics. Our success rate for chest infections has been less spectacular. There are a number of reasons for this. Firstly, it can be extremely difficult to obtain sputum specimens – especially from female residents. Secondly, because chest infection can be so serious in older adults our GPs tend to prescribe 'when in doubt' or to prevent secondary bacterial infection. They are more likely to 'watch and wait' than previously. Each case is reviewed individually.

Infection control programmes do enable older people to lead more fulfilling lives and reduce nursing workload.

References

1   Wilson, J. (1995) Epidemiology of infection. In: *Infection Control in Clinical Practice*. Balliere Tindall, London.

2   Emmerson, A.M., Griffin, M. & Kelsley, C. *et al.* (1996). The second national prevalence study of infection in hospitals. *Journal of Hospital Infection*, **32**(3), 175–190.

3   De Week, A.L. (1992) Immune response and ageing. Constitutive and environmental aspects. In Munro, H. & Schlief, G. (eds) *Nutrition and the Elderly*. Raven Press, New York.

4   Goode, H.P., Penne, N.D., Kelleher, J. & Walker, B.E. (1991) Evidence of cellular zinc depletion in hospitalised but not in healthy elderly subjects. *Age & Ageing*, **20**, 345–348.

5   Laing, W. (2000) *Laing's Review of Private Healthcare*. Laing & Buisson, London.

6   Davey, P.G., Bax, R.P. & Reeve, D. (1996) Growth of the use of antibiotics in the Community in England and Scotland (1989–1993). *British Medical Journal*, **312**, 613.

7   Williams, E.I., Savage, S., McDonald, P. & Groom, L. (1992) Residents of private nursing homes and their care. *British Journal of General Practice*. **42**, 477–481.

8   Valigra, I. (1994) Engineering the future of antibiotics. *New Science*, **142**(1923), 25–27.

9   John, J.E. & Ribner, B.S. (1991) Antibiotic resistance in long term care facilities. *Infection Control & Hospital Epidemiolgy*, **12**(4), 245–250.

10 Kelly, J. & Chivers, G. (1996) Built in resistance. *Nursing Times*, **92**(2), 50–54.

11 De Week, A.I. (1992) Immune response and ageing. Constitutive and environmental aspects. In: Munro, H. & Schlierf G. (eds) *Nutrition and the Elderly*. Raven Press, New York.

12 Bastow, M.D., Rawlings, J. & Allison, S.P. (1982) Benefits of supplementary tube feeding after fractured neck of femur: a randomised control trial. *British Medical Journal*, **287**, 1589–1592.

13 Department of Health (1992) *The nutrition of elderly people*. Report on Health and Social Subjects. The Stationery Office, London.

14 Chandra, R.K. (1992) Effect of vitamin and trace element supplementation on immune response in elderly subjects. *Lancet*, **340**, 1124–1127.

15 McWhirter, J.P. & Penningtpon, C.R. (1994) Incidence and recognition of malnutrition in hospitals. *British Medical Journal*, **306**, 945–948.

16 Rowe, J.W. (1988) Renal system. In: Rowe, J.W. & Besedine, R.W. (eds) *Geriatric Medicine* (2nd edn) pp. 231–245. Little Brown & Company, Boston.

17 DuBeau, C.E. & Resnick, N.W. (1991) Evaluation of the causes and severity of geriatric incontinence; a critical appraisal. *Urological Clinics of North America*, **18**(2), 243–256.

18 Reardon, M. (1996) Transfers to nursing homes. *Elderly Care*, **8**(5), 16–18.

19 Nazarko, L. (1997) The whole story. *Nursing Times*, **93**(43), 63–68.

20 Garibaldi, R.A., Burke, J.P., Dickman, M. & Smith, C.B. (1974) Factors predisposing to bactinuria during indwelling urethral catheterisation. *New England Journal of Medicine*, **291**(5), 215–219.

21 Mulhall, A. (1991) Biofilms and urethral catheter infections. *Nursing Standard*, **5**(18), 26–28.

22 Burke, J.P., Garibaldi, R.A., Britt, M.R., Jacobson, J.A., Conti, M. & Alling, D.W. (1981) Prevention of catheter associated urinary tract infection. *American Journal of Medicine*, **70**, 655–658.

[23] Dance, D.A.B., Pearson, A.D., Seal, D.V. & Lowes, J.A. (1987) A hospital outbreak caused by a chlorhexideine and antibiotic resistant proteus mirabilis. *Journal of Hospital Infection*, **10**, 10–16.

[24] Ouslander, J.G., Greengold, B. & Chen, S. (1987) External catheter use and urinary tract infections among incontinent nursing home patients. *Journal American Geriatrics Society*, **35**(12), 1063–1070.

[25] Nazarko, L. (1995) The therapeutic uses of cranberry juice. *Nursing Standard*, **9**, 33–35.

[26] Ayliffe, G.A.J., Noy, M.E. & Davis, J.G. (1990) *Hospital Acquired Infection – Principles and Prevention*, 2nd edn. Butterworth, London.

[27] Tomlinson, D. & Bullock, D. (1992) To clean or not to clean. *Nursing Times*, **88**(34), 66–68.

[28] Hutchinson, J.J. & Lawrence, J.C. (1991) Wound infection under occlusive dressings. *Journal Hospital Infection*, **17**, 83–84.

[29] Lock, P.M. (1979) The effects of wound temperature on mitotic activity at the edge of experimental wounds. *Symposium on wound healing*. (Ed. N. Sundell). Espoo, Finland.

[30] Gilchrist, B. (1997) Should iodine be reconsidered? *Nursing Times*, **93**(32), 70–76.

[31] Schmidt, R. (1996) Redox homeostasis and microbial colonisation of healing wounds: new insights into the energy economy of healing wounds. *Journal Anasthesie und Intensivbehandlung*, **3**(3), 26–31.

[32] Danielson, L., Westh, H., Balselv, E., Rosdahl, V. & Doring, G. (1996) Pseudomonas aeruginosa exotoxin A antibodies in rapidly deteriorating chronic leg ulcers. *Lancet*, **347**(8996), 265.

[33] Thomas, S., Andrews, A.M. & Jones, M. (1998) The use of larval therapy in wound management. *Wound Care*, **7**(10), 521–524.

[34] Thomas, S., Andrews, A.M. & Hay, N.P. (1999) The anti-microbial activity of maggot secretions: results of a preliminary study. *Journal Tissue Viability*, **9**(4), 127–132.

[35] Thomas, S. & Andrews, A.M. (1999) The effect of hydrogel dressings on maggot development. *J Wound Care*, **8**(2), 75–77.

[36] Rayner, K. (1999) Larval therapy in wound debridement. *Professional Nurse*, **14**(5), 329–333.

[37] Sherman, R.A., Hall, M.J. & Thomas, S. (2000) Medicinal maggots: an ancient remedy for some contemporary afflictions. *Annu. Rev. Entomol.*, **45**, 55–81.

[38] MacIntosh, C.A., Marples, R.R. & Kerr, G.E. (1991) Surveillance of MRSA in England & Wales 1986–90. *Journal Hospital Infection*, **18**, 279–292.

[39] Beedle, D. (1993) Beating the bug. *Nursing Times. Journal of Infection Control Nursing (supplement)*, **89**(45), 2–6.

[40] Nue, H.C. (1992) The crisis in antibiotic resistance. *Science*, **257**, 1064–1073.

[41] Shanson, D.C. (1992) Antibiotic resistance in *Staphylococcus aureus*. In: Cafferty, M.T. (ed.) *Methicillin Resistant Staphylococcus Aureus Clinical Management and Laboratory Standards*. Marcel Dekker, New York.

[42] Waldvogel, F.A. (1990) *Staphylococcus aureus*. In: Douglas, R.G. (JR) Bennett, J.E. (eds) *Principles and Practices of Infectious Diseases*. Churchill-Livingstone, Edinburgh.

[43] Boyce, J.M. (1991) Patterns and prevalence of methicillin resistant *Staphylococcus aureus. Infection Control and Hospital Epidemiology*, **12**(2), 79–82.

[44] Cookson, B.D. (1990) Mupirocin resistance in staphylococci. *Journal of Antimicrobal Chemotherapy*, **25**, 497–503.

[45] Boyce, J.M. (1992) Methicillin resistant *Staphylococcus aureus* – detection,

epidemiology and control measures. *Infection Control and Hospital Epidemiology*, **13**, 725–737.

[46] Hsu, C.C.S. (1991) Serial survey of methicillin resistant *Staphylococcus aureus* nasal carriage among residents in a nursing home. *Infection Control and Hospital Epidemiology*, **12**(7), 416–421.

[47] Waldvogen F.A. (1990) *Staphylococcus aureus*. In: Douglas, R.G. (JR) Bennett, J.E. (eds) *Principles and Practices of Infectious Diseases*. Churchill-Livingstone, Edinburgh.

[48] Boyce J.M. (1991) Patterns and prevalence of methicillin resistant *Staphylococcus aureus*. *Infection Control and Hospital Epidemiology*, **12**(2), 79–82.

[49] Goodall, B. & Tompkins, D.S. (1994) Nursing homes act as a reservoir. *British Medical Journal*, 308–358.

[50] Nazarko, L. (1994) Infection control in nursing homes. *Elderly Care*, **6**(4), 13–16.

[51] Ansari, S.A., Spinthorpe, U.S. & Sattar, S.A. *et al.* (1991) Comparison of cloth, paper and warm air in eliminating bacteria and viruses from washed hands. *American Journal of Infection Control*, **8**, 243–249.

[52] Gould, D. (1993) Assessing nurses hand decontamination performance. *Nursing Times*, **89**, 47–50.

[53] Gould, D., Wilson Barnett, J. & Rean, E. (1996) Nurses infection control practice; hand decontamination, the use of gloves and sharp instruments. *International Journal of Nursing Studies*, **33**(2), 143–159.

[54] Report of the Combined Working Party of the British Society for Antimicrobal Chemotherapy and Hospital Infection Society (1995) Guidelines on the control of Methicillin Resistant *Staphylococcus Aureus* in the Community. *Journal of Hospital Infection*, **31**(1), 1–12.

[55] Beedle D (1993) Beating the bug. *Nursing Times. Journal of Infection Control Nursing (supplement)*, **89**(45), 2–6.

Individual infection Risk Assessment Tool

NAME: _____
DATE ADMISSION _____

HOW TO USE THIS FORM
Please tick one box for each category. Add the points together to calculate infection risk. Plan care to eliminate or reduce risk. Document your aims, objectives, actions, and evaluation in the care plan.

Age
☐ 74-84 =1
☐ 85+ =2

Nutritional status
☐ Feeds self, good appetite =0
☐ Poor appetite =1
☐ Dependent on nursing staff =2
☐ Nasogastric feeding = 3
☐ Gastrostomy feeding =4

Continence
☐ Continent = 0
☐ Urinary incontinence = 1
☐ Urinary sheath =2
☐ Urinary catheter =3
☐ Faecally incontinent =5

Skin integrity
☐ Intact skin =0
☐ Skin ulcer 1-4 dependent on size/depth
☐ Pressure sore 1-4 dependent on size/depth

Smoking
☐ No =0
☐ Yes =1

Hospital admission/Treatment
☐ Within last 28 days = 4
☐ Minor surgery, e.g. cataract, =2
☐ Major surgery, e.g. repair of fractured femur, =4
☐ Chemotherapy or radiotherapy =4

Medication
☐ Steroid therapy = 2
☐ Antibiotic therapy =2
☐ Sedatives = 2
☐ Anti-inflammatory =2

Social factors
☐ Sharing a room = 1
☐ Sharing with a catheterised patient = 2
☐ Sharing a room with a faecally incontinent patient =2
☐ Sharing a room with a patient with a skin lesion =2

Mobility
☐ Mobile with help =1
☐ Wheelchair bound = 2
☐ Immobile = 3
☐ Bedfast =4

Enter total score in box ☐
Please note the higher the score the more vulnerable the person is to infection.

Comments:

Date of assessment _____

Assessment completed by _____

Protocol for suspected urinary tract infection

Definition
Inflammation of one or more urinary tract structures.

Physiology and Aetiology
Decrease in strength of bladder muscle leading to incomplete bladder emptying.
Establishment of Gram-negative bacteria in residual urine. Altered antigen antibody
response leading to age-related reduction of resistance to infection.
Benign prostatic hypertrophy, bladder diverticulae, bladder stones, faecal contamination,
immobility, constipation, indwelling catheter or urinary sheath.

Symptoms
Urinary urgency and/or frequency. Burning or pain on urination. Perineal, suprapubic or
back pain. Pain can be less severe or absent in older adults. Blood, protein and nitrate
present in urine. Fever and chills – this response can be impaired in older adults.
Urinary incontinence, confusion and restlessness may be presenting symptoms in some
older adults.

Agreed protocol
Check individual's temperature, pulse, respirations and blood pressure.
Call GP if: Temperature is above 37.5°C, respirations are above 20, the individual is
hypotensive – for example a fall of 20 mmhg below normal diastolic measurement – the
person is in severe pain, or you are in any way concerned about the individual's condition.
If observations of TPR and BP are not within normal limits they should be monitored four-
hourly. The GP should be called if you have any concerns at any time.

Check urine for the presence of blood, protein and nitrite. The presence of blood and
protein is not necessarily indicative of urinary tract infection. The presence of nitrite is a
reliable indicator for infection. If nitrite is present send a urine specimen to microbiology at

. . . .

Information regarding nursing actions and any specimens sent should be recorded in the
care plan and nursing notes. A record of the specimen sent should be entered in the
infection control record.

*Nursing note: The presence of a heavy mixed growth often indicates contamination and
not infection. An infection which shows predominant growth of one bacteria for example
E. Coli at a concentration of 10^6 indicates infection and is normally treated with antibiotics.*

Check that the resident's condition remains stable and satisfactory. When the result of urine
culture and sensitivity arrives inform the GP immediately if antibiotics are recommended
by microbiology. If antibiotics are not required then the GP can be informed on his next
routine visit.
See nursing procedures for details of elements of essential nursing care relating to UTI.

This protocol has been agreed with

. . . .

. . . .

Protocol for suspected wound infection

Definition
Inflammation and invasion of the skin by bacteria.

Physiology and aetiology
Age related atrophic changes, a break in skin integrity caused by trauma or pressure. Altered antigen antibody response leading to age related reduction of resistance to infection. Cellulitis, impetigo, chronic venous or arterial ulceration, pressure sore, immobility.

Symptoms
Wound discharge, hot inflamed skin, presence of swelling or pain. Pain can be less severe or absent in older adults. Fever and chills – this response can be impaired in older adults. Confusion and restlessness may be presenting symptoms in some older adults.

Agreed protocol
Check individual's temperature, pulse, respirations and blood pressure.
Call GP if: Temperature is above 37.5°C, respirations are above 20, the individual is hypotensive – for example a fall of 20 mmhg below normal diastolic measurement – the person is in severe pain, or you are in any way concerned about the individual's condition. If observations of TPR and BP are not within normal limits they should be monitored four-hourly. The GP should be called if you have any concerns at any time.

Take swab before cleansing wound. Send wound swab – ensuring that swab is sent in culture medium. Send to microbiology at . . . .
Information regarding nursing actions and any specimens sent should be recorded in the care plan and nursing notes. A record of the specimen sent should be entered in the infection control record.

Nursing note: Research indicates that the majority of chronic wounds culture a mixed growth. This is normal and does not impair wound healing. A culture where the growth of one organism predominates is indicative of infection.

Check that the resident's condition remains stable and satisfactory. When the result of culture and sensitivity arrive inform the GP immediately if antibiotics are recommended by microbiology. If antibiotics are not required then the GP can be informed on the next routine visit.
See nursing procedures for details of elements of essential nursing care relating to wound infections.

This protocol has been agreed with

. . . .

. . . .

Protocol for suspected chest infection

Definition
Inflammation of the lungs that is accompanied by exudation and consolidation.

Physiology and aetiology
Multiplication of micro-organisms in pulmonary tissue followed by oedema and other inflammatory changes. Blood flow is initially increased but capillary blood flow is reduced to affected areas. The lungs gradually stiffen.
Viral and bacterial infection. Poor chest expansion, shallow breathing, chronic bronchitis, asthma and other chronic respiratory diseases.

Symptoms
Confusion, restlessness and changes in behaviour may be presenting symptoms in some older adults. The classic presenting symptom is 'going off the legs', i.e. becoming prone to falls and less mobile. Pleuritic pain may be absent in older adults. Pyrexia may be absent or present late. Cough, increased respiratory rate, tachycardia.

Agreed protocol
Check individual's temperature, pulse, respirations and blood pressure.
Call GP if: Temperature is above 37.5°C, respirations are above 20, resting pulse is above 80 per minute, the individual is dyspnoeic, the individual is hypotensive – for example a fall of 20 mmhg below normal diastolic measurement – the person has pleuritic or chest pain, the person is expectorating green or purulent sputum, there is any sign of blood in sputum, or if you are in any way concerned about the individual's condition. If observations of TPR and BP are not within normal limits they should be monitored four-hourly. The GP should be called if you have any concerns at any time.

Whenever possible obtain and send a sputum specimen. Send to microbiology at
. . . . If it is not possible to obtain a sputum specimen call the doctor immediately if observations are not within normal limits. If observations are within normal limits but the person appears unwell call the doctor within eight hours of onset of presenting symptoms.
Information regarding nursing actions and any specimens sent should be recorded in the care plan and nursing notes. A record of the specimen sent should be entered in the infection control record.

Nursing note: Older adults present atypically when they develop chest infections. Complications include congestive cardiac failure, pleurisy, hypotension, shock, hypoxia and septicaemia. Observe older adults with suspected chest infection very closely and do not hesitate to call doctor.

Check that the resident's condition remains stable and satisfactory. When the result of culture and sensitivity arrive inform the GP immediately if antibiotics are recommended by microbiology. If antibiotics are not required then the GP can be informed on the next routine visit.
See nursing procedures for details of elements of essential nursing care relating to chest infections.

This protocol has been agreed with

. . . .

. . . .

Chapter 6

Wound Care

Introduction

The commonest types of wounds cared for by nurses within nursing homes are leg ulcers and pressure sores (decubitus ulcers); fungating lesions and surgical wounds are less common. Wound care within nursing homes is generally the responsibility of the nurse. Leg ulcers in particular can be chronic and simply caring for the wound is not enough. Research indicates that individuals can suffer from recurrent leg ulcers over periods ranging from 10[1] to 50 years[2]. Many nurses have seen leg ulcers heal only to see them break down again.

There has been a revolution in wound care in recent years and we now know more about the anatomy and physiology of wound healing than ever before. Research within nursing homes demonstrates that nurses use modern dressings such as hydrocolloids and alginates appropriately in the majority of cases and often go to considerable trouble to obtain dressings not currently available on FP10 prescription for individuals in nursing homes. Nurses report feeling isolated and find it difficult to obtain access to study days and courses dealing with wound care. There are many articles in the nursing journals that provide guidance on choosing dressings and there are a few which examine the underlying causes of leg ulcers and help nurses to treat the resident who has a leg ulcer, rather than simply the ulcer. This chapter aims to assist the nurse to provide holistic treatment for the individual with a chronic wound, and by correcting, wherever possible, factors which predispose to chronic wounds, to prevent tissue breakdown in the future.

Chronic wounds can present many problems. They can take a long time to heal and are vulnerable to infection and complications until healing has taken place.

This chapter aims to enable you to:

- Understand how wounds heal
- Understand the fundamentals of wound assessment
- Assess the person with the wound
- Act on factors that impede wound healing
- Assess the wound
- Choose appropriate dressings to facilitate wound healing

How do wounds heal?

There are three main layers of skin: the epidermis, the dermis and sub-cutaneous tissue.

The epidermis is the outer layer of the skin. The cells of the epidermis are dead and contain no blood cells. The epidermis is constantly being shed and replaced by cells from the deep layers.

The dermis is the middle layer of the skin. It supports and attaches firmly to the epidermis. Complex protein fibres called collagen in the dermis provide strength and elasticity. The skin's blood vessels, nerve endings, hair follicles, sweat glands and lymphatic drainage vessels are situated in the dermis. The blood vessels carry blood that contains the nutrients required to keep the skin healthy. The blood vessels also regulate heat – dilating to increase blood flow and allowing heat loss; constricting to reduce blood flow and to conserve body heat. The dermis cannot regenerate if it is destroyed. It heals by forming granulation tissue which is eventually replaced by scar tissue.

The subcutaneous or fatty layer carries the larger blood vessels that supply the skin. Its thickness varies enormously depending on the area of the body and the individual. It acts as a thermal barrier and energy store for fats and water in the body and disperses localised pressure protecting the superficial skin from the effects of sharp internal bony prominences. The subcutaneous layer adheres to muscle. The muscle covers bone.

Surgical wounds and wounds where only a small area of tissue has been lost heal by primary intention. The two skin edges knit together and heal quickly.

A wound extending into the dermis or deeper tissues results in a greater loss of tissue. These wounds heal from the wound bed up. The lost tissue is replaced by new tissues and covered with epithelium. Secondary healing takes weeks or months depending on the factors relating to the wound and the factors relating to the person.

Wound healing consists of four phases that overlap:

(1)   Inflammatory phase – lasting 1–3 days
(2)   Destructive phase – lasting 3–5 days
(3)   Proliferation phase – lasting 5–24 days
(4)   Maturation phase – lasting 24 days to up to a year.

The first response to tissue damage is inflammation. This is a normal part of wound healing. It is a protective mechanism causing increased capillary permeability and oedema and the stimulation of pain fibres. The five signs of inflammation are:

(1)   Heat
(2)   Redness
(3)   Pain
(4)   Swelling
(5)   Loss of function

The inflammatory response is essential for healing. It can be prolonged in large wounds. During the destructive phase polymorphs and macrophages remove dead tissue and stimulate the multiplication of fibroblasts. During the proliferation phase fibroblasts begin to produce fibres of collagen. New capillary loops grow into the collagen and form granulation tissue. During the maturation phase more collagen fibres are produced and reorganised strengthening the scar. Finally epithelial tissue covers the wound.

Wound assessment

Wound assessment should aim to assess not only the wound but also the person who has the wound. This enables you to assess the extrinsic factors – the factors affecting the person who has the wound and the intrinsic factors such as the site, size and stage of healing of the wound. The extrinsic factors you should assess are:

- Age
- Medication: steroid therapy, non steroidal anti-inflammatory drugs
- Anaemia
- Diabetes
- Cardiac disease
- Hypertension
- Thyroid disease
- Nutrition
- Fluid intake
- Mobility
- Chronic diseases

The following sections examine how the factors relating to the person affect wound healing, and discuss what we can do to enable wounds to heal.

Ageing

Ageing slows the rate of wound healing and the skin of older people is more prone to damage than that of younger people[3]. Although we cannot reverse the ageing process we can take note of it and avoid further damage to skin by not applying dressing tape directly to vulnerable skin. It is best to use bandages or tubular bandages to secure dressings.

Medication

Some medications such as steroids and non-steroidal anti-inflammatory drugs (NSAIDs) can impair healing by reducing the normal inflammatory response required in wound healing. Sometimes older people have been on steroids for a long time and have not been reviewed. It is worth asking medical staff if it is possible to reduce or tail off steroid therapy. It may be possible to reduce or discontinue NSAIDs. Pain can sometimes be controlled using simple analgesia that will not impair wound healing.

Anaemia

Haemoglobin transports oxygen around the body. Wounds require high levels of oxygen in order to heal. Anaemia reduces the ability of the body to transport oxygen to the wound and delays wound healing[4]. Iron deficiency anaemia is common in some older people because they do not have a balanced diet. Medications such as steroids or non-steroidal anti-inflammatory drugs (NSAID) can cause gastric ulceration and gastric bleeding. This bleeding can be either acute or chronic. Chronic slow gastric bleeding can cause severe anaemia over a period of time. Around 40–70% of people taking long term NSAID have micro erosions of the stomach muscoa and have blood loss of 2–6 ml daily. Chronic ulceration of the mucosa may also cause malabsorption[5] of vitamin C and vitamin B_{12} and protein loss. Pernicious anaemia is caused by a lack of intrinsic factor and is treated with vitamin B_{12} injections.

If the person has a deep cavity wound it is important to ask medical staff if you can take blood for a full blood count. If the person is anaemic the underlying cause can be treated and the anaemia treated. Treatment of anaemia will improve wound healing by increasing the amount of oxygen at the wound surface[6].

Diabetes

Diabetes can compromise circulation and hyperglycaemia can delay healing[7]. The presence of a wound, especially an infected wound, can lead to poor diabetic control and can further inhibit healing[8]. It is important that you monitor blood glucose carefully. If diabetic control is deteriorating you should consult medical staff. The person may require additional medication to control diabetes. Good diabetic control is essential because high glucose levels will inhibit healing and increase the risk of infection. Diabetes can compromise circulation, and hyperglycaemia can delay healing[9].

Cardiac disease

If cardiac disease is not treated effectively, blood flow throughout the body is reduced. The amount of oxygen and nutrients available to the wound is reduced. Checking the person's pulse and informing medical staff of any abnormalities is an important part of wound assessment. Treatment of cardiac disease often leads to more efficient cardiac output and this improves wound healing[10].

Hypertension

High blood pressure leads to decreased blood flow to the wound. This impairs healing. It is important that you check blood pressure and inform medical staff of any abnormality. Treatment of hypertension improves wound healing. In obese individuals hypertension often resolves with weight loss. In some individuals medication is required.

Thyroid disease

Thyroid disease becomes more common as we age. The thyroid gland is responsible for controlling metabolic rate. An underactive thyroid gland (hypothyroidism) will slow down wound healing. It is important to check for clinical signs of an underactive thyroid and to refer the person to medical staff if you detect signs. Treatment with thyroxine will restore normal metabolic function and facilitate wound healing.

Nutrition and wound healing

It is important to weigh the person and calculate the BMI. This will enable you to work out if the person is underweight or overweight. Nutrition is one of the most important factors in healing wounds. Healing is impaired in obese individuals because blood supply to adipose tissue is poor. This affects blood supply to the wound. Underweight individuals usually lack the protein reserves required to repair tissues. Both underweight and obese individuals normally have a poor diet and this affects the supply of nutrients available to the wound.

Individuals with wounds require a high calorie diet as healing increases the metabolic rate and additional calories are required to enable the body to repair damaged tissues. It is recommended that individuals with wounds have at least 2500 calories per day. The more extensive the wound the greater the individual's calorie requirement; in some cases as many as 5000 calories per day are required. If the person is underweight you may be asked to take blood to check serum albumen. This can be measured to check nutritional status. Individuals who do not consume sufficient calories initially utilise body fat stores and when these are exhausted begin to loose protein from muscle tissue. An adequate diet containing a mixture of carbohydrate, fat and protein is required if wounds are to heal. Carbohydrates provide energy for cell metabolism, fats are essential if cells are to regenerate, and protein is required to enable a blood supply to be established to growing cells and to build collagen which is necessary for tissue repair.

Vitamins and trace elements

These are required to enable wound healing. Vitamin A is required to repair tissues. Vitamin C is essential in wound repair and enables the body to fight infection. Sometimes high doses of vitamin C, 500 mg or more, are prescribed to help wounds to heal. Vitamin B complex is required if cells are to reproduce. Vitamin K is required to enable blood clotting to take place and enable wounds to heal.

Zinc deficiency delays wound healing[11]. It can be difficult to measure zinc levels and sometimes zinc is prescribed to help enable wounds to heal.

Ensuring that older adults consume a diet with sufficient calories and nutrients to enable optimal wound healing can be difficult. Many individuals with wounds may require dietary supplements to ensure an adequate diet. Many dietary supplements are available on prescription and contain a balance of fat, carbohydrate, protein and vitamins. A range of supplements are available including ready-made puddings and drinks. If you need advice on how to meet an individual's dietary requirements you must ask the person's GP to refer the person to the local community or hospital-based dietician. Dieticians do not accept referrals from nurses.

Fluid intake

Healthy adults require 1.5 to 2 litres of fluid per day. If the person has an infection and fever additional fluids will be required. If the person has a heavily exuding wound additional fluids are required. If the individual becomes dehydrated this will reduce the flow of fluid and nutrients to the wound bed and slow the rate of wound healing.

Mobility

The ability to move around or change position unaided is important. We all make tiny adjustments to our posture when seated or in bed. If the person is unable to change position with assistance you must assess pressure risk. When you have assessed pressure risk you can then use appropriate equipment such as pressure relieving overlays and mattress replacements to reduce the pressure. You will also need to document how often the person's position is to be changed, and monitor skin condition.

Chronic diseases

People with rheumatoid arthritis are at increased risk of developing leg ulcers[12]. When ulcers do develop they take longer to heal than venous ulcers[13]. Drugs used to treat arthritis (steroids and non-steroidal anti-inflammatory drugs) slow the rate of healing because they damp down the normal inflammatory response.

Intrinsic factors

Having assessed the person, you can then begin to assess the wound itself. The information you should obtain is:

- Site of the wound
- Size of the wound
- Nature of the base of wound
- Grading of the wound using a grading system
- Appearance of wound
- Duration of wound
- Condition of surrounding skin
- Smell of wound.

The easiest way to document the site of the wound is to mark it on a dermal diagram. It can be difficult to determine if a wound is healing when you see the wound almost every day. Using a grid to trace the outline of a wound can enable you to check how quickly healing is taking place. It is important to remember that if you are debriding a necrotic wound it can appear larger when the hard black necrotic tissue known as eschar is removed.

You may wish to photograph the wound. You can measure the depth of a wound by using a wound probe. There are two widely used methods of classifying wounds. One classifies wounds in five categories[14] while another uses four categories. It is important that you decide which classification system you will use and ensure that all staff use this classification. The classification should be recorded. Table 6.1 gives details of the Torrance classification.

Table 6.1   Torrance classification of pressure sores.

Stage	Description
1	Reddening is present. Light finger pressure causes the skin to whiten. This is referred to as 'blanching hyperaemia'. The whitening indicates that capillary circulation is intact and undamaged.
2	Reddening remains when light finger pressure is applied. This is referred to as 'non-blanching hyperaemia' and indicates that capillary circulation is damaged. The skin may be broken.
3	The skin is ulcerated and subcutaneous tissue is ulcerated.
4	The ulcer extends into subcutaneous fat. Underlying muscle is inflamed and swollen.
5	The ulcer extends into muscle or bone.

Principles of wound healing

Wounds heal best in a warm moist environment with low levels of oxygen tension. Exposing wounds to the air or cleaning them reduces the temperature of the wound. Cooling a wound reduces the rate of healing[15]. You can avoid cooling wounds by:

- Choosing an appropriate dressing and avoiding unnecessary dressing changes
- Avoiding routine cleaning of wounds
- Using a warmed solution if wound cleansing is necessary
- Replacing a dressing as soon as it is removed. Do not leave dressings off so that a doctor or specialist nurse can see the wound.

Research by Winter proved that wounds covered with an occlusive dressing healed twice as fast as wounds allowed to dry out[16]. Occlusive dressings prevent moisture evaporating and the wound bed remains moist. It is important that you choose a dressing that will prevent the wound drying up but will not lead to excess moisture as this can damage skin.

In the 1980s researchers compared healing rates of wounds left exposed, wounds covered in gauze soaked in saline, wounds covered with a film dressing and wounds covered with a hydrocolloid dressing. Those covered with a hydrocolloid dressing healed fastest, followed by those covered with a film, those soaked in saline and finally those that had been left exposed. The different rates of wound healing were due to oxygen tension. Occlusive dressings such as hydrocolloid and film dressings create a very low oxygen tension. This leads to high levels of oxygen at the capillaries and low levels of oxygen at the wound edges. This provides the ideal environment for wound healing because granulation and wound healing are stimulated[17].

Choosing appropriate dressings

Cavity wounds heal from the base upwards. It is important to prevent the wound healing from the edges as a sinus can develop. The usual way to prevent this is to pack the wound and cover it with a suitable dressing. The ideal dressing will:

- Maintain a moist environment without causing maceration
- Maintain wound temperature
- Maintain low levels of oxygen to aid healing
- Remove excess exudates without drying the wound bed
- Remove necrotic tissue and slough
- Protect the wound from damage
- Protect the wound from bacteria
- Control odour
- Be cheap
- Cause no pain or trauma on removal.

Unfortunately the ideal wound dressing does not exist[18,19]. Nurses are faced with a huge range of dressings to choose from. No single dressing is suitable for all wounds. The same wound may require very different dressings at different stages of healing[20]. Nurses are accountable for their practice. Nurses must use evidence-based practice and have the ability to explain why certain wound care products have or have not been used[21,22,23]. In order to meet professional standards you need to be aware of the properties of different dressings so that you can choose a suitable dressing for the stage of wound healing. The following paragraphs look at the different types of dressings available and when they should and should not be used.

Alginates

Alginates are made from seaweed. They contain differing amounts of calcium and sodium salts of alginic acid. Alginate dressings are dry and interact with the wound. When the alginate fibres come in contact with exudates they form a gel. When alginates come in contact with blood or exudates and gel is formed the wound has a warm moist environment that facilitates healing. Alginates draw excess fluid away from the wound and help to prevent maceration. The gel prevents the slough from drying out and enables the body to break down the slough. Alginates should be cut or folded to the shape of the wound to prevent maceration of surrounding skin. Alginate ropes are available and these are suitable for packing cavity wounds. It is important not to pack the wound too tightly as the dressing swells when it absorbs fluid, and if the wound is packed tightly it can cause pressure on the wound bed when it swells[24]. A secondary dressing is required. Kaltostat has haemostatic properties and is useful if you wish to stop bleeding.

Examples of alginate dressings: Kaltostat, Sorbsan, Sorbsan Plus, Algosteril.

Indications: Can be used on exuding and sloughy wounds

Contraindications: They should not be used on dry or necrotic wounds. If the dressing has dried out use warm tap water or saline to moisten the dressing and then remove.

Film dressings

Adhesive coated vapour permeable film dressings are thin dressings. They are permeable to water vapour and oxygen but impermeable to micro-organisms. They reduce the amount of water and oxygen escaping from the wound. This provides a moist environment with low levels of oxygen tension. Film dressings can be used alone on shallow wounds with low amounts of exudates. They can be used as secondary dressings to enable you to maintain a moist wound environment.
Example of film dressings: Opsite.
Indications: Can be used to protect reddened or blistered skin. Can be used on shallow, lightly exuding wounds. Can be used as a secondary dressing.
Contraindications: They should not be used alone on heavily exuding wounds. It is important to stretch the film to break the adhesive bond when removing the dressing.

Foam dressings

There are two types of foam dressings – those designed to fit into a cavity wound and flat sheets of foam.

Cavi-Care and Allevyn cavity dressings are designed to fit into the cavity. Cavi-Care is a silicone foam dressing that is mixed and poured into the wound. The foam then takes up the shape of the wound. It is covered with a secondary dressing and left in place for 24 to 48 hours. It is then removed and cleaned before being placed back in the wound. It is suitable for clean, granulating, cavity wounds. It is not suitable for narrow cavities or sinuses[25]. Allevyn cavity dressings are available in a range of shapes and sizes. They consist of an outer membrane and hydrophilic foam chips. Exudate is absorbed into the centre of the dressing where it is locked into the foam chips[26]. The dressing can be left in place until it is saturated. The manufacturers recommend that it is changed at least every five days. It is suitable for granulating cavity wounds.

Flat foam dressings absorb fluid and provide a warm moist environment for exuding healthy granulating wounds. Foam dressings such as Allevyn and Lyofoam Extra have three layers and fluid is absorbed into the layers. Foam dressings (apart from Allevyn adhesive) should be cut to size. They should be 1.5–2 cm smaller than the wound. Foam dressings can be left in place for several days. A secondary dressing is required.
Examples of foam dressings: Allevyn, Allevyn Adhesive, Lyofoam, Lyofoam Extra, Spyrosorb, Allevyn Cavity, Cavi-Care.
Indications: Can be used on healthy granulating wounds that are exuding. Cavity dressings can be used in cavities.
Contraindications: Film dressings should not be used as secondary dressings as this affects the ability of the dressing to absorb fluid.

Hydrocolloids

Hydrocolloid dressings are made of a film coated with an absorbent mass containing methylcellulose, gel forming agents, elastomers and adhesive. Hydrocolloids interact with the wound surface. Fluid is absorbed into the dressing and a gel is formed. Hydrocolloids can reduce wound pain because they cause changes to the oxygen tension in the wound bed. They stimulate healing by changing oxygen tension and providing a warm moist environment. When hydrocolloids were first introduced in the 1980s there were fears that the warm moist environment they provided would encourage bacterial growth and raise infection rates. We now know that hydrocolloids have a bacteriostatic effect on some organisms such as pseudomonas[27,28]. The rate of infection is reduced from 5% when using traditional dressings to 2% when hydrocolloids are used[29]. Infection rates may be reduced because occlusive dressings provide a more effective barrier to bacteria and prevent contamination of the wound. Hydrocolloids can be left in place for up to seven days. It is important that the dressing covers the wound plus a margin of 1.5 to 2 cm to reduce the risk of leakage.

Examples of hydrocolloid dressings: Granuflex, Comfeel, Tegasorb.

Indications: Can be used on necrotic, sloughy or granulating wounds.

Contraindications: Hydrocolloid dressings are not suitable for use on infected wounds. They can cause overgranulation.

Hydrogels

Hydrogels are 80% water and 17% glycol, and around 3% is a gel-forming ingredient such as carboxymethylcellulose. Hydrogels are applied to the wound and a secondary dressing is applied. When wounds are very dry a film dressing prevents evaporation and moisture loss. Hydrogels prevent water evaporating from the necrotic tissue and help the necrotic tissue to rehydrate. The glycol in the hydrogel softens the necrotic tissue and the water in the gel moves into the necrotic tissue causing it to soften[30]. When the tissue is softened the body can begin to break it down and healing can begin.

Examples of hydrogel dressings: Intrasite gel, Granugel, Sterigel, Nu-gel. Granugel is a combination of a hydrocolloid and a hydrogel. Nu-gel contains an alginate and a hydrogel.

Indications: Can be used on necrotic sloughy or moderately exuding granulating wounds. Can be used in cavity wounds and sinuses.

Contraindications: Hydrogel dressings are not suitable for use when anaerobic infections such as pseudomonas are suspected.

Hydropolymer dressings

Hydropolymer dressings consist of an island dressing and a secondary dressing. The island dressing absorbs fluid but allows excess fluid to evaporate through the back of the dressing. This enables the wound to remain moist but reduces the risk of maceration. Apply water to the dressing to allow the adhesive bond to be broken. Tielle dressings have a unique advantage as you can reapply them and if they do not require changing, they can be left in place for up to seven days.

Indications: Can be used on superficial or moderately exuding granulating wounds.
Contraindications: Not suitable for heavily exuding wounds.

Impregnated dressings

Gauze dressings impregnated with paraffin tulle are rarely used these days because granulating tissue can grow into the gaps in the dressing, causing pain and trauma on removal. Inadine is a viscose fabric impregnated with 10% providone iodine. It is designed specifically for infected or contaminated wounds and can be left in place for up to five days.
Indications: Can be used on sloughy and infected wounds.
Contraindications: Check for sensitivity to iodine before use. The iodine in the beads can be absorbed systemically. This can affect thyroid function and should not be used if the person is hypothyroid.

Larval therapy

Larvae or maggots have been used to treat infected, gangrenous and necrotic wounds for thousands of years. Before antibiotics were discovered they were used on battlefields to clean wounds[31]. Larvae secrete enzymes that liquefy necrotic tissue[32]. The larvae then eat this necrotic tissue. The larval secretions promote healing and destroy bacteria[33].

Blowfly larvae are normally used in the UK. These larvae only feed on necrotic tissue. They can remove 10–15 g of necrotic tissue a day and will not harm healthy tissue. Sterile blowfly larvae can be obtained from the biosurgical research unit in Wales. The larvae are supplied with fine mesh and full instructions. Normally a hydrocolloid dressing with a space cut out to expose the wound is applied to the person's skin. The larvae are applied and a fine mesh is placed over the wound. This is taped in place. An absorbent dressing is then applied. The absorbent dressing absorbs liquefied eschar and wound secretions. This is changed as often as necessary. When the larvae are applied to the wound they look like very fine, almost invisible, pieces of thread. The larvae should be removed from the wound after three days. At this stage they look like fat maggots. A further application of larvae can be applied when the first application is removed.

Larvae clean wounds rapidly, reduce odour and treat infection[34]. Larvae are not yet available on prescription and have to be purchased from the biosurgical research unit in Wales.

Xerogel dressings

Xerogel dressings consist of hydrophilic polysaccharide beans and cadexomer iodine. The beads draw excess fluid away from the wound. The iodine is released into the wound as the fluid is absorbed by the beads. A secondary dressing is required. The dressing should be changed when it has become saturated.

Examples of xerogel dressings: Iodosorb, Iodoflex.
Indications: Can be used on sloughy and infected wounds.
Contraindications: The iodine in the beads can be absorbed systemically. This can affect thyroid function and should not be used if the person is hypothyroid. Xerogels should not be used on dry wounds.

Table 6.2 illustrates suitable dressings for different types of wounds.

Table 6.2   Suitable dressing types for different wounds.

Classification	Suitable dressings
Epithelialising	Film or hydrocolloid dressing
Granulating	Film, foam or hydrocolloid dressings
Sloughy	Debrisan, Iodosorb, Iodoflex, hydrocolloids, hydrofibre, alginates and larvae
Necrotic	Hydrogels with film dressing, hydrocolloids, larval therapy with secondary dressing

Leg ulcers

The risk of developing a leg ulcer rises with age. Many of these ulcers heal slowly if at all. Assessment enables you to identify the reasons why the ulcer has occurred and to offer treatment that promotes wound healing.

Causes of leg ulcers

A leg ulcer is defined as: 'a loss of skin below the knee on the leg or foot which takes more than six weeks to heal'[35]. Older people are more likely to develop leg ulcers and 3.6% of people over the age of 65 have leg ulcers. Women over the age of 85 are ten times more likely to develop leg ulcers than men. For half of all individuals with leg ulcers, the ulcers have failed to heal within a year[36].

Discovering the factors that contributed to the development of the ulcer and, wherever possible, eliminating them helps existing wounds to heal more rapidly and prevents recurrence. The major causes of leg ulcers are:

- Venous disease – 70%
- Arterial disease – 22%
- Rheumatoid arthritis – 8.5%
- Diabetes – 5.5%
- Burns – 2.5%

Venous ulcers

Venous ulcers are the most common type of leg ulcers and are the cause of 70% of all leg ulcers. Most venous ulcers are secondary to long established disease in the deep veins[37]; they develop because valves in the deep and perforating veins become incompetent or damaged. This causes back-flow of blood into the thin walled superficial veins. The superficial veins become stretched and dilated. This causes further back-flow of blood and increased pressure in the superficial veins. This increased pressure is transferred to the capillaries. Capillaries have walls only one cell thick; when they become stretched fluids leak into the skin and tissues. The effects of increased capillary permeability are:

- Oedema caused by the loss of plasma and water into the tissues
- Leakage of red blood cells releasing haemoglobin as they break down
- Skin irritation and eczema caused by haemoglobin breakdown
- Skin staining caused by haemoglobin breakdown
- Fibrin layer around the capillaries of the person is associated with impaired tissue oxygenation and impaired healing.

Mixed arterial/venous ulcers

Some people who appear to have straightforward venous ulcers actually suffer from arterial problems as well. Compression in such circumstances reduces already poor blood flow and can lead to tissue damage and in extreme cases to the development of gangrene and death[38]. Department of Health guidance on the treatment of leg ulcers recommends that Doppler ultrasound investigations be performed to exclude arterial disease before compression therapy is commenced.

Arterial/ischaemic ulcers

Arterial or ischaemic ulcers are caused by a blockage to one of the smaller arteries. This arterial disease may be part of general arterial disease affecting large and small arteries. It may however be small vessel disease affecting only the smaller arteries. Arterial disease causes blood flow to be reduced or completely interrupted to an area of tissue. This reduction or interruption of blood flow results in an area of tissue becoming starved of the nutrients and oxygen required to maintain healthy tissue, and that tissue will break down.

Chronic vascular ulcers can be associated with rheumatoid arthritis. They are common complications of connective tissue diseases and are extremely difficult to heal. Recent research suggests that applying nerve growth factor for eight weeks heals such ulcers[39].

Embolism

If ischaemic ulcers suddenly develop then embolism is the probable cause and urgent medical attention must be sought. Embolism of a large vessel such as the femoral artery can result in rapid tissue death if not treated urgently. Normally, if the resident is well enough, femoral embolectomy is carried out in hospital and anticoagulant therapy is normally given thereafter. Embolism of small vessels can also lead to rapid tissue death but embolectomy is usually not possible because the vessels are too small to operate on.

Anticoagulant therapy and treatment to dilate non-affected arterial vessels are usually given.

Peripheral arterial disease

Peripheral arterial/vascular disease is caused by the deposit of fatty sub-stances known as artheroma within the lining of the arteries. These plaques cause narrowing of the arteries and arterioles and can lead to the eventual blockage of vessels. Onset is more gradual.

Assessment

Assessment is the most important aspect of wound management[40]. Assessment enables nurses to treat and manage wounds effectively[41]. Assessment should have three components: assessment of the wound and surrounding tissue, assessment of the person with the wound and vascular assessment.

The first part of wound assessment is to examine the wound. Asking the person how the wound feels and checking the past medical history enables you to identify the clinical features of different types of leg ulcers.

The clinical features of *venous ulcers* are:

- Usually in the gaiter area of leg
- Usually large
- Oval in shape
- Have shallow diffuse edges
- Generalised oedema is often present
- Varicose veins may be present
- Skin staining often visible around ulcer
- Eczema often present
- May complain of itching especially over veins
- History may include:
  Previous fracture of leg
  Surgery or injection of varicose veins
  Deep vein thrombosis
- Pedal pulses are normal
- Pain is described as 'aching' or 'throbbing'
- Elevating legs relieves pain.

Arterial ulcers have a different appearance and the clinical features and medical history are very different. The clinical features of *arterial ulcers* are:

- Occur on any part of leg – often below ankle
- Usually small
- Deep punched out appearances
- Dry – do not exude
- Any oedema is localised around the edges of the wound
- Skin is shiny and white
- Absence of hair on leg
- Foot cold and bluish
- Pedal pulses not palpable
- History of heart disease, stroke, intermittent claudication, diabetes, rheumatoid arthritis, previous arterial surgery
- More likely to be male
- More likely to be smokers or ex-smokers

- Pain is acute especially at night – will wake the resident
- Pain brought on by elevating leg
- Pain relieved by dangling legs over the edge of bed.

The next phase of assessment is to find out about any medical condition that the person has that might impair wound healing. This has been explored earlier in the chapter.

Mobility

Mobility is an important and little understood factor in wound healing. Individuals who are suffering from venous ulceration benefit from exercise which encourages venous drainage and reduces oedema. Gentle exercise helps improve the circulation of people with vascular disease. People who are immobile are more likely to be at risk of developing deep vein thrombosis and postural oedema than those who are mobile. Walking or moving around in a chair increases general blood flow and general health. This exercise improves appetite and makes nutritional deficiencies less likely. Improved morale also affects general health and helps wounds to heal.

Vascular assessment

Vascular assessment checks that the person has an adequate blood supply to the legs. Doppler ultrasound is an important part of vascular assessment. It enables nurses to determine the cause of leg ulcers and to treat them appropriately. Doppler ultrasound bounces sound off moving red blood cells and amplifies sound so that it can be heard. It enables trained and experienced nurses to check the ankle and brachial pressure indices (ABPI). Blood pressure readings are taken from both arms and both legs to calculate the ABPI. An index of 1.0 indicates that arterial flow is 100%. An index of 0.8 indicates a 20% reduction in arterial flow. ABPIs should be interpreted with caution in people with diabetes as calcification of the arteries can give misleadingly high readings.

Compression bandaging is the treatment of choice. The vast majority of venous ulcers treated with compression therapy heal within 12 weeks of treatment. Compression bandaging can safely be used if the ABPI is 0.8 or above[42]. Compression bandaging reduces oedema and venous congestion and increases arterial blood flow[43]. If the ABPI is 0.5 to 0.8, reduced compression therapy can be used if the person is able to tolerate this[44]. If the ABPI is less than 0.5 the person should not have compression applied under any circumstances. An immediate and urgent referral should be made to the vascular surgery department at the local hospital.

The benefits of assessment

An individual who has a chronic wound can suffer pain and discomfort that affects quality of life. Leg ulcers can take months or years to heal. Assessment enables you to identify the factors that lead to the ulcer developing and to work with medical staff to treat these factors. Doppler ultrasound enables you to determine the most effective way to treat the ulcer and enable it to heal.

Compression bandaging

Compression bandaging is now recommended in the treatment of venous ulcers. Compression reduces the superficial venous pressure, improves venous return, reduces oedema and relieves the feelings of aching and heaviness which affect individuals with venous ulceration[45]. Compression therapy should never be used without a thorough assessment to exclude arterial problems. The use of compression therapy in individuals who suffer from arterial problems can cause tissue damage that can lead to the development of gangrene. Community nurses have pioneered the use of Doppler ultrasound; increasingly nursing home staff are developing such skills and using compression bandaging appropriately.

It has been proved that the use of high compression bandaging dramatically improves healing in venous ulceration[46]. There are four different levels of compression therapy:

(1) Light compression is achieved by using crepe or short stretch compression bandages
(2) Moderate compression is achieved by the use of paste bandages and an outer bandage
(3) High compression is achieved by the use of compression bandages or compression stockings
(4) Extra high compression is achieved by the use of three or four layer bandaging techniques.

Bandages should be applied early in the morning, ideally before the individual is up and about as this is when oedema is least pronounced. Bandages should not be applied so tightly that they impair circulation.

Individuals suffering from venous ulcers should be encouraged to elevate their legs. Using a footstool is not normally sufficient; individuals should be encouraged to lie down on their bed and the legs can be elevated on several pillows so that the legs are higher than the heart. The pillows should be placed lengthwise to avoid calf pressure which could impede venous circulation. This elevation aids venous return and assists healing.

Treatment of ischaemic and mixed aetiology ulcers

The individual's doctor should be asked to refer them to a vascular clinic. Vascular specialists will carry out investigations and determine if it is possible to improve blood supply by the use of drugs or surgery. They may decide that surgical treatment of the wound is required. If this is not indicated they can provide advice on caring for ischaemic wounds and can monitor progress.

The nurse who wishes to provide the best possible care to individuals with wounds must become a 'wound detective'. The nurse has a duty to carry out a comprehensive assessment of the individual who has a wound. Assessment enables the nurse to identify problems that might not have been discovered otherwise. The role of nutrition is critical if wound healing is to occur, and assessment may identify that Mrs Davis has a poor diet because her dentures no longer fit and her mouth is sore. Few nurses would think of calling a dentist when a wound was failing to heal. Mrs Hill may suffer from marked postural oedema and no longer walks about because she cannot get her shoes on. The nurse can organise a referral to an orthotist who can supply shoes to accommodate oedema. Mrs Hill can be encouraged to walk around and walking will improve venous return and reduce oedema. The nurse should adopt a problem solving approach to wound care and should identify and rectify wherever possible the factors which contributed to the development of the wound. Nurse and resident can work together to identify problems and find solutions that enhance the older person's quality of life.

Preventing recurrence

Many nurses have seen wounds heal only to break down again weeks or months later. Recurrence of chronic wounds can cause individuals to become upset and depressed and nurses can become demoralised asking, 'Why? Was it my fault? Was it something I did? Or something I didn't do?'.

Using a holistic approach to wound management lessens the chance of wounds breaking down again. Individuals who have not benefited from a holistic approach to wound management are more prone to recurrence. The individual whose iron deficiency anaemia remains undetected and untreated is more at risk than the individual who has received treatment

The individual who has a poor diet lacking in nutrients is more at risk than the individual who is having a healthy diet. The immobile individual is more at risk of recurrence than the individual who has been encouraged and helped to regain mobility.

Compression hosiery

Two thirds of all people with leg ulceration have two or more episodes of ulceration and 21% have more than six episodes of ulceration. Compression hosiery plays a vital role in preventing recurrence[47]. Individuals with venous ulcers should wear support stockings or tights to aid venous return and prevent recurrence. Support stockings can be obtained by asking the doctor to refer the individual to the orthotist at the local hospital, the individual is then measured for stockings. There are three different types of compression stockings available, as shown in Table 6.3.

Many individuals are reluctant to wear compression stockings and only around half of people prescribed compression stockings actually wear them[48]. Women complain that the colours are awful and the stockings look

Table 6.3 Classes of compression stockings.

Class	Pressure applied	Recommended use
1	14–17 mmhg	Varicose veins and mild oedema
2	18–24 mmhg	Moderate to severe varicose veins and recurrent ulceration
3	25–35 mmhg	Gross varices, post phlebetic limb recurrent ulceration, lymphoedema

dreadful, but it is now possible to obtain compression stockings in a range of colours. It is important that you help ensure the person gets a colour she will be happy with, otherwise the stockings will not be worn and the risk of ulcer recurrence rises. Men usually object to wearing stockings, but thick black compression stockings that look like knee length socks are now available and most men find these acceptable if you refer to them as compression socks.

Two pairs of stockings are normally supplied. Laundered carefully each pair will last three to six months. Further supplies can be obtained on FP10 prescription from the local pharmacist. It is important to keep a record of the size, colour, level of compression and the measurements supplied by the orthotist as the pharmacist will require these.

Compression stockings do not survive normal nursing home laundering. They should be washed by hand in a mild detergent such as washing up liquid. Biological washing powders ruin the carefully selected colour and can irritate delicate newly-healed skin. On no account should elastic stockings be dried in the tumble dryer or put on a hot radiator as they will shrink. They can be dried on a washing line outside or in a warm room. Compression stockings can be difficult to get on. A little talcum powder applied to the leg can help. It is possible to get a special steel frame known as a medi-valet to help put stockings on. The stocking is stretched over the frame and the individual slides the foot into the stocking and pulls the frame up the leg, so applying the stocking.

Problem wounds

Some wounds fail to heal despite your best efforts.. You may lack the expertise to deal with some wounds such as fistulas and ulceration around stoma sites. You may not have access to Doppler ultrasound machinery or may lack the skills to perform ultrasound measurements. You have a duty to act within your sphere of competence. Admitting that you do not possess specialist skills to care for individuals who have problem wounds is a sign of strength not weakness. You should be aware of what help is available in your local area, who has the skills and knowledge to advise in certain cases, and how to gain access to that person.

Where to get further information and help

Some years ago there was confusion over whether homes should access hospital or community-based specialists. Now it is generally accepted that homes access community-based specialists. If there is not a community-based specialist then you will have to access the hospital-based specialist. You may need to consult the stoma care nurse if you are dealing with problem fistulae or ulceration around stoma sites. The diabetes nurse specialist and the tissue viablility nurse may also be invaluable if you need advice. Many health authorities also employ hospital and community-based wound care specialists.

You should find out how to contact these nurse specialists and should note their names and contact numbers. Do not hesitate to contact them; they will welcome enquiries from nurses keen to give the best possible research-based care. It is often possible for the nurse working in a nursing home to arrange to spend a day with the nurse specialist, learning about her work and gaining information and skills that can be applied on return to work. Nurse specialists often run or are involved in study days and national board courses. Getting to know your nurse specialists is a good way of ensuring that you are informed of any relevant study days or courses that you might wish to attend.

Conclusion

Wound care is more than a matter of dressing a wound. The health status of the whole person has contributed to the development of the wound. The nurse who assesses the individual with the wound can identify the factors that contributed to the development of the wound. The nurse can work with the individual, the individual's doctor, nurse specialists and other relevant professionals to help the individual to heal physically and mentally from the effects of the wound.

As nurses we have a duty to do the resident no harm. An awareness of the actions of wound cleansing agents and dressings enables the nurse to make informed choices and select appropriate cleansing agents and dressings. The use of compression bandaging is harmful in individuals with arterial disease and of benefit to individuals with venous ulcers. An ability to discover the causes of ulceration enables the nurse to provide appropriate care. The nurse has a duty to remain professionally up to date. Contact with clinical specialists and other professionals can prevent professional isolation and ensure that she is aware of relevant courses and study days.

Useful addresses and telephone numbers

Stoma care nurse

Wound care specialist nurse

Key points

- Venous problems cause 70% of all leg ulcers and the remainder are arterial, mixed, diabetic and rheumatoid in origin
- Nurses are normally responsible for treating venous leg ulcers
- Compression therapy is the most effective way to treat venous ulcers

- Medical staff are responsible for treating arterial ulcers although nurses have an important role to play in caring for people with arterial ulcers
- Doppler ultrasound investigations enable nurses to verify that it is safe to apply compression therapy. Compression therapy should not be applied if arterial disease is suspected.

Further reading

RCN Institute, University of York and School of Nursing Midwifery and Health Visiting University of Manchester (1998) *Clinical Practice Guidelines: The Management of Patients with Venous Leg Ulcers*. RCN Publishing, Harrow, Middlesex. Details available on the website: www.rcn.org.uk

SIGN guidelines (Scottish Intercollegiate Guidelines Network) – In 1993 Scotland developed a national initiative to produce and disseminate multidisciplinary guidelines. Over 40 SIGN guidelines have now been published. *The SIGN Guideline: The Care of Patients with a Chronic Leg Ulcer* was published in 1998. It is available on the SIGN website: www.sign.ac.uk

References

[1] Callan, M.J., Harper, D.R., Dale, J.J. & Rucklye, C.V. (1987) Chronic ulcer of the leg; clinical history. *British Medical Journal*, **294**, 1389–1391.

[2] Negus, D. & Friedgood, A. (1983) Effective management of venous ulceration. *British Journal of Surgery*, **70**, 623–627.

[3] Jones, P.L. & Milman, A. (1990) Wound healing and the aged patient. *Nursing Clinics of North America*, **25**, 263–267.

[4] Bryant, R. (1987) Wound repair; a review. *Journal of Enterostomal Therapy*, **14**, 262–266.

[5] Davis, N. *et al.* (2000) Detection and prevention of NSAID induced enteropathy. *Journal of Pharmacy and Pharmaceutical Science*, **3**(1), 137–155.

[6] Casey, G. (1998) Three steps to effective wound care. *Nursing Standard*, **12**(49), 49–54.

[7] Rosenburg, C.S. (1990) Wound healing in the resident with diabetes mellitus. *Nursing Clinics of North America*, **25**, 247–261.

[8] Krentz, A.J. (2000) *Churchill's Pocket Book of Diabetes*. Harcourt Publishers, London.

[9] Rosenburg, C.S. (1990) Wound healing in the resident with diabetes mellitus. *Nursing Clinics of North America*, **25**, 247–261.

[10] Jones, P.L., & Milman, A. (1990) Wound healing and the aged patient. *Nursing Clinics of North America* **25**, 263–267.

[11] Papantonia, C.T. (1988) Holistic approach to healing. (part 2) *Home Healthcare Nurse*, **6**(6), 31–35.

[12] McRorie, E.R. (2000) The assessment and management of leg ulcers in rheumatoid arthritis. *Journal of Wound Care*, **9**(6), 289–292.

[13] Browse, N. *et al.* (1998) *Diseases of the Veins: Pathology, Diagnosis and Treatment*. Edward Arnold, London.

[14] Torrance, C. (1983) *Pressure Sores Aetiology Treatment and Prevention*. Croom Helm, Beckenham.

[15] Lock, P.M. (1979) The effects of wound temperature on mitotic activity at the edge of experimental wounds. *Symposium on wound healing* (ed. N. Sundell) Espoo, Finland.

[16] Winter, G.D. (1962) Formation of a scab and the rate of epithilisation of superficial wounds in the skin of a young domestic pig. *Nature*, **193**, 293–294.

[17] Alvarez, O.M., Mertz, P.M., & Eaglestein, W.H. (1983) The effects of occlusive dressings on collagen synthesis and re-epithialisation in superficial wounds. *Journal of Surgical Research*, **35**, 142–148.

[18] Turner, T.D. (1985) Which dressing and why? In: *Wound Care* (Ed. S. Westby). Heinman Medical Books, London.

[19] Morgan, D. (1994) *Formulary of Wound Management Products*, 6th edn. Euromed Communications, Hazelmere.

[20] Turner, V. (1991) The standardisation of wound care. *Nursing Standard*, **5**(19), 25–28.

[21] United Kingdom Central Council (UKCC) (1992) The Code of Conduct, 3rd edition. UKCC, London.

[22] United Kingdom Central Council (UKCC) (1992) The Scope of Professional Practice. UKCC, London.

[23] United Kingdom Central Council (UKCC) (1996) Guidelines for Professional Practice. UKCC, London.

[24] Fowler, E. *et al.* (1991) Evaluation of an alginate dressing for pressure ulcers. *Decubitus*, **4**(3), 47–53.

[25] Williams, C. (1995) Cavi-Care. *British Journal of Nursing*, **4**(9), 526–528.

[26] Butterworth, R. *et al.* (1992) Comparing Allevyn cavity dressings and silastic foam. *Journal of Wound Care*, **11**, (1), 10–12.

[27] Gilchrist, B. & Reed, C. (1989) The bacteriology of of chronic venous ulcers treated with occlusive hydrocolloid dressings. *British Journal of Dermatology*, **121**, 337–344.

[28] Hutchinson, J.J. (1992) Influence of occlusive dressings on wound microbiology. In: *Proceedings of the 1st European conference on wound management* (eds Harding, K.G., Leaper, D.L. & Turner, T.D.) McMillan, London.

[29] Hutchinson, J.J. (1990) The rate of infection in occluded wounds. In: *International Forum on Wound Microbiology* (eds Alexander, J.W., Thompson, P.D. & Hutchinson, J.J.). Excerpta Medica, Princeton.

[30] Thomas, S. & Hay, N.P. (1996) In vitro investigations of a new hydrogel dressing. *Journal of Wound Care*, **5**(3), 130–131.

[31] Church, J.C. (1996) The traditional use of maggots in wound healing, and the development of larva therapy (biosurgery) in modern medicine. *J Altern Complement Med*, **2**(4), 525–527.

[32] Bunkis, J., Gherini, S. & Walton, R. (1985) Maggot therapy revisited. *West J Med*, **142**(4), 554–556.

[33] Thomas, S., Jones, M., Shutler, S. & Andrews, A. (1996) All you need to know about maggots. *Nursing Times*, **92**(46), 63–76.

[34] Weil, G.C., Simon, R.J. & Sweadner, W.R. (1993) A biological, bacteriological and clinical study of larval or maggot therapy in the treatment of acute and chronic pyogenic infections. *American Journal of Surgery*, **19**(1), 36–48.

[35] Dale, J.J., Callam, M.J., Ruckley, C.V., Harper, D.R. & Berry, P.N. (1983) Chronic ulcers of the leg; a study of prevalance in a Scottish community. *Health Bulletin*, **41**, 310–314.

[36] Dale, J. & Gibson, B. (1986) The epidemiology of leg ulcers. *Professional Nurse*, **1**(8), 215–216.

[37] Burnard, K.G. & Browse, N.L. (1982) The post phlebetic limb and venous ulceration. *Recent Advances in Surgery*. Churchill Livingstone, London.

[38] Callam, M.J., Ruckley, C.V., Dale, J.J. & Harper, D.R. (1987) Hazards of compression treatment of the leg; an estimate from Scottish surgeons. *British Medical Journal*, **295**, 1382.

39 Tuveri, M. *et al.* (2000) NCF a useful tool in the treatment of chronic vasculitic ulcers. *Lancet*, **356** (9234), 1739–1740.

40 Gibson, B. (1998) The nursing assessment of patients with leg ulcers. In: Cullum, N. & Roe, B. eds: *Leg Ulcers: Nursing Management*. Balliere Tindall, London.

41 Jones, J. (2000) The use of holistic assessment in the treatment of leg ulcers. *British Journal of Nursing*, **9**(16), 1040–1052.

42 RCN Institute, University of York and School of Nursing Midwifery and Health Visiting University of Manchester (1998) *Clinical Practice Guidelines: The Management of Patients with Venous Leg Ulcers*. RCN Publishing, Harrow, Middlesex.

43 Moffat, C.J. (1992) Compression Bandaging – state of the art. *Journal of Wound Care*, **1**(1), 45–50.

44 Dealy, C. (1999) *The Care of Wounds: A Guide for Nurses*, 2nd edn. Blackwell Science, Oxford.

45 Burnard, K.G. *et al.* (1988) How effective and long lasting are elastic stockings? In: *Phlebology* (eds D. Negus & G. Janter). John Libbey, London.

46 Moffatt, C.J., Franks, J.P., Oldroyd, M. & Bosanquet, N. *et al.* (1992) Community clinics for leg ulcers and impact on healing. *British Medical Journal*, **305**, 1389–1392.

47 Moffat, C.J. & O'Hare, L. (1995) Graduated compression hosiery for venous ulceration. *Journal Wound Care*, **4**(10), 459–462.

48 Sarafino, E.P. (1998) *Health, Psychology: Biopsychosocial interactions*, 3rd edn. John Riley and Sons, New York.

Chapter 7

Continence Promotion

Introduction

Urinary incontinence is a major problem in nursing homes. There is little research into the level of urinary incontinence within nursing and residential homes but social services and health authority entry criteria are so restrictive that only the most frail are eligible for admission to homes.

People admitted to homes are now more frail and dependent than ever before, yet it is still possible in many cases to enable the person to regain bladder control. When it is not possible to promote continence, assessment enables you to manage incontinence effectively and to avoid the complications of poorly managed incontinence.

This chapter is divided into five sections: continence and ageing, continence and disease, why incontinence occurs, continence assessment, and continence promotion programmes.

This chapter aims to enable you to:

- Understand how ageing offers the abillty to remain continent
- Understand how the person's abilities affect continence
- Understand how nursing practice affects continence
- Develop your skills in promoting continence

Continence and ageing

What is incontinence?

Incontinence has been defined as: 'A condition in which involuntary loss of urine is a social or hygienic problem and is objectively demonstrable'[1]. Incontinence is a common problem and affects large numbers of frail elderly people[2]. Traditional continence promotion strategies are often ineffective in this group. I believe that this is because continence strategies fail to recognise that older people are different.

Ageing affects every aspect of the mind and body. Ageing causes physiological changes to all body systems. Ageing also affects the person psychologically. Older people are more vulnerable to the effects of illness than younger people. Older people take longer to recover after illness. Sometimes it can be difficult to work out what changes are caused by old age and what changes are caused by illness. The age related changes we have to live with and work around. The changes caused by illness can often be treated but sometimes we have to work around those as well. Before we can decide what can be treated and what we have to work around, we need a basic working knowledge of the ageing urinary system. This section aims to enable you to understand how ageing affects the urinary system.

This section will explore:
- How ageing affects renal function
- How ageing affects uretic function
- How ageing affects the bladder
- How disease affects the ability to remain continent
- How medication affects continence

Why continence problems are more common in old age

Most nursing home residents are women and are in their eighties and nineties. Ageing leads to normal and pathological changes in the urinary system. Ageing diminishes the ability of the body to maintain homeostasis. An acute illness or the worsening of chronic disease can place a strain not only on the urinary system that may be unable to respond to the increased demands placed on it, but also on other previously unaffected systems. Diseases in older adults frequently display multi-system involvement. The urinary system plays an important part in maintaining health in old age. In older people, the urinary system normally functions adequately; however illness and injury can impair the already reduced homeostatic capacity of older adults. Basic knowledge of age-related changes assists in understanding potential problems and their implications.

The ageing urinary system

This section examines how ageing affects the kidney's ureters, bladder, prostate and urethra.

Function of the kidneys

The kidneys have four functions: to maintain fluid, pH and electrolyte balance; to excrete end products of metabolism and drugs; to secrete hormones; and to produce vitamin D. A quarter of cardiac output goes to the kidneys. The kidneys filter 170 litres of fluid a day. Water, salt, glucose, bicarbonate, amino acids and calcium are reabsorbed into the blood. Waste products are filtered out; these are hydrogen ions, ammonium salts, phosphates and potassium. Urea, uric acid and creatinine, the waste products of protein metabolism, are excreted in the urine. Many drugs are broken down and excreted by the kidneys.

How ageing affects the kidneys

The kidneys become smaller and lighter with age; the weight of the average kidney decreases from 250 grams to 200 grams between the ages of 20 and 80. The majority of cells lost are in the renal cortex, which contains the largest number of functioning glomeruli. It is estimated that the decrease in functioning glomeruli is between 30% and 50% in extreme old age. These changes do not normally cause problems in older adults unless diseases cause further stress. The surface area of the remaining glomeruli is reduced and there is thickening of the glomerular basement membrane. These structural changes affect the blood flow through the nephrons and decrease the ability to concentrate urine and to maintain pH balance.

Blood flow
In old age, the blood flow to the kidneys falls dramatically. The blood flow to the kidneys is affected by arteriosclerotic changes. Research has demonstrated that renal bloodflow decreases from 600 ml per minute at the age of 40 to 300 ml per minute at the age of 80. It has been suggested that this reduction is caused partly by decreased cardiac output and the decreased renal vascular bed.

Glomular filtration rates
Glomular filtration rates (GFR) have been shown to decline significantly with age. One study of healthy men living in the community demonstrated a decline of 30 50% in GFR in two thirds of the men studied, but a third showed no decline in GFR with age. The age related decline in GFR is of great significance to nurses caring for older adults. Many older adults are less able to excrete drugs normally excreted rapidly from younger kidneys that are more efficient. Older adults are more at risk of the toxic effects of many drugs such as digoxin, cimetidine and cephalosporins that are excreted from the kidney and are affected by changes in GFR. Illness can further lower GFR and can lead to elevated levels of phosphate, uric acid and potassium, and lower levels of bicarbonate.

Concentrating urine
The ability of the kidneys to concentrate urine declines with age. There are several theories to explain this. There is not thought to be any change in the levels of anti-diuretic hormone (ADH) produced in old age but it is thought that kidney response to ADH diminishes with age. Rennin activity is diminished with age and this leads to a reduction in aldosterone. This can lessen the kidney's ability to reabsorb sodium, potassium and water in the distal tubule. Because of these changes older adults are more at risk of electrolyte imbalance. This risk can be increased by the use of diuretic therapy that is currently widespread among the elderly population. The use of potassium sparing diuretics and of potassium supplementation with diuretics such as frusemide is not without its hazards. One study found that 73% of cases of hyponatraemia in elderly people were caused by diuretic therapy. Older adults are less able to dispose of large fluid loads and run the risk of cardiac failure resulting from increased blood volume if too much fluid is given too rapidly. Intravenous fluids must be given with particular care because of this risk.

How ageing affects bladder function
Ageing decreases bladder capacity, makes the bladder less sensitive, and leads to an increase in the amount of residual urine. When we empty our

bladders a small amount of urine is left in the bladder. This is known as the residual urine. The amount of residual urine rises with old age. This reduces the working capacity of the bladder. The bladder muscle – the detrusor – is smooth muscle that expands and contracts in all directions. The detrusor is primarily under parasympathetic control. Parasympathetic stimulation releases acetylcholine causing detrusor contraction and assisting bladder emptying. Sympathetic control is via the beta-adrenergic receptors that are situated in the body and fundus of the detrusor. Stimulation of these receptors assists in bladder relaxation and filling. The main age related bladder changes are all intrinsically linked. The afferent sensors in the bladder become less sensitive with age. Older adults are not aware of the desire to void until their bladders are 90% full; younger adults are aware of the desire to void when their bladders are 50% full. This means that older people have less time to find a toilet and when combined with disabilities that impair mobility this can lead to incontinence. There is a reduction in the contractability of the bladder muscle; it no longer stretches and contracts as efficiently as before, the amount of fibrotic tissue in the bladder increases and this further decreases bladder capacity.

How ageing affects the urethra

There are also age related changes to the urethra that can affect an older adult's ability to maintain continence. The female urethra may become de-oestrogenated with age and this can lead to decreased urethral closing pressures and in some cases to stress incontinence. It must be emphasised that many women are able to produce sufficient oestrogen to maintain adequate urethral closing pressures throughout their lives. Lack of oestrogen can cause stress incontinence.

How ageing affects the prostate

Older men have larger prostate glands than younger men do, as the prostate gland enlarges with age. This change is not pathological in many men but if prostatic growth is into the bladder neck (this is common in prostatic malignancy) this can lead to decreased sphincter control. Benign prostatic enlargement can lead to an increased amount of residual urine because of urethral obstruction. This residual urine, if in excess of 350 ml, can cause back-flow to the kidneys, renal damage and infection. Older men are much more at risk of urinary tract infections because as they age the prostate produces less prostatic bactericide that prevents urinary infections.

Summary of age-related changes

Ageing affects every aspect of the urinary system. The age-related changes outlined above make it more difficult for older adults to maintain continence. For many older people maintaining continence is like walking a tightrope; the smallest of physiological or psychological changes can send the person crashing down into incontinence. Age related changes can be summarised as:

- The kidneys become less efficient at concentrating urine, metabolising drugs and maintaining pH balance

- Bladder capacity is reduced, and bladder sensitivity is reduced so 'warning time' is lessened.
- Urethral changes caused by age related reduction of collagen and oestrogen leads to decreased closing pressures
- Prostatic enlargement can lead to increased residual urine, lower working bladder capacity and increased risks of infection.

Compensating for age-related changes

The role of the nurse is to protect residents from harm. The onset of urinary incontinence can have a devastating effect on the lives of older adults. Urinary incontinence or the fear of urinary incontinence can lead an individual to become worried about odour or fear loss of control in the presence of family or friends. In many cases, older people withdraw from company because of this fear. The majority of individuals acquire bladder control in early childhood and its acquisition is one of our first rites of passage – the transition from babyhood to childhood. We learn to become clean and dry and in control of our body functions and we are praised for being 'good and clean'.

The loss of control over such a basic function as bladder control is a taboo subject among adults. Urinary incontinence is still regarded as a shameful, dirty, sordid little secret[3]. Individuals who suffer from urinary incontinence often cut back on fluid intake; this can predispose to infection, electrolyte imbalance, macerated skin and even sores[4]. Older adults can withdraw completely from friends and family and become depressed and less mobile than before. Immobility, isolation and depression can lead to self-neglect, illness, infection, falls and hospital admission[5]. Hospital admission can cause anxiety and fear that can lead an older person to disregard bladder signals until they become urgent. Hospitals can be busy and understaffed, an older person's request for assistance to the toilet may not be answered immediately, and urinary incontinence can result. Research from the US indicates that continence status plays a major part in the decision to suggest nursing home care to older adults. Older adults do not want to end up wet and smelly. Good nursing, the best of nursing, recognises that older people find it more difficult to remain continent. Recognising how age-related changes affect continence enables nurses to protect residents and promote continence.

Compensating for renal changes
Renal capacity is reduced in extreme old age. If we treat older adults in the same way as younger adults, we can inadvertently contribute to continence problems. Table 7.1 outlines how nursing action can compensate for renal problems.

Compensating for bladder changes
The bladder becomes less efficient with age. Compensating for those changes enables older adults to retain or regain continence. Table 7.2 outlines bladder changes and nursing action.

Table 7.1   Compensating for the ageing renal system.

Change and consequences	Nursing action
Increased amount of urine produced	Aware that older person needs to use toilet more often
Reduced ability to concentrate urine, increased risk of dehydration	Provide extra fluids when it is hot to reduce risk of dehydration
Reduced ability to concentrate urine at night as ADH less effective	Aware that it is normal to get up to the toilet twice in an eight-hour night when you are 85, and provide appropriate support
Reduced ability to concentrate urine, diuretics hazardous and can cause hyponatraemia	Review diuretics. Ensure diuretics reduced to smallest possible dose. Titrate diuretics. Be vigilant to risks of hyponatraemia
Reduced ability to clear drugs from the system. At risk of adverse effects of medication especially digoxin, cimetidine and cephalosporins	Avoid the risks of polypharmacy[6]. Ensure that only essential medicines are prescribed. Ensure dosage takes account of reduced ability to metabolise drugs because of declining renal function. Monitor individuals for adverse effects of medication

Table 7.2   Compensating for the ageing bladder.

Change and consequence	Nursing action
Bladder becomes fibrotic and stiff. Bladder capacity is reduced	Recognise that older adults need to pass smaller amounts of urine more often
Residual urine increases. Working capacity of the bladder is reduced	Recognise that older people may need to go more frequently
Residual urine increases. The reservoir of stale urine provides breeding ground for bacteria. Risk of infection increases	Encourage fluids. Reinforce good hygiene, such as wiping front to back. Ensure infection treated. Recommend cranberry juice, 200 ml BD if recurring infection a problem[7,8]
Bladder less sensitive. There is less warning of the need to void	Responds to requests for the toilet promptly

Summary

Older people have greater difficulty in maintaining continence because ageing affects the urinary system and reduces its efficiency. Nurses can compensate for many of these age related changes and enable the older person to remain continent.

Older people can find it difficult to maintain continence because of physical changes. The next section will examine how illness can lead to incontinence.

Continence and disease

Maintaining continence is for many older people like walking a tightrope. The urinary system in older people is more finely balanced than in younger people. Homeostasis is maintenance of a stable physiological state by autoregulatory processes of the body. Age related changes affect every body system. These changes affect the older person's ability to maintain homeostasis. Illness places an additional strain on the older person's body and can easily lead the person tumbling into incontinence. This section aims to enable you to understand how disease affects continence and how to promote continence in spite of the disease.

This section will explore:

- How to maintain continence
- How illness affects the ability to remain continent
- How stroke affects continence
- How dementia affects continence
- How Parkinson's disease affects continence
- How osteoporosis affects continence

Maintaining continence

The bladder fills while the detrusor muscle is relaxed and the urethra is closed. When the detrusor is relaxed, parasympathetic action is inhibited. Urethral closure occurs because of pudental nerve control and an increase in alpha-adrenergic tone. When the bladder is partially full (the degree is age related) the afferent sensors in the detrusor alert the area of the brain that deals with micturition (this is probably located in the pons) and it informs us that our bladder is filling up. We are not normally aware of any sensation of bladder fullness until the bladder contains about 300 ml of urine. The micturition centre in the frontal lobe allows us to inhibit micturition; the bladder muscle relaxes and capacity is increased. Micturition is delayed until a socially acceptable place is located and the individual is ready to void. When it is convenient the cortical centre inhibits the sympathetic system and stimulates the parasympathetic. The detrusor contracts the pudental nerve and relaxes the urethra, and urine is released. Continence is thus dependent on a complex system of hormonal, muscular and neurological controls. The causes of incontinence are equally complex. There is no one single cause of incontinence and continence cannot be viewed in isolation from other aspects of physical and mental well-being.

The effect of illness on continence

Illness can cause incontinence for four reasons:

(1)   Physiological changes caused by the illness
(2)   Neurophysiological changes affecting bladder function
(3)   Factors relating to medical and nursing care and hospitalisation
(4)   The effects of medication given to treat the illness.

Research indicates that many people who suffer from neurological diseases such as multiple sclerosis, stroke and dementia become incontinent not because of the effect of the disease on their neurological system but because they become immobile and lose the ability to use the toilet unaided. The ability to move around unaided or with limited help improves morale, appetite and bowel and bladder function[9].

Stroke and continence

Strokes can cause loss of function, loss of mobility, loss of communication skills, loss of cognitive function and loss of bladder control. Individuals who develop bladder and bowel problems after stroke are usually the people who have been most disabled by stroke[10]. The person is often admitted catheterised. Many nurses, and even continence advisers, think it is futile to consider continence promotion strategies with such individuals. Fortunately they are mistaken; skilled nursing care can enable many people to regain continence after stroke.

Why people develop continence problems after stroke

Most people are incontinent immediately after a stroke[11]; within eight weeks most have spontaneously regained continence[12]. However, people who suffer severe strokes tend to have ongoing continence problems. Three factors affect continence after strokes:

- Physiological changes caused by the stroke
- Neurophysiological changes affecting bladder function after stroke
- Factors relating to medical and nursing care and hospitalisation.

Physiological changes – Physiological changes range from the mild to the severe. Short-term memory can be affected. Communication difficulties can include difficulty understanding speech (receptive dysphasia) and problems with speaking (dysphasia and dysarthria). Some individuals lose complete function on one side of the body (hemiplegia); others experience weakness (hemiparesis). Vision is often impaired and visual fields are affected. The individual may lose the ability to move unaided, read or communicate needs. These changes can often lead to depression and feelings of despair.

Neurophysiological changes – Normally bladder control is maintained by the parasympathetic system. We are unaware of any sensation of bladder fullness until the bladder contains around 300 ml of urine. Then we can postpone the need to void until it is convenient. The micturition centre in the brain stem informs us that our bladder is filling up. The micturition centre in the frontal lobe allows us to inhibit urination. The bladder muscle relaxes and capacity is increased. The urethra remains tightly closed preventing leakage. The autonomic nervous system and both micturition centres must function properly, otherwise we will be unable to maintain continence. Stroke can directly or indirectly affect either the frontal or brain stem micturition centres, coming them to malfunction. The level of damage sustained is related to the severity of the stroke. Damage to the frontal lobe causes urge incontinence. Parietal and basal ganglia lesions cause bladder dyssynergia[13].

Contributing factors – Medication can cause incontinence[14]. How medication affects continence is discussed later in this chapter. Insufficient toilets or commodes, and lack of privacy can also lead to incontinence. In the first days or weeks after stroke individuals have little warning of the need to pass urine. It is vitally important that nurses respond promptly to their calls for assistance when the toilet is required. Unfortunately, the individual may have difficulty communicating this to nursing staff. Hospitals and homes are busy places and it may not always be possible to respond immediately. As a result incontinence can occur.

Helping people regain continence following a stroke

Awareness of the effects of stroke can enable nurses to plan holistic care that enables the stroke resident to regain abilities.

Catheterisation should be avoided unless the individual is in urinary retention. Most people will regain continence naturally as they recover from stroke – this is not possible if there is a catheter in place. Catheterisation inevitably leads to infection. Infection normally persists for some time after the catheter is removed. Urinary tract infection can cause urinary incontinence[15]. Over three-quarters of people catheterised for three months or more develop inflammatory bladder changes. Catheterisation also makes it more difficult for individuals to regain continence because it rapidly leads to a reduction in bladder capacity[16]. If there are indications for catheterisation, using a catheter valve to drain the bladder at regular intervals may prevent bladder contraction. There is little research evidence on the use of catheter valves. When the catheter is removed, the stroke resident usually has not only to regain bladder control but also to contend with the effects of infection, inflammatory bladder changes, and a reduced bladder capacity.

Fluid intake requires careful monitoring. Fluid deficits of 10% can cause serious illness. The average person requires 1.5 litres of fluid daily. Fluid requirements rise during illness to two or three litres. An intake of three litres daily prevents urinary tract infection.

When Burns conducted a study on a small group of elderly catheterised women, their mean fluid intake was less than 500 ml[17]. So monitor intake carefully – it could be lower than you think.

Communication is vital if we are to meet physical and psychological needs. Be creative. Use cards with large pictures and words. Individuals can waste vital minutes searching for the right sign to indicate that the toilet is required. Making up a special toilet card with a picture and the word toilet on a sheet of brightly coloured paper or card can save time and prevent accidents. The person can wait a few moments for tea but not for the toilet!

Watch your language. We all speak too quickly and our sentences are too long for many people with communication problems to follow. Try to use five word sentences. Bring up one idea at a time. Offer one choice. Be patient – wait for the person to answer. Enabling the person to communicate with you makes an enormous difference to morale. The person can again develop some control over his or her life.

Mobility – Immobility is common after stroke. Immobility increases the risk of urinary tract infection – and the risk of incontinence. The ability to walk unaided is the most important factor in regaining continence. It is vital that nurses work with the individual and other professionals to enable the person to regain mobility as soon as possible after stroke. The ability to move around unaided or with limited help improves morale, appetite and bowel and bladder function[18]. Mobilisation, elevation of the feet when sitting out and the use of support stockings can virtually eliminate the use of diuretics to control limb oedema after stroke.

Bowel problems after stroke

Bowel care receives less attention than it used to. The bowel book has been consigned to the nursing history books. Bowel care though is very important. Constipation and faecal impaction can cause or worsen existing urge incontinence. Nursing measures to enable the person to maintain or re-establish normal bowel patterns can virtually eliminate the use of laxatives and enemata[19]. Constipation is the most common bowel problem after stroke, although some people develop faecal incontinence.

Many stroke patients suffer from constipation; normally a laxative is prescribed. Millions of pounds are spent each year on laxative prescriptions. Constipation and laxative use are highest in older adults; 79% of those in hospitals, 59% in nursing homes, and 38% living at home are prescribed laxatives regularly[20]. Constipation is *not* a disease, it is a symptom. Every time a laxative is prescribed without investigating the causes of constipation, a health promotion opportunity is lost and the cycle of laxative misuse perpetuated.

Ageing does not lead to constipation. A healthy 85-year-old is no more likely to be constipated than a healthy 20-year-old is[21]. Older people are more likely to suffer from ill health than younger people are. Illness, limited mobility, medication and other factors associated with illness can increase the risk of constipation. Offering holistic research-based care can often effectively prevent constipation and promote good health without using laxatives or enemas.

Specialist treatment

Individuals who have not regained continence within eight weeks of stroke should be investigated. Investigation need not be intrusive or distressing to the individual. Careful history taking and basic investigations can be carried out by appropriately experienced and qualified nursing staff. Most individuals will suffer from urge incontinence. In many instances, this can be treated without medication. Some individuals do require drug therapy and must be referred to a medical practitioner. My own experience is that almost three-quarters can be enabled to regain continence within six weeks. Cognitively impaired individuals and those with severe strokes are less likely to respond to treatment. However, two-thirds of such individuals can remain dry using individual prompted voiding schedules.

Key points

- 80% of people develop bladder problems after stroke
- If left uncatheterised most people will regain bladder control
- Urinary incontinence is a symptom, not a disease

- The usual causes of urinary incontinence post stroke are urge incontinence and bladder dyssynergia
- Skilled nursing care can enable many people to regain continence following stroke
- Bowel problems are common in the most disabled stroke survivors
- Constipation is the most common bowel problem following stroke
- Bowel management programmes enable you to discover the causes of bowel problems and develop treatment plans.

Dementia and continence

Research indicates that 25% of people over the age of 85 suffer from dementia. Dementia is defined as: 'A global impairment of cognitive function that is usually progressive and that interferes with normal social and occupational activities.' Dementia is a global term used to describe a group of diseases that affect the brain. It describes a syndrome or group of symptoms. These have been defined as intellectual losses, personality losses, planning losses and lowered stress threshold.

Intellectual losses lead to loss of memory, initially for recent events. Sense of time is lost and the individual becomes unable to make choices or to problem solve. Judgement is affected and the individual loses the ability to express his or her thoughts. The individual develops profound difficulties in processing information, language abilities decline, and they have difficulty expressing themself and understanding others. Intellectual losses may make it difficult for the individual to find their way around the home independently. They may have difficulty in recognising their room and may go into other residents' rooms. They may go into the kitchen or leave the taps on and cause a flood.

Personality losses lead to a decreased attention span and the individual with Algheimer's type dementia (ATD) is easily distracted. Inhibitions are reduced. The individual may take off clothing in public. Emotional liability becomes more marked as the dementia progresses. The individual loses the ability to be tactful and may lose the ability to control temper and delay gratification – wants it now! The individual withdraws socially – mixes and converses less and becomes increasingly preoccupied with self and uninterested in others. They avoid overwhelming or complex stimuli, and develop antisocial behaviour, confabulation and perseveration (recurrent thoughts, ideas, or actions).

Planning losses lead to an individual with ATD initially losing the ability to plan their day. They become unable to carry out activities which require thought to set goals, organise, and complete a task, and develop functional losses starting with tasks such as handling money, shopping, etc. As the disease progresses the ability to plan and carry out activities of daily living are lost, usually in the following order:

- Increased fatigue on exertion or mental exertion, loss of energy reserve
- Frustration, refusal to participate, or expression of helplessness

- Bathing, grooming, choosing clothing
- Dressing, walking, using the toilet
- Communicating
- Eating independently.

It is important to note that worry about ability tends to worsen performance. *Progressively lowered stress threshold*, which is characteristic of individuals with ATD, can lead to catastrophic behaviours, confused or agitated night waking, purposeful wandering, violent, agitated or anxious behaviour, withdrawal and belligerence, noisy behaviour, purposeless behaviour, compulsive repetitive behaviour and other socially unacceptable behaviours. This can lead to individuals becoming unwilling to get up, bathe, dress, use the toilet, and becoming agitated if the carer insists. These symptoms worsen if the ATD sufferer becomes very tired or becomes anxious.

Promoting continence in people with dementia

Traditionally doctors considered that people with dementia developed continence problems because of detrusor instability. Treatment has focused on drug treatment to control detrusor instability and toileting. These approaches have had limited success[22]. This is discussed later in the chapter. When promoting continence in people with dementia we need to develop an individualised problem-solving approach. This often compensates for the difficulties the person faces and enables the person to retain continence for longer.

Osteoporosis

Advanced osteoporosis is endemic in elderly Caucasian women living in advanced industrialised societies. It is now, for the first time, being seen in elderly Afro-Caribbean women who were born and brought up in advanced industrialised societies[23]. Osteoporosis leads to weakening of the structure of the bones. The spine can crumble and vertebral collapse can lead to differing continence problems. Osteoporosis can also impair mobility. The person with osteoporosis can develop urinary retention, overflow incontinence, or urgency. Continence promotion strategies must be tailored to the individual[24]. Improving mobility, treating pain and preventing constipation are important aspects of continence promotion.

Parkinson's disease

Parkinson's disease can affect the micturition centre in brain stem. Impulses from the bladder are relayed via the spinal cord to the micturition centre when the bladder is full. Parkinson's disease disrupts this pathway so the person with Parkinson's may be unaware that the bladder is full until it is too late. Drugs prescribed to treat Parkinson's disease increase bladder tone and reduce bladder contractions. This can cause urinary retention[25]. People with Parkinson's disease are vulnerable to continence problems because of the disease and because of the treatment.

There are three stages of Parkinson's disease:

(1) Early Parkinson's
(2) Fluctuating Parkinson's
(3) Non-fluctuating Parkinson's[26].

Continence promotion strategies vary according to the stage of the disease and individual factors. In the first two stages, prompted voiding may enable the person to remain continent. In the third stage, nurses must work with doctors to balance medication to alleviate symptoms with strategies to enable voiding to take place.

Summary

Illness affects the older person's ability to remain continent. Illness can directly affect the urinary tract or the neurological mechanisms that enable us to remain continent. Illness can indirectly affect continence by preventing the person responding to the needs of the bladder. Medication prescribed to treat illness can cause incontinence.

Conclusion

Maintaining continence is a complex function. Older people have greater difficulty maintaining continence because of age. Illness puts an additional burden on older people and can cause continence problems to develop. In the next section we will explore the reasons why some people develop continence problems in old age or because of illness, while others do not.

Why incontinence occurs

If we are to promote continence, we need to know why it occurs. We need to have the answers in order to find the solutions. Doctors seek the answers in the urinary tract. Nurses seek the answers in the toilet. Many factors can lead to a person developing incontinence. This section aims to examine some of the often-overlooked reasons that incontinence occurs.

Prevalence of urinary incontinence in nursing homes

The incidence of urinary incontinence rises with age. Unfortunately, little research into continence has been carried out in UK nursing homes. We do know that the average nursing home resident is female and in her mid eighties. However, to find out more about nursing home residents with continence problems we have to examine research from other countries. Urinary incontinence is more common in elderly women than in men. Hellstrom's study[27] found that 83% of 85-year-old nursing home residents suffered from urinary incontinence. Ouslander's study of urinary incontinence indicated urinary incontinence rates of 50% but excluded catheterised patients. American research suggests that nurses working in nursing homes tend to accept urinary incontinence as 'normal'. Palmer[28] discovered that despite high rates of urinary incontinence, fewer than 3% of nurses had identified urinary incontinence as a problem on care plans. Researchers have identified urinary incontinence as a major problem within nursing homes.

Medical research

Many researchers in other countries have studied the incidence of urinary incontinence among nursing home residents. Medical researchers tend to focus on finding 'the cause' of urinary incontinence. Often medical researchers have looked to the urinary tract for answers. They have looked for abnormalities that can be treated. Traditionally doctors considered that the cause of urinary incontinence in most nursing home residents was detrusor instability. Now attitudes are slowly changing and medical researchers are, at last, beginning to realise that promoting continence in the frail elderly is more than simply a matter of medical treatment. One study of 133 incontinent nursing home residents with an average age of 86 found that[29]:

- 88% had dementia
- 41% had normal bladder function
- 38% had detrusor instability (unstable bladder)
- 16% had stress incontinence
- 5% had overflow incontinence.

The researchers concluded that incontinence was not solely related to detrusor instability (DI). Another research study found that 64% of incontinent nursing home residents with dementia had DI but 47% of lucid continent residents had the same problem! They stated: 'It is no longer tenable to assume the incontinence in residents with dementia is due merely to detrusor hyper-reflexia.'

Nursing research

Nursing research tends to concentrate on toileting. The implication is that if only nursing home nurses could be bothered to organise toileting schedules continence problems would be greatly reduced.

One US trial involved changing the prompted voiding schedules on 41 nursing home residents with dementia. The rate of urinary incontinence fell by 22% during the trial[30]. Another US trial demonstrated a reduction of 26%[31]. Another US trial using a combination of toileting and medication to treat DI led to a reduction of 26% in incontinence rates. However, numerous researchers have complained bitterly that the nurses fail to maintain these improvements. Why?

One thing the researchers fail to make clear is that it is impossible to introduce a continence promotion programme and treat 34 or 41 people all at once, unless you bring in extra staff – and that is what the researchers do. Most of the funding on these research programmes is spent on employing toileting assistants. The research assistants toilet the residents – sometimes hourly – to achieve these dramatic results. What sort of life is it when you have to use the toilet hourly? Is it worth it? When the researchers and their assistants depart, nursing homes revert to their normal staffing patterns. Most US nursing homes are so poorly staffed that it is impossible to offer adequate care. Minimum US staffing levels stipulate one registered nurse on duty for eight hours each day. Licensed practical nurses (LPNs) with one

year's training provide 24 hour cover. Care assistants, with minimal training, provide the bulk of care. Care assistant to resident ratios vary from 1:12
to 1:18 on day shifts[32].

UK nursing homes have better staffing levels and skill mixes than those in
the US. However, dependency is rising in UK nursing homes and many do
not have sufficient staff in relation to dependency. If we are to promote
continence, we need to be able to do it within our existing staffing levels. Can
it be done? Can residents be helped to regain continence? Palmer's study[33]
indicates that individuals who are incontinent two weeks after admission will
remain incontinent. However, my own work indicates that a holistic
approach can enable individuals with established incontinence to regain
bladder control[34].

Why do nursing home residents have continence problems?

As we have seen, much of the research on urinary incontinence has been
carried out by medical staff. It concentrates on the rates of urinary incontinence and on medical diagnosis. The findings are often inconsistent because
medical staff fail to take a holistic view of urinary incontinence. They seek to
find medical causes that can be treated. Continence is a complex skill
dependent on hormonal, muscular and neurological control. It involves an
elaborate interplay between the individual and the environment. As nurses,
we are all too aware that for many older adults maintaining continence is like
walking a tightrope. The smallest change can set the individual tumbling into
incontinence and a host of other problems. Promoting continence in older
adults suffering from the effects of acute and long-standing illness and who are
physically or mentally impaired, is a *specialised skill*. It is a skill that
experienced nursing home nurses can acquire.

Holistic continence care

The most effective way of promoting continence is to use a holistic
approach. It is very difficult to teach nurses how to use a holistic approach
because it is so individual. I have developed what academics would term a
conceptual model, which is simply a summary of the factors involved in
maintaining or restoring continence (Box 7.1).

Functional abilities

Individuals who are immobile depend on staff to take them to the toilet.
Hospital and nursing home admission can cause anxiety and fear that can
lead an older person to disregard bladder signals until they become urgent.
Hospitals and nursing homes can be busy and understaffed. An older person's request for assistance to the toilet may not be answered immediately
and urinary incontinence can result. If staff do not help immobile individuals
use the toilet, they become incontinent. Schnelle[35] found that staff did not
take immobile individuals to the toilet frequently enough.

Impaired mobility has serious psychological and physical consequences.
Impaired mobility is associated with increased risk of bowel dysfunction,
including constipation. Bowel dysfunction increases the risk of urinary tract

Box 7.1   Factors affecting continence in older adults (a conceptual model)

Urinary incontinence in older adults living in nursing homes is a result of factors relating to the individual and factors relating to the environment. Factors relating to the individual are:

- Functional abilities of the individual
- Degree of mental impairment
- Psychological state
- Existing disease
- Medication

Factors relating to the environment are:

- The abilities of other residents
- The design of the home
- The quality of nursing care
- The attitude of the nursing home manager
- The quality of medical care
- The involvement of staff trained in continence promotion.

infection and urge incontinence. The ability to use the toilet unaided is of great importance if individuals are to regain and retain continence. A study carried out in a US nursing home found that mobile individuals were less likely than immobile individuals to suffer continence problems *regardless of cognitive impairment*. Hoists were used in the study to enable staff to toilet immobile residents – it took on average 18 minutes to toilet each individual. No details of any attempts to improve mobility are given in the study. Another study found that individuals who retained the ability to dress (even partially) and transfer were more likely to retain continence. In this study researchers found that dementia doubled the risk of incontinence but losing the ability to transfer and dress increased the risk of incontinence 13 times.

It is so easy through our practice to disable older adults in nursing homes and reduce their mobility. Enabling individuals to regain mobility enhances quality of life and reduces nursing workload to manageable levels. This enables nursing staff to toilet the individuals who remain immobile.

Factors relating to the environment

Older adults often model the activity levels and status of other residents[36]. This desire to 'fit in' and be accepted is part of being human. As children, we want to wear similar clothes to our friends; as young adults we wear the same clothes and have the same hairstyles as our friends. We dress and act differently in different situations; our roles may include child, parent, employee, employer, student and teacher. In homes where most people are wheelchair bound, many individuals who can walk ask for wheelchairs. In homes where incontinence levels are high, people who are admitted continent rapidly become incontinent. In nursing homes with high levels of urinary incontinence, it is all too easy for urinary incontinence to be viewed, by staff and residents, as 'normal'. Every chair is plastic. Every bed is protected; pads are put on 'just in case' and the message is that incontinence is expected. Such environments actively promote incontinence.

The design of the home

Many nursing homes are converted buildings. If there are insufficient toilets, it is more difficult to maintain continence. Nursing home residents are now more disabled than before. Toilets should be large enough for disabled individuals and nursing staff to enter. Ensuring that toilets are designed to enable individuals to use them independently whenever possible is essential. Homes with long corridors and lots of confusing, poorly marked doors make it difficult for the person to find her way around and can encourage inappropriate urination – such as urinating in waste bins and showers. Some ways that you can enable people to identify and use toilets are:

- Paint toilet doors a certain colour. Residents can easily identify the toilet in a corridor if all toilet doors are bright red or yellow. People with severe visual problems see red and yellow most easily.
- Use pictures of toilets to enable residents who are no longer able to read to identify toilets
- Use tape or cut out footprints to lead people to toilets
- Use black or red toilet seats to enable people to see the toilet more easily
- Remove or hide clutter in cupboards if the person is easily distracted
- If the person is urinating in the waste bin in the room consider replacing it with a chamber pot.

The quality of nursing care

The quality of nursing care is affected by a number of factors. These include the number of registered nurses employed, their educational level and their attitudes to continence promotion. Nursing home residents who suffer from urinary incontinence are likely to be the most disabled, the least mobile and the most cognitively impaired residents in the nursing home. Incontinent nursing home residents will place much greater demands on nursing staff than continent residents will. In many UK nursing homes the rate of urinary incontinence is more than 75% and affects staff workload and morale.

Nursing staff faced with such overwhelming needs from residents feel powerless and as though they are on a treadmill of constantly washing and changing residents. Staff feel guilty and stressed in such situations and react by providing functional care, washing and changing the resident but failing to seek nursing or medical treatment for the incontinence. Nursing staff caring for incontinent residents can feel overwhelmed by the futility of endlessly changing the same residents. Many nursing home nurses, like their colleagues working in hospitals, are not aware of the causes, investigations and treatments available to help older people suffering from continence problems. Introducing continence promotion strategies can enable nurses to take control. Quality of care is enhanced and workload reduced.

The nurse manager

The manager's attitude is of crucial importance. A 'hands on' manager with up-to-date clinical skills, good knowledge and a positive attitude to continence promotion can reduce the rate of urinary incontinence and increase the morale of staff and residents.

The quality of medical care

If individuals are to retain the highest possible level of function and enjoy quality of life, medical care must be of the highest quality. If medical care is poor, it is all too easy to ignore treatable conditions. In the 1930s, the pioneering work of Marjorie Warren demonstrated how medical care could enhance the lives of older adults. Reports from across the UK indicate that many GPs do not regularly review medications or examine individuals to diagnose treatable physical illness. There are three possible solutions to this problem: providing geriatrician input, encouraging GPs to gain specialist skills in gerontology or developing the role of the specialist gerontological nurse.

Continence advisers

In 1993 I carried out a research project and sent questionnaires to every UK continence adviser. Then few continence advisers offered continence promotion services to older people living in nursing homes. Continence advisers had an extremely heavy workload. Some lacked the time or resources to offer a service to nursing homes. Some continence advisers considered the frail elderly 'untreatable', although thankfully their numbers are diminishing. Continence advisers reported that nursing home staff seldom consulted them. Research carried out in Leicester nursing and residential homes found that staff received poor levels of support, although 39% of residents had severe but treatable problems. The researchers called for urgent action to support nursing home nurses in their efforts to promote continence and manage incontinence[37]. In the last year, a number of continence advisers have been appointed specifically to promote continence in nursing and residential homes. This is in line with government guidance[38].

Drugs and their effect on continence

Medication can have a profound effect on continence. It is policy on some elderly care units for doctors to discontinue all medication, monitor resident condition carefully, and prescribe only when absolutely necessary. Some nursing home residents do not benefit from a radical review of medication but merely have each doctor caring for them treat problems symptomatically by prescribing more medication. Drugs prescribed to cure one problem can lead to another problem – urinary incontinence.

How medication can cause urinary incontinence

Diuretics are often prescribed. One study showed that 48% of patients were prescribed diuretics, often for swollen ankles. Diuretic therapy can lead to urgency, frequency and urinary incontinence. Postural oedema can be treated by encouraging exercise (wherever possible), elevation of legs and the use of support stockings and tights. Diuretic therapy can, because of the fear of incontinence, cause older people to become less mobile. If diuretic therapy is required, it is important to work with doctors and pharmacists to ensure that diuretics prescribed have a minimal effect on continence. If diuretics are interfering with a person's ability to maintain continence, ask the doctor if the person can be prescribed diuretics that work gently throughout the day, such as Moduretic, rather than those that act by producing a rapid diuresis, such as Frumil.

Hypnotics use is widespread; research indicates that 33–45% of patients regularly receive night sedation. Hypnotics decrease the level of awareness and increase the risk of nocturia, reduced ability to metabolise drugs rapidly can prolong drug half-lives, and the older person may be less alert during the day, increasing the risk of incontinence. Measures such as increasing exercise and occupational therapy, providing milky drinks at bedtime and having realistic expectations about how much sleep an adult requires, would reduce reliance on hypnotics and improve continence for many older adults.

Psychotropic drugs are prescribed to 35–45% of nursing home residents. These can cause urinary retention with overflow. They can also reduce alertness and this can lead to incontinence. It is important to minimise the use of psychotropic drugs, giving them only when clinically indicated, in the smallest possible dose and for the shortest possible time. You will need to work with the resident's GP and other clinicians to ensure that this happens.

Muscle relaxants such as dantrolene and baclofen are frequently prescribed to treat spasticity following strokes. They frequently relax the urethral sphincter and lead to urinary incontinence. Exercise and passive movements can often effectively treat spasticity without adverse effects on continence; unfortunately muscle relaxants are more readily available than community physiotherapists.

Antihypertensives can affect continence. The alpha-adrenergic receptors in the bladder are affected by drugs that can reduce detrusor contractions and affect continence. They can lead to postural hypotension, which can lead to falls; falls and the fear of falling can lead to loss of mobility and incontinence. Hypertension may be improved by weight loss and patients on hypotensives require regular monitoring.

Anticholinergics are often prescribed in an effort to treat incontinence and they can be effective. They can however cause urinary retention or, if given mistakenly to older adults in urinary retention with overflow, can worsen the situation[39]. It is important that anticholinergics are not prescribed unless the person has a continence assessment and these are clinically indicated. It is also important to monitor the effectiveness or otherwise of such medication and liaise with the person's GP on this.

Many drugs indirectly affect continence, for example iron can cause constipation which can lead to faecal impaction, and faecal impaction can lead to urinary incontinence. Analgesics can cause similar problems. The greater number of drugs prescribed, the greater the risk of drug interaction. Table 7.3 gives a list of drugs and how they affect continence.

Summary

Many factors can lead to the development of incontinence. The design of the home, prescribed medication, and nursing and medical practice can all encourage or discourage continence.

Table 7.3 Some medications that affect continence.

Category	Examples	Effects	Results	Solutions
Benzodiazepines	Nitrazepam Temazepam	Half-lives of 7–48 hours are extended in elderly with impaired renal function	Build up of drugs – increased sedation and lower levels of alertness	Review and eliminate routine use of night sedation
Sedatives	Thioridazine (Melleril) Haloperidol	Half-lives of 12–48 hours are extended in elderly with impaired renal function	Build up of drugs – increased sedation and lower levels of alertness	Review and work towards eliminating; use other methods to control behaviour
Tricyclics (anti-depressants)	Amitryptiline	Extended half-lives, postural hypotension, cardiac arrhythmias	Increased sedation, reduced mobility, loss of abilities	Review need for anti-depressants; if essential suggest newer preparations
Diuretics Loop diuretics	Frumil, frusemide	Rapid action large diuresis in short period, usually given in morning	Older people and busy staff cannot cope with rapid diuresis = incontinence	Do not give before breakfast; split dose
Thiazide diuretics	Moduretic, bendrofluazide	Gentle diuresis but action prolonged in elderly	Delayed and prolonged action can lead to nocturnal enuresis	Consider giving at bedtime if develops nocturnal enuresis
Cardiac glycosides	Digoxin	Increases smooth muscle tone and bladder pressure = reduced bladder capacity	Reduced renal function = increased risk of toxicity and side effects	Review regularly, eliminate or reduce where possible Digoxin levels to give lowest possible dose. May be possible to discontinue

Analgesics	Co-proxamol Co-dydramol	Cause constipation and increase in faecal loading rectum and sigmoid colon	Faecal mass causes pressure and often causes urge incontinence	Pain assessment, review medication and bowel management programme
Iron	Ferrous sulphate Ferrous fumerate	Cause constipation and increase in faecal loading rectum and sigmoid colon	Faecal mass causes pressure and often causes urge incontinence	Check HB, discontinue if FE not required. If required give with orange juice to increase absorption
Antihypertensives	Nifedipine	Reduce detrusor contractions	1. If person has urgency can improve continence 2. If person has outflow obstruction or voiding problems can cause retention with overflow 3. Postural hypotension. Falls, reduced mobility	Monitor BP, discontinue if BP has stabilised
Anticholinergics and calcium channel antagonists	Oxybutinin Propantheline	Dry mouth, constipation, cardiac arrhythmias, constipation	Urinary retention, cardiac arrhythmias, loss of functional abilities, incontinence	Use only after assessment and when other methods have failed and in the smallest possible dose
Muscle relaxants	Dantrolene, baclofen, diazepam	Relax muscles including the bladder (detrusor)	Can cause incontinence	Find other ways to deal with spasticity such as exercise splints

Conclusion

General measures to enable older people to remain mobile, to identify toilets and to prevent adverse drug reactions can enable many older people to remain continent or to regain continence. Nurses can create an environment that actively promotes continence. In this environment, continence is viewed as normal. If incontinence occurs it is investigated and wherever possible treated. The next section examines the different types of incontinence.

Continence assessment

Assessment is the key to continence promotion. Before we can promote continence, we need to ask:

- What are the problems?
- What does the resident want to achieve?
- What do we want to achieve?
- How can we meet the resident's needs and meet our objectives?
- What needs to be done?
- How can it be done?
- Who is the best person to do this?
- How will we know when we have achieved our aims?

The first step is to identify the problems. In earlier sections of this chapter we discussed how we could treat general problems. The aim of this section is to help you identify the different types of urinary incontinence.

This section will explore the features of:

- Urge incontinence
- Overflow incontinence
- Stress incontinence
- Mixed incontinence
- Functional incontinence
- Transient incontinence

The aims of assessment

The aims of assessment are to discover why the incontinence has occurred. You need to find the reasons for it before you can work out the solutions. If you skip the assessment stage, your answers will not only be ineffective but may actually make the problem worse. You may end up working terribly hard and achieving very little. A few years ago an article on continence promotion in nursing homes was published. The author concluded that it made little difference whether you toileted two hourly or four hourly – it was equally ineffective. Unfortunately, the article gave the impression that toileting was all there was to continence promotion and that even that was a waste of time. Effective assessment appears to be time consuming but it is time well spent. Assessment aims to find answers to important questions – when you have found the answers you can begin to work out solutions.

Assessment forms

It is easier to find the answers if you have an assessment form. Assessment forms are tools. They remind you to ask the right questions and find out why incontinence has occurred. An assessment form should be simple and easy to use; many are not. There is no right or wrong way to draw up an assessment form so do not be afraid to draw up your own. Assessment forms for the frail elderly may be different from those used on new mothers. Your assessment form should obtain the following information:

- History of incontinence
- When did it start?
- Did it start suddenly or slowly?
- What brings it on or makes it worse?
- How do you feel about it?
- What would you like to achieve?
- What are the problems?
- Medical history
- Medications
- Ability to use toilet, walk to toilet, understand what toilet is for.

Obtaining information

Your assessment form gives you some of the information you need in order to find out what the problem is, but you need further information. You need to find out how much the person is drinking and how much urine is being passed. Maintaining a fluid balance chart for a week enables you to work out the person's intake and output. You can use a frequency volume chart at the same time. This enables you to see how often the person is urinating, how much urine the person is passing, and how often the person is incontinent. You can then begin to work out the causes of incontinence. When you have worked out the causes, you can plan effective treatment. The following sections discuss the different types of incontinence and how they can be treated.

Case history

Annie is 85 and has had a stroke. She walks with a tripod and the help of one nurse. Annie is lucid. Until recently Annie was continent but now she has started having little accidents. When Annie asks for the toilet, you walk her there. Usually when you close the door and help Annie pull down her pants she wets all over your shoes. What do you think Annie's problem is? What do you do?

Urge incontinence

Urge incontinence is also called bladder dysreflexia, detrusor instability, or the unstable bladder. This is also referred to as 'key in the door incontinence'. People who have urge incontinence are the ones who ask you to take them to the toilet. You get there and just as you get in the door of the toilet or as you are helping pull down pants, the person wets. Nurses respond by taking the person to the toilet earlier. If you take Annie every two hours and you get wet shoes, you respond by taking her every hour and a half. Then because your shoes are still wet you take her hourly. Eventually you decide that the situation is hopeless and supply Annie with incontinence pads. Annie's problems are caused by urge incontinence and inability to respond to the demands of her bladder. If Annie did not have to rely on you to get to the toilet, she would probably manage to get there on time. If Annie could walk faster, she would make it.

Why urgency occurs

Normally bladder contractions are suppressed while the bladder is filling. The micturition centre in the frontal lobe inhibits bladder contractions.

People suffering from an unstable bladder suffer from uncontrolled bladder contractions. The bladder contracts while it is filling up. This means that although the bladder might have a capacity of 500 ml, contractions might start to occur at 250 ml. The working capacity of the bladder is reduced. Strokes affecting the frontal lobe affect the ability of the micturition centre to inhibit bladder contractions. One research study found that 95% of people who suffered from urinary incontinence after stroke had urge incontinence. People with Alzheimer's type dementia, disseminated sclerosis, spinal cord injury or cerebrovascular accidents can develop urgency. Older people are more likely to suffer from urgency than younger people are.

Researchers discovered that 47% of nursing home residents who had unstable bladders were continent. Other factors can make bladder instability worse and lead to incontinence. Constipation can increase pressure on the bladder and make bladder instability worse. This can lead to incontinence. Infection can make instability worse.

Symptoms of urgency

The unstable bladder does not necessarily lead to incontinence. If the person retains the ability to use the toilet independently then she can retain continence, but at a price. The resident who sits nearest the toilet when in the dining room, the resident who chooses the seat nearest the toilet when in the lounge, the resident who bangs on the door if anyone is using the toilet, may well have an unstable bladder. She is only managing to cope because she can respond to the demands of the bladder. One minor problem may send this person tumbling down into incontinence. The symptoms of an unstable bladder are:

- Increased frequency of passing urine
- Urgency – having to rush to use the toilet
- Urge incontinence
- Nocturnal enuresis

Treatment of urgency

There are three ways of treating urgency:

- Treat factors that are making the urgency worse
- Enable the person to respond to the demands of the bladder
- Treat the urgency.

Factors making urgency worse

Constipation – If the person is constipated, a large mass of hard faeces can press on the bladder. This makes the bladder even more irritable and makes the problem worse. Treating constipation removes the mass of faeces and helps resolve the problem.

Infection – Infection makes the irritable bladder more irritable. Treating the infection can often restore continence. If the infection recurs then incontinence can recur. Reinforce good hygiene, wiping from top to bottom not bottom to top. Ensuring that the person has a good fluid intake prevents recurrence. If recurrent infection is a problem offer cranberry juice, 200 ml, twice a day.

Medication – Powerful diuretics can make urgency worse. Encourage GPs to prescribe the smallest possible dose. Give diuretics at sensible times, not when staff will not have time to cope with the effects. If the person is having two Frumil, divide the dose and give one with breakfast and one with lunch. Drugs that cause drowsiness make problems worse so eliminate them whenever possible.

Enabling people to cope with demands of the bladder

Often the key to treating an unstable bladder is to enable people to cope with its demands.

Mobility is one of the most important skills. Do everything that you can to enable the individual to remain mobile or to regain mobility. Recent research suggests that 78% of people admitted to nursing homes are unable to transfer from bed to chair unaided[40]. Evidence to the Royal Commission reveals that if the person is to be transferred to a nursing home physiotherapy is often not offered. Many people admitted to nursing homes can be helped to regain mobility.

Dressing and undressing – The ability to remove or adjust clothing quickly is essential if you have difficulty holding on. Ensuring that the person has easy-to-manage clothes can help. Helping the person practise dressing and undressing can prevent incontinence.

Treating urgency

There are two methods of treating urgency: bladder retraining and medication.

Bladder retraining – People who suffer from urgency often get into the habit of using the toilet very frequently to avoid accidents. This leads to a reduction in bladder capacity. Over time the bladder becomes smaller and smaller and the problem worsens. Bladder retraining aims to enable the person to take control of the bladder. Bladder retraining aims to teach the resident to 'hold on' for longer periods and gradually increase the time between voiding *without incontinence occurring.*

If the person holds on, bladder capacity increases and the person learns how to dampen down bladder contractions. Success breeds success, the bladder capacity becomes larger and the person spends less time thinking about the toilet. As the individual becomes less anxious and begins to enjoy life bladder control improves. It is important to start slowly; ask the person to hold on for five minutes at first and then build up the time between using the toilet. Give the person something to do or something else to think about.

Medication – If toileting programmes are unsuccessful or only partially successful, drug therapy can be considered. Medication acts by 'damping down' bladder contractions[41]. This increases bladder capacity and allows individuals to hold on longer. The drugs used to treat urge incontinence are anticholinergics, antispasmodics and calcium channel antagonists[42]. The drugs act directly on the bladder to reduce bladder contractions. The most commonly used drugs are oxybutinin, imipramine, and propantheline. These drugs should be used with caution because of the danger of side effects.

Propantheline – One study showed that 30 mg four times a day was required to obtain therapeutic results. Half of the volunteers in the trial suffered major side effects and had to have the medication withdrawn. The side effects were dry mouth, difficulty in swallowing, bradycardia followed by tachycardia, palpitations, arrythmias, urinary retention and constipation.

Imipramine and other tricyclic antidepressants – One study found no significant difference between using an average dose of 54 mg and a placebo. Side effects included postural hypotension, sedation and cardiac arrythmias.

Oxybutinin – One study showed that the therapeutic dose was 2.5 mg to 5 mg three times a day. Two-thirds of people taking this experienced side effects but only 16% of people had to have medication withdrawn. Side effects included urinary retention, dry mouth and constipation. Doses of 2.5 mg twice a day can be effective and reduce the risk of side effects[43].

Medication should be given in the smallest possible dose in older people to minimise side effects. Anticholinergics can cause urinary retention; maintaining a fluid balance chart in the first three weeks of use or if the dosage is increased will alert nurses to this side effect. Other side effects include a dry mouth. A holistic approach enables you to treat all the factors that lead to incontinence.

Acupuncture

Acupuncture affects the autonomic nervous system. Acupuncture can effectively treat nocturnal enuresis (one of the main symptoms of the irritable bladder)[44]. In 1988, researchers found 76% of patients with irritable bladder symptoms were cured by acupuncture[45]. Acupuncture has been proven to be as effective as anticholinergics in managing irritable bladder problems.

Stress incontinence

Stress incontinence was first described in 1928 to describe urine lost as a result of coughing. Stress incontinence is a symptom. Genuine stress incontinence is a diagnosis. The difference between the two terms is that genuine stress incontinence is stress incontinence in the absence of unstable bladder contractions. The International Continence Society define stress incontinence as: 'the involuntary loss of urine when the intravesical pressure exceeds the maximal urethral pressure in the absence of detrusor activity'[46]. Small amounts of urine leak if a woman sneezes, coughs, laughs or jumps.

Causes of stress incontinence

It is common in pregnant and postmenopausal women and rare in men, usually only occurring after prostatectomy[47]. The causes of stress incontinence are thought to be:

- Abnormal descent of the bladder neck and proximal urethra. The bladder neck should sit on the symphsis pubis. When the bladder neck falls this affects the urethral closing pressures and leads to leaks.
- Poor muscle support[48].
- Damage to the pudental nerve. The pudental nerve supplies the pelvic floor and urethral sphincter[49]. The pudental nerve is traumatised during vaginal delivery. The bigger the baby and the longer the delivery, the greater the risk. The risk increases with each subsequent delivery.
- Oestrogen deficiency. Normally when intra-abdominal pressure is raised the urethra remains tightly closed and no leakage occurs. Ageing can lead to de-oestrogenation of the urethra and this causes tissues to become thinner and unable to close so effectively.
- Reduction in collagen.
- Other risk factors include pelvic fracture, fractured hip or hip surgery.

Treatment of stress incontinence

Several factors can lead to stress incontinence. These include coughing, uterine prolapse, weakness of the pelvic floor and oestrogen deficiency.

Coughing raises the abdominal pressure. This can cause stress incontinence. Treating chest infections can restore continence. Individuals with chronic chest conditions can be referred to physiotherapists who can teach a method of coughing which does not raise intra-abdominal pressure as much as a 'normal' cough.

Uterine prolapse can be treated surgically but the risks of surgery are high so conservative treatments are normally used.

Ring pessaries

Ring pessaries act by supporting the uterus; they relieve abdominal pressure and treat incontinence. Ring pessaries can be inserted by GPs with family planning training or by a nurse specialist with family planning or continence training. Family planning nurses can usually be persuaded to visit the nursing home once they have recovered from the shock of being asked to see someone in their eighties or nineties. You may be able to spend time with your local family planning nurse or in the urogynaecological clinic of the hospital gaining the skills to change pessaries yourself. Pessaries are normally changed every six months.

Pelvic cones

The pelvic floor can be strengthened by using pelvic floor exercises. Vaginal cones can also be used to strengthen the pelvic floor. The resident has a set of pelvic cones of differing weights, ranging from 20 g to 100 g. The resident starts with the heaviest weight that can be held in the vagina without falling out. The cone is worn for 10–15 minutes each day. If the resident can hold that weight for two days, she progresses to the next weight. Researchers have found a 70% cure rate within a month[50]. Women report that they find cones easier to use and more effective than pelvic floor exercises[51]. Obviously great sensitivity must be used when suggesting vaginal cones. Some frail older women would be horrified by the thought, while others will be prepared to try them.

Oestrogen deficiency

Many nurses think that the urethra is like the anal sphincter. It is very different. The urethra is a series of plump folds of skin. After the menopause, oestrogen levels fall. Many women maintain oestrogen levels sufficiently high to maintain a plump urethra that does not leak. Some women though suffer a deoestrogenated urethra. The urethra becomes thinner and less able to close tightly and keep urine in the bladder. Oestrogen treatment plumps up the urethra. Oestrogen can treat urgency, urge incontinence, dysuria and nocturia[52]. Oestrogen also prevents urinary tract infection in older women[53]. Doctors normally prescribe oestrogen cream that is applied vaginally. This is usually given daily initially and then reduced to weekly or monthly as a maintenance dose. Anticholinergic drugs can help some individuals.

Injections

Injections to bulk out the bladder neck and prevent slippage were first used in 1938[54]. In 1964, doctors began to use Teflon; cure rates varied from 11% to 60%[55]. Side effects included urinary obstruction, pulmonary emboli, migration of Teflon and cancer[56]. In 1992, Bard launched the contigen implant. This is purified bovine collagen. It is injected into the tissue around the bladder neck under local anaesthetic. The injected collagen begins to break down after 13 weeks but stimulates the body to produce collagen[57]. Three months after surgery 86% of patients consider themselves cured; this falls to 68% two years later. Side effects include short-term urinary retention; there are no reports of BSE or other major complications. Collagen injections effectively treat genuine stress incontinence when conservative measures have failed. The average cost of a contigen implant is £900.

Male stress incontinence

Men suffering from stress incontinence following prostatectomy should be referred back to the surgeon who performed the operation for investigation or treatment. Research indicates that collagen implants can effectively treat post prostatectomy stress incontinence[58].

Case history

Kate has Parkinson's disease. She depends on you to meet all her needs. You do your best to keep Kate continent but you are having problems. Kate is never incontinent at night but every morning when you get her up to help her onto the commode she wets. Every time you move Kate, she wets. What do you think the problem is? What would you do about it?

Overflow incontinence

Overflow incontinence is a condition where the bladder fails to empty properly and the individual leaks small amounts of urine on movement. It can easily be confused with stress incontinence. The commonest cause is faecal impaction. Other causes include enlarged prostate, urethral stricture, Parkinson's disease, diabetes and spinal cord compressions. When the bladder fails to empty properly this condition is known as hypotonic bladder. There are several reasons why the bladder fails to empty properly.

Causes of overflow incontinence
The bladder stretches in all directions. When the bladder is reaching normal capacity, the stretch receptors send a signal to the brain that the bladder is becoming full. We can then delay urination for a while. When the bladder becomes hypotonic this signalling mechanism fails to work and the bladder becomes over-stretched, big and floppy. A hypotonic bladder can hold between 500 ml and 2 litres. The causes of hypotonic bladder are:

- Lesions to the micturition centre in the pons. These are rare but can occur after stroke or head injury.
- Spinal cord lesions in the area between the pons and the sacral nerves can disturb the normal voiding mechanism.
- Cauda equina lessions can damage the sacral nerve roots at S2–S4 and can lead to loss of bladder sensation and the inability to pass urine. The commonest causes of cauda equina lesions in older people are osteoporosis and protruding lumbo-sacral discs. Spinal tumours and secondaries can also damage the sacral nerves. Fracture of the femur, pelvis or hip can lead to temporary voiding difficulties. The swelling and bruising that follow the injury and the surgery to repair injury can affect the sacral nerves. When the swelling settles down, voiding returns to normal – if the resident has not acquired a long-term catheter or become impacted or immobile in the meantime.
- Diabetic peripheral neuropathy can damage the motor pathways and reduce bladder sensation.
- Multiple sclerosis and Parkinson's disease can lead to bladder dyssynergia and voiding difficulties. Box 7.2 outlines the features of bladder dyssynergia.

Treatment of overflow incontinence

Many doctors consider that the only possible treatment of overflow incontinence is catheterisation[59]. That is not necessarily true. Sometimes the cause of overflow incontinence is a simple one.

If the person is faecally impacted, dissimpaction can often treat the problem. The individual enjoys a better quality of life uncatheterised and with normal bowel function. Sometimes medication can cause retention. If the

Box 7.2   Bladder dyssynergia.

Normally the bladder contracts and the urethral sphincter relaxes on urination. In individuals with dyssynergia, the urethral sphincter fails to relax and complete bladder emptying is not possible. If untreated the bladder becomes overstretched and loses tone (hypotonic bladder), residual urine increases and infection is almost inevitable. Symptoms include:

- Incomplete bladder emptying
- Passing small frequent amounts of urine
- Leakage on standing
- No leakage in bed
- No nocturnal enuresis.

person is on antidepressants, especially amitryptiline, discontinuing the antidepressants can solve the problem. Sometimes antihypertensives can prevent voiding; a change of medication can solve the problem.

Sometimes draining off the residual urine with an in-out catheter and helping the person to void can help. Tapping the bladder, applying a warm flannel to the abdomen or stroking the inside of the thighs (the resident can do this) can stimulate bladder contractions. Medication can be used to stimulate the bladder but this should be used with caution because of side effects. Diazepam (given at night to reduce daytime drowsiness) can help. This should be given for a short period only as it can impact on the person's ability to carry out the activities of daily living, increase the risk of falls and cause dependence.

Intermittent catheterisation once a day or once every other day can keep overflow incontinence at bay[60]. If these strategies fail then you will have to use an indwelling catheter.

Mixed incontinence

Mixed incontinence is a combination of stress and urge incontinence. You need to use the methods of treatment outlined in the sections on urge incontinence and stress incontinence to tackle these problems.

Functional incontinence

Functional incontinence is incontinence that occurs in people with normal bladder function. It is common in people with advanced dementia and head injury. People who suffer from functional incontinence are often unaware that they have passed urine or that they are wet.

Managing functional incontinence

People who have functional incontinence are not able to interpret bladder signals or respond appropriately to a full bladder. People with functional incontinence are the most disabled of nursing home residents. It is not possible to treat functional incontinence, but with careful management you can keep some people with functional incontinence dry. Use a chart to identify the times that the person is wet. If you keep the chart for a week you can, with luck, identify a pattern. Take the person to the toilet before the incontinence occurs and you will be able to keep the person dry. Keeping the person dry is totally dependent on nursing staff taking the person to the toilet. If you forget, the person will be incontinent. In my experience around two-thirds of people with functional incontinence will display a pattern and can be kept dry if you use an *individual* toileting pattern. Routine two-hourly toileting will not work. You may find that the person uses the toilet twice in two hours in the morning and three-hourly in the afternoon. Only an individual schedule will enable you to keep the person dry. A third of people with functional incontinence do not display a pattern and you need to work out ways to manage the incontinence.

Transient incontinence

Many older adults or their families say that the incontinence has only just started. Often the resident (or relative) can tell nurses exactly when and often why incontinence began. 'I was fine until the doctor changed my water tablets'. 'I was managing until my arthritis got so bad I couldn't get to the toilet in time.' 'She was fine until her stroke.' This is known as 'transient incontinence' and older people suffering from transient incontinence can often be helped to regain continence. Resnick identified the causes of transient incontinence using the acronym DIAPPERS, which is rather patronising but does make the causes easy to remember:

Delirium/confusional state
Infection
Atrophic urethritis/vaginitis
Pharmaceuticals
Psychological – especially depression
Endocrine
Restricted mobility
Stool impaction

Treatment of transient incontinence

Treatment of transient incontinence is straightforward and very rewarding. Identify the causes and work to eliminate them. Ensure infection is treated; prevent further urinary tract infection by giving sufficient fluids, promoting good hygiene and giving cranberry juice if infection recurs. Urethritis and vaginitis can be treated by oestrogen cream. Review medications to ensure they are not contributing to continence problems. Make people feel that they have come to the home to live and not to die, and depression often resolves. If the person has diabetes ensure it is treated. If the person is slow, has crêpy skin, is constantly cold and is overweight and puffy, think thyroid. Treating myxoedema resolves continence problems, improves the hair and skin, and resolves depression. If the person has mobility problems do everything you can to improve mobility. Look after bowels. Bowel care is deeply unfashionable; the bowel book has been ditched. If you do not have one reintroduce it – tell the inspectors it is an auditing tool. Auditing tools are 'where it's at' in nursing and no one in their right mind would argue with an auditing tool.

These simple nursing measures will enable people to regain continence. Relatives and care managers will think you are a saint and a miracle worker and the inspector may think long and hard before mentioning continence in your presence because your expertise is obvious to all. Gaining those skills and making a real difference was not that difficult.

Conclusion

Continence promotion, like anything else in life, is easy when you know how. This chapter has aimed to equip you with the know-how to promote continence easily and effectively. There is no need to break into a sweat promoting continence, if you know how.

Continence promotion programmes

This section aims to discuss how to introduce a continence promotion programme in your home.

This section aims to discuss:
- Managing change
- Managing your GPs
- Managing the nursing home environment
- Educating staff and residents

Managing change

Introducing a continence promotion programme involves changing practice within the home. Change can be frightening and threatening. Change can make staff feel that they are doing it wrong and are not good at what they do. Nurses feel stressed and guilty about incontinence so the last thing you want to do is make things worse.

Sell the idea to staff. If you can, get someone else to think it was their idea. Tell everyone what a brilliant idea Mary has had. Support and guide Mary and everyone else who supports the idea. Introduce changes carefully and sensitively and gain the co-operation of colleagues when making these changes. Make sure everyone is aware of the reasons for introducing change and sell the staff's ability to introduce change as a sign of strength – not an admission that they were doing everything wrong before. Tell the staff that they are brilliant and that they are doing a superb job. Make the staff feel that they are stars and they will behave like stars. Do not impose change – get staff to 'own' the changes; then they will give their heart and soul to changes. If you try to impose changes without their consent or co-operation, they will block you every step of the way. The atmosphere will become hostile and instead of improving things, you will have made them worse. Make change something that you do hand in hand without fear. Do not make change a fearful push; it does not work.

It is important when managing change to begin slowly and to break the work down into small manageable units. Management texts refer to this as 'small bite-sized chunks'.

Managing the nursing home environment

Before implementing a continence programme, take some time to look at your home. Look at the factors that contribute to people developing urinary incontinence. These factors will include the environment, staffing levels and nursing practice. You may be able to change some of these factors easily, some with great difficulty, and some may be completely outside your control. Begin by tackling the easy tasks first.

Timing of medication

If large numbers of your residents are on diuretics your long-term aim will be to have these medications reviewed and if they are not essential (e.g. for treatment of congestive cardiac failure or other disease) but are merely to treat trivial symptoms like oedema, find other ways of controlling oedema such as exercise, elevation and elastic stockings. In the meantime, look at when diuretics are given out. If they are given early in the morning by night staff, consider giving them later, perhaps with breakfast. Then there will be more nursing staff on duty to help residents go to the toilet. Do not be afraid to split diuretics. Most of us would struggle to cope with the effects of two Frumil. Try giving one at breakfast and one at lunchtime. If the person is struggling to maintain continence on one Frumil it can be halved (or the GP can prescribe Frumil LS) and one half can be given at breakfast time and the other at lunchtime. If the person is on a slow acting diuretic such as Moduretic and night time incontinence is a problem, consider giving it at bedtime. Slow acting diuretics can take so long to act in frail elderly people that they have their maximal effect when the person is fast asleep. If you give it at night, it will have its maximal effect during the day when the person is awake.

Environment

Consider what time residents normally go to bed. Do they go early and stay in bed for a long period? Consider encouraging people to go to bed later. Encourage friends and relatives to visit in the evening. Introduce evening activities including film shows and bingo. Can residents easily get out of bed to use the toilet at night? Are all the lights out? Is it too dark? Consider using night lights so that people can find their way to the toilet. Is it too cold? Make sure windows are closed and the heating is on. Do you use cotsides? Do the residents need these or is this just normal practice? Are shoes and walking aids within easy reach or have they been tidied out of reach?

Managing your GPs

You need to gain the co-operation of GPs if the programme is to succeed. You will need to review medication with them. You should aim wherever possible to eliminate the use of hypnotics and minimise the use of sedatives and diuretics.

You will need to gain their co-operation when you send off urine specimens, to find out what the appropriate antibiotic is to treat a urinary tract
infection. Urine culture costs £7 and is charged to the GP. Explain what you
are attempting. Sell the changes to the GP and explain the benefits. The
drugs bill will be reduced. Admittedly you will be spending more on support
stockings and special shoes, but the GP will see a reduction in spending and
resident quality of life will be enhanced. If you spend some time selling your
ideas to the GP, you will seldom have problems.

Educating staff and residents

Before you can begin to promote continence, you have to convince staff that
it can be done. You may also need to convince relatives that you are not
being cruel when you encourage mother to walk rather than wheeling her.
You many need to provide leaflets, books, articles and videos to educate and
encourage people. At the end of this section you will find a list of leaflets,
articles, videos and books that will help you do this.

Beginning the programme

When you introduce change, there is always the temptation to try to
change the world before lunch. Slow down or it will end in tears. Start
slowly and build up. Before you decide how many residents to begin to
work with, be realistic. If you are busy and short of staff it is better to
begin with two residents and succeed, rather than try to work with five
residents and fail because you have taken on too much. Discuss this with
staff. Choose residents who can co-operate (the degree of co-operation
will vary from home to home) and who you have the greatest chance of
succeeding with.

A person who is mobile and lucid will normally have more chance of
regaining continence quickly than an immobile and cognitively impaired
resident. It is important when managing change to tackle the least challenging aspects first as there is more likelihood of success. Success builds
momentum and raises morale and if there are problems later earlier success
can be pin-pointed to boost flagging morale.

Ways to promote continence

- Find out why the incontinence has occurred
- Do everything you can to eliminate the causes of incontinence
- Work with the person to improve mobility; you may need to order special
  shoes, organise physiotherapy, etc.
- Help the person regain the ability to dress and undress if this has been
  lost
- Work with the GP to review medication and when possible discontinue
  or reduce medication that affects continence to the smallest possible
  dose
- Maintain a bladder chart so that you can measure success
- Praise residents and staff and ensure that you appreciate their efforts.

Conclusion

Continence promotion programmes can change people's lives. Continence promotion can make an older person think that life is worth living. Continence promotion can make relatives feel confident enough to have mum home for Sunday lunch. Continence promotion can make nurses feel that working in the home is not just one long slog and clean-up job. Nurses are busy and there never seems to be enough time to do all that you want to do. Continence promotion enables you to take control and reduce your workload.

Further information

Association for Continence Advice (ACA), 102a, Astra House, Arklow Road, New Cross, London SE14 6EB. Tel. 020 8692 4680. Fax 020 8692 6217. website: www.aca.uk.com email: info@aca.uk.com

Incontact, United House, North Road, London N7 9DP. Tel. 0870 770 3246 Fax 0870 770 3249 website: www.incontact.org email: edu@incontact.org

Leaflets

The Alzheimer's Disease Society produce a number of useful leaflets. Advice sheet 1 – Incontinence, sheet 2 – How Professionals Can Help, and sheet 3 – Later Stages of Dementia, are particularly useful. All of this information can be downloaded from: www.alzheimers.org.uk/carers/advice incontinence

The Continence Foundation have a help line 020 7831 9831 Monday to Friday, 9.30AM to 4.30PM. Their website: http://www.continence-foundation.org.uk contains a wealth of useful leaflets and resources. The following are especially useful:

The Misbehaving Bladder This highly popular leaflet with amusing illustrations is about urgency and urge incontinence. It includes a descriptive introduction, a suggested plan of management and a five-day bladder chart.

Bladder training charts Three one-week sheets, with instructions. A5 size.

Advice for Relatives of People in Residential and Nursing Homes Causes of incontinence and prevention, assessment, treatment and management in the care home setting.

You can also write (preferably enclosing a large SAE) to: The Helpline Nurse, The Continence Foundation, 307 Hatton Square, 16 Baldwin Gardens, London ECIN 7RJ.

Videotapes

Understanding and Treating Incontinence (part 1) is for professionals and gives information on causes, investigations and treatment of urinary incontinence

Understanding and Treating Incontinence (part 4) is for professionals and gives details of bladder re-education and prompted voiding

Both can be obtained from The King's Fund, 11–13 Cavendish Square, London W1G OAN. Tel. 020 7307 2400. Fax 020 7307 2801.

Guidelines for Continence is a set of three videos available from Molynke. Contact your local Molynke representative for details.

Books

Nursing for Continence, 2nd edn (1996) Edited by Christine Norton. Beaconsfield Publishers, Beaconsfield, Bucks. A great introduction to continence promotion.

In Control – Help with Incontinence (1990) Mares, P. Age Concern, London. This is a simple resident centred book aimed at older people with continence problems. It has a positive outlook and the print is large enough to be read by those with less than perfect eyesight.

Staying Dry – A Practical Guide to Bladder Control (1989) Burgio K., Pearce, K.L. & Lucco, A.J. John Hopkins Press, Baltimore, USA. The authors have successfully translated their work at John Hopkins medical school into a self-help programme that can be followed at home. This book is aimed at the more educated and motivated individuals with continence problems.

Bladder re-education for the promotion of continence (1992) Kennedy A. In: *Clinical Nursing Practice – The promotion and management of continence.* Roe, B. (ed.). Prentice Hall, New Jersey. This a detailed well referenced chapter for professionals

Inappropriate Urination (1990) Stokes, G. Winslow Press, Bicester. This is a useful book for newly qualified staff.

Not such private places (1992) Council and Care, London. This is a report by a charity who are committed to promoting excellence within nursing and residential homes. It highlights areas where dignity and privacy are of paramount importance.

Exchanging Ideas (1991) Alzheimer's Disease Society, London. This booklet for carers is full of helpful hints on caring for individuals with Alzheimer's.

Articles

Brocklehurst, J., Dickinson E. & Windsor, J. (1999) Laxatives and faecal incontinence in long term care. *Nursing Standard*, **13**(52), 32–36.

Fonda, D. (1990) *Improving management of urinary incontinence in geriatric centres and nursing homes. Australian Clinical Review*, **10**(2), 66–71. This one-day census of 1659 older adults in elderly care wards and nursing homes revealed that only 43% of hospital patients and 23% of nursing home residents were able to attend to their own toileting needs. This work identifies patients whose continence is dependent on nursing staff and concludes that urinary incontinence is more common in these settings than previous studies indicate.

Frewen, W. K. (1990) A reassessment of bladder training in detrusor dysfunction in the female. *British Journal of Urology*, **54**, 372–3.

References

[1] Anderson *et al.* (1988) The standard terminology of the lower urinary tract function. *Scandinavian Journal of Urology and Nephrology*, supplement, **114**, 5–19.

[2] Koyano, W., Shibata, H., Haga, H. & Sumaya, Y. (1986) Prevalence and outcome of low ADL and incontinence among the elderly: Five years follow-up in a Japanese urban community. *Archives of Gerontology & Geriatrics*, **5**, 197–206.

[3] Nazarko, L. (1993) Solving incontinence through assessment. *Nursing Standard*, **8**(8), 44–45.

[4] Palmer, M.H., German P.S. & Ouslander, J.G. (1991) Risk factors for urinary incontinence one year after nursing home admission. *Research in Nursing and Health*, **14**(6), 405–412.

[5] Thom, D.H., Haan, N.M. & Van Den Eeden, S.K. (1997) Medically recognised urinary incontinence and risks of hospitalisation, nursing home admission and mortality. *Age, Ageing*, **26**(5), 367–374.

[6] Shepherd, M. (1998) The Risks of Polypharmacy. *Nursing Times*, **94**(32), 60–62.

[7] Nazarko, L. (1993) The therapeutic uses of cranberry juice. *Nursing Standard*, **9**(34), 33–35.

[8] Avorn, J., Monane, M., Gurwitz, J.H. & Glyn Robert, J. (1994) Reduction of bactinuria and pyuria after ingestion of cranberry juice. *Journal American Medical Association*, **271**(10), 751–754.

[9] Nazarko, L. (1996) Power to the people. *Nursing Times*, **92**(41), 48–49.

[10] Ouslander, J.G., Morishita, L. & Blaustein, J. (1987) Clinical, functional and psychosocial characteristics of an incontinent nursing home population. *Journal of Gerontology*, **42**(6), 631–637.

[11] Brocklehurst, J.C., Andrews, K., Richards, B. & Laycock, P.J. (1985) Incidence and correlates of incontinence in stroke patients. *Journal of the American Geriatrics Society*, **35**, 540–542.

[12] Borrie, M.J., Campbell, A.J., Caradoc-Davis, T.H. & Spears, F.S. (1986) Urinary incontinence after stroke: a prospective study. *Age & Ageing*, **15**, 177–181.

[13] Rottkamp, B. (1985) A holistic approach to identifying factors associated with an altered pattern of urinary elimination in stroke patients. *Journal of Neurosurgical Nursing*, **17**(1), 37–44.

[14] Nazarko, L. (1994) Drugs, continence, elderly people. *Primary Health Care*, **4**(1), 19–22.

[15] Mollander, U. et al. (1990) An epidemiological study of urinary incontinence and related urogenital symptoms in elderly women. *Maturitas*, **12**, 51–60.

[16] Kristiansen, P., Pompiers, R. & Wadtrrom, L.B. (1983) Long term bladder drainage and bladder capacity. *Neurology and Urodynamics*, **2**, 135–143.

[17] Burns (1992) Working up a thirst. *Nursing Times*, **88**(26), 45–47.

[18] Nazarko, L. (1996) Power to the people. *Nursing Times*, **92**(41), 48–49.

[19] Nazarko, L. (1996) Preventing constipation. *Professional Nurse*, **11**(12), 816–818.

[20] Kinnunen, O. (1991) Study of constipation in a geriatric hospital, old people's home and at home. *Age & Ageing*, **3**(2), 161–170.

[21] Heaton, K.W., Radvan, H. & Cripps, H. et al. (1992) Defecation frequency and timing and stool form in the general population; a prospective study. *Gut*, **33**, 818–824.

[22] Skelly, J. & Flint, A.J. (1995) Urinary incontinence associated with dementia. *Journal American Geriatrics Society*, **43**(3), 286–294.

[23] Miller, K.L. (1996) Hormone replacement therapy in the elderly. *Clinics of Obstetrics and Gynaecology*, **39**(4), 912–932.

[24] Cobbs, E.L. & Ralapati, A.N. (1998) Health of older women. *Medical Clinics of North America*, **82**(1), 127–144.

[25] Holthoff-Detto, V.A., Kessler, J., Herholtz, K., Bönner, H., Poetrzyk, U., Würker, M., Ghaemi, M., Wienhard, K., Wagnr, R. & Heiss, W.D. (1997) Functional effects of striatial dysfunction in Parkinson's Disease. *Archives Neurology*, **54**(2), 145–150.

[26] Manyam, B.V. (1997) Practical guidelines for the management of Parkinson's disease. *Journal American Board Family Practice*, **10**(6), 412–424.

[27] Hellstom, L., Elkeland, I.M. & Mellstrom, D. (1990) The prevalence of urinary incontinence and the use of incontinence aids in 85-year-old men and women. *Age and Ageing*, **19**, 383–389.

[28] Palmer, M.H., German, P.S. & Ouslander, J.G. (1991) Risk factors for urinary incontinence one year after nursing home admission. *Research in Nursing and Health*, **14**(6), 405–12.

[29] Yu, L.C., Rohner, T.J. & Kaltreider, D.L. (1990) Profile of urinary incontinent elderly in long term care institutions. *Journal American Geriatrics Society*, **38**, 433–439.

30 Burgio, L.D., McCormack, K.A. & Sheeve, A.S. (1994) The effects of changing prompted voiding schedules in the treatment of incontinent nursing home residents. *Journal American Geriatrics Society*, **42**, 315–320.

31 Hu, T.W., Igou, J.F. & Kaltreider, L. (1989) A clinical trial of a behaviour therapy to reduce urinary incontinence in nursing homes. *Journal of the American Medical Association*, **261**, 2656–2662.

32 Wunderlich, G.S., Sloan, F.A. & Davis, C.K. (1996) *Nursing Staff in Hospitals and Nursing Homes. Is it adequate?* Institute of Medicine, National Academy Press, Washington.

33 Palmer, M.H., German, P.S. & Ouslander, J.G. (1991) Risk factors for urinary incontinence one year after nursing home admission. *Research in Nursing and Health*, **14**(6), 405–412.

34 Nazarko, L. (1993) Solving incontinence through assessment. *Nursing Standard*, **8**(6), 25–27.

35 Schnelle, J.F. *et al.* (1988) Reduction of urinary incontinence in nursing homes: does it reduce or increase costs. *Journal American Geriatric Society*, **36**, 34–39.

36 Selikson, S., Damus, K. & Hamerman, D. (1988) Risk factors associated with immobility. *Journal American Geriatrics Society*, **36**, 707–712.
Yu, L.C. & Kaltreider, D.L. (1987) Stressed nurses dealing with incontinent patients. *Journal of Gerontological Nursing*, **13**(1), 27–30.

37 Peet, S.M., Castleden, C.M., McGrother, C.W. & Duffin, H.M. (1996) The management of urinary incontinence in residential and nursing homes for older people. *Age, Ageing*, **25**(2), 139–143.

38 Department of Health (2000) *Shaping the Future NHS: Long Term Planning for Hospitals and Related Services*. Consultation Document on the Findings of the National Beds Enquiry. Department of Health, London. This document can be found on the website:
http://www.doh.gov.uk/pub/docs/doh/nationalbeds.pdf

39 Keever, M.F. (1990) An investigation into recognised incontinence within a health authority. *Journal of Advanced Nursing*, **15**(10), 1197–1207.

40 Readerdon (1996) Transfers to nursing homes. *Elder Care*, **8**(5), 16–18.

41 Nazarko, L. (1996) A matter of urgency. *Nursing Times*, **92**(32), 63–65.

42 Wein, A.J. (1990) Pharmacological treatment of incontinence. *Journal American Geriatric Society*, **8**, 317–325.

43 Malone-Lee, J.G., Lubel, D. & Szonyi, G. (1992) Low dose oxybutinin for the unstable bladder. *British Medical Journal*, **304**, 1053.

44 Song, Baozhu & Wang Xiyou (1985) Short term effect in 135 cases of enuresis treated by wrist ankle needling. *Journal Traditional Chinese Medicine*, **5**, 27–28.

45 Philp, T., Shah, P.J.R. & Worth, P.H.L. (1988) Acupuncture in the treatment of bladder instability. *British Journal of Urology*, **61**, 490–491.

46 Abrams, P., Blaivas, J.G., Stanton, S.L. & Anderson, J. (1988) Standardisation of terminology of lower urinary tract function. *Scandinavian Journal Urology and Nephrology*, **114**(9 suppl.) 5–19.

47 Delancy, J.O. (1990) Functional anatomy of the female urinary tract and pelvic floor. *CIBA Foundation Symposium*, **151**, 57–76.

48 De Lancy, J.O.L. (1992) Three dimensional analysis of urethral support; the hammock thesis. *Neurological Urodynamics*, **11**, 306–308.

49 Allen, R.E., Hosker, G.L., Smith, A.R.B. & Warrell, D.W. (1990) Pelvic floor damage and childbirth; a neurophysiological study. *Journal Obstetrics and Gynaecology*, **97**, 770–779.

50 Haken, J., Benness, C., Cardozo, L.D. & Cutner, A. (1991) A randomised trial of

vaginal cones and pelvic floor exercises in the management of genuine stress incontinence. *Neurolol Urodynamics*, **10**, 393–394.

[51] Wilson, P.D. & Borland, M. (1990) Vaginal cones for the treatment of genuine stress incontinence. *Australian and New Zealand Journal of Obstetrics and Gynaecology*, **30**, 157–160.

[52] Henna, S.M., Hutches, C.J., Robinson, P. & Macular, J. (1989) Non operative methods in the treatment of genuine stress incontinence. *British Journal of Obstetrics and Gynaecology*, **9**, 222–225.

[53] Kirkengen, A.L., Andersen, P., Gjersoe, E., Johanssen, G.R., Johnsen, N. & Bodd, E. (1992) Oestriol in the prophylactic treatment of recurrent urinary tract infection in post menopausal women. *Scandanavia Journal Primary Health Care*, **10**, 139–142.

[54] Murless, B.C. (1938) The injection treatment of stress incontinence. *Journal Obstetrics and Gynaecology British Empire*, **45**, 67–73.

[55] Politano, V.A. (1992) Transurethral polytef injection for post prostatectomy incontinence. *British Journal of Urology*, **69**, 26–28.

[56] Dewan, P.A. (1992) Is injected PTFE (Polytef) carcinogenic? *British Journal of Urology*, **69**, 29–33.

[57] Stanton, S.L., Monga, A.K. & Robinson, D. (1994) Periurethral collagen for female genuine stress incontinence; results at 3-year follow up. *Neurology and Urodynamics*, **13**, 449–450.

[58] Martins, F.E., Bennett, C.J., Dunn, M., Filho, D., Kelleher, T. & Lieskovsaky, G. (1997) Adverse prognostic features of collagen injection therapy for urinary incontinence following radical retropubic prostatectomy. *Journal Urology*, **158**(5), 1745–1749.

[59] Jolleys, J.V. (1994) Urinary incontinence. *Reviews in Contemporary Pharmacotherapy*, **5**(3), 53–162.

[60] Nazarko, L. (1999) Assess all areas. *Nursing Times*, **95**(6), 68–71.

Chapter 8

Management of Incontinence

Introduction

Some older people maintain continence until the last few days of life. Others, because of the effects of disease or disability, become incontinent. Before you decide that someone is incontinent carry out a continence assessment. If a person has six months to live and you can get that individual to remain continent for four of those months, then you have enhanced quality of life. In some circumstances it is obvious that continence promotion is inappropriate so you must move your focus to managing incontinence. Then the aims of care are:

- To contain incontinence
- To avoid the complications of poorly managed incontinence
- To enable the person to maintain dignity.

This chapter aims to:

- Examine methods used to contain incontinence
- Explain the benefits and problems associated with each method
- Enable you to choose an appropriate method to contain incontinence
- Enable you to avoid complications of poorly managed incontinence
- Enable you to use research to guide your practice

Choosing the right method to contain incontinence

If the person is incontinent you must choose a suitable method to contain incontinence. You have a number of options. You can use incontinence pads, sheaths (for males) and catheters. Every collection device has advantages and disadvantages. It is important to choose the right collection device for each person. You may find it useful to use the continence assessment even on people who have no prospect of regaining continence. If you understand the reasons why incontinence is occurring then you will be in a better position to choose the most effective method of containing incontinence. The following sections look at the options and discuss their advantages and disadvantages.

Incontinence pads

Incontinence pads are used for three different types of urinary incontinence[1]:

- Light – stress incontinence (Type 1)
- Moderate to heavy – daytime incontinence (Type 2)
- Heavy – night time incontinence (Type 3)

Categories of pads

Pads can be divided into two categories – reusable and disposable. Disposable pads consist of a plastic backing, paper fluff pulp and a one-way liner. Most pads contain absorbent powder or crystals. The absorbent material gels on contact with urine and 'locks' urine into the core of the pad, keeping the person's skin dry.

Type 1 incontinence – Type 1 incontinence can be effectively contained using either disposable or reusable body worn pads. Some companies produce pants with integral washable pads. Pants are available for men and women. The ladies briefs are available in a variety of styles and patterns. The capacity of the integral pad varies from 60 to 200 ml. Using fabric conditioner ruins the ability of the pads to absorb urine.

Type 2 incontinence – People with type 2 incontinence may require a body worn pad. You can of course choose other methods of containing urine such as sheaths or catheters for people with type 2 incontinence. The next section looks at how to choose suitable pads for containing type 2 incontinence. Urinary sheaths will be discussed later.

Choosing the right incontinence pad for the individual

Research has shown that no one pad is right for all people[2]. Research findings can enable us to discover the features to look for in pads and to order pads that will suit each individual. In October 2001 all people living in nursing homes who fund their own care and require incontinence pads became entitled to receive their pads from the NHS. This entitlement is being implemented in different ways in different areas. In some areas the NHS is supplying pads; in others the NHS is providing a cash sum to enable pads to be purchased. Regardless of how the system works, it is important that you are able to assess the individual and ensure that he or she receives the most suitable pad.

Research indicates that the following features reduce leakage, minimise skin problems and maintain the older person's dignity and comfort:

- Shaped pads are more effective in reducing leakage
- Pads with elasticated sections around the legs reduce leakage[3]
- Adequate absorbent material in the central section of the pad reduces leakage
- Pads fitted closely to the body, e.g. using net pants, reduce leakage
- Rapid absorption of liquid into the core of the pad reduces skin problems and leakage
- Absorbent crystals or powder reduce leakage and skin problems
- Kanga pads and pants are inadequate for heavy incontinence[4]. Some individuals are admitted from home with Kanga pads and pants; you may have to wean them off these if incontinence is heavy.

Advantages of disposable pads

- Can reduce laundry costs
- No cross infection risks – each pad is new
- Enable people who are incontinent to remain dry and comfortable.

Disadvantages of disposable pads

- They can take up a lot of storage space
- They can be misused by staff
- They may be ineffective – leakage can be a problem. Ineffective pads do not reduce laundry costs
- Storage and disposal of used pads can be unpleasant and costly
- They are not environmentally friendly. Over 9 million disposable nappies are used in the UK every day. It takes between 200 and 500 years for a disposable nappy to decompose. Those with environmentally friendly pulp take six years to decompose[5].

Body worn reusable pads

Interest in body worn reusable pads originated in the US. There were two main reasons why nurses began to consider their use in long-term care. Firstly, laundry companies in the US offered to supply, launder and return pads (possibly because their traditional market nappy service was declining due to falling birth-rates and increased use of disposables by mothers). The second factor was an increasing interest in environmental issues. Concern about pollution caused by the use of dioxin (an extremely carcinogenic substance) to bleach paper used in pads, and disposal of used pads, led many nurses to consider reusable body worn pads[6].

Costs and effectiveness of reusables

Research (sponsored by the makers of disposables) concludes that the environmental costs of disposables and reusables are roughly equal[7]. This research takes into account the costs of heating water, drying and detergents which all have an environmental impact. Research has been carried out in long-term care settings using reusables and comparing them with disposables. In one study nurses found that with disposables leakage was reduced and the amount of laundry was halved. But after the trial nursing staff went back to using reusable pads because they felt that disposables had caused more skin problems[8].

Further research found that leakage was a greater problem with reusable pads and the cost savings associated with reusables were outweighed by increased laundry costs. The costs of both systems were roughly equal when laundry costs were taken into account; however the cost of nursing time spent in changing patients who were wet was not costed into the study[9]. Another study found no differences between disposables and reusables; both products were effective and there was no difference in skin health. This report concluded that disposables were more expensive[10]. Dealing with urinary incontinence and its consequences in terms of washing and changing patients and bed linen can account for 20–34% of nursing staff time. Incontinence pads that fail to contain urine and lead to leakage are a false economy as the costs of nursing time, laundry, domestic time and cleaning materials far exceed the cost of pads.

Research has demonstrated that older people with continence problems are likely to be immobile[11]. Many older people who are immobile require two members of staff (and often equipment such as hoists) to move, wash and change them. On average it takes two staff members 15 minutes to deal with an episode of incontinence. Each episode of incontinence costs between £3.05 and £4.19 in staff salaries. If a pad has leaked and the individual requires a change of clothes, the time taken to fetch clean clothing and wash the individual rises on average to 25 minutes and costs between £5.08 and £6.98. Domestic and laundry costs arising from the incontinence total a further £1.50 (laundry costs 87p, domestic costs 63p). The cost of an episode of incontinence rises to between £6.68 to £8.48. If an older person has five episodes of incontinence in 24 hours this costs between £15.25 and £20.95 in staff time if no leakage occurs.

Advantages and disadvantages of reusable pads

There are over 30 reusable products available in the UK. Few accounts of research have been published. There are few trials comparing different types of reusables. Trials that compare a disposable with a reusable rarely identify which disposable or reusable have been used. It is difficult to judge if the trials compare like with like; a high quality disposable will score well against a poor quality reusable and vice versa. It is not currently possible to identify which features make certain reusables more effective. Reports of cost savings are dependent on the costs of laundry and nursing time (which few researchers consider). Little research is available about the infection control risks of reusable pads. Manufacturers of reusables do not recommend their use when people are doubly incontinent.

Type 3 incontinence

Type 3 incontinence can be managed by using either body worn pads, disposable or reusable underpads. You can choose to manage type 3 incontinence using urinary sheaths or catheters. This section will concentrate on using bed sheets.

Until the 1970s the traditional way of managing night time incontinence was using a plastic draw sheet and a cotton draw sheet. In 1977 the Kylie bed sheet, the first reusable underpad, was introduced. The Kylie bed sheet was designed in Australia and Kylie is the aboriginal word for nappy. Initial research demonstrated that Kylies kept patients drier, reduced odour and skin problems and reduced bed changing by half[12]. Research carried out in the UK found that Kylies were more effective than draw sheets, reduced laundry costs and their use improved the skin condition of people who suffered from incontinence. The main disadvantage of Kylie bed sheets was the time they took to dry. In the mid 1980s the manufacturers introduced a new lightweight 300 g Kylie. Pottle carried out a study that only involved six patients, and she concluded that the 300 g Kylie was not sufficiently absorbent to contain incontinence in six hospital patients[13].

Research comparing Kylie bed sheets, disposable draw sheets and a polyweb pad indicated that the Kylie had greater absorption properties, was kinder to skin and reduced odour and costs[14]. Since those trials, many manufacturers have produced bed protectors which they claim offer a superior performance and are more economical than the Kylie bedsheet. There are more than 30 similar products on the market now, although few have been subject to controlled trials. It is difficult to make informed choices about the effectiveness of such products without unbiased information about their performance[15].

Urinary sheaths and collection devices

Urinary sheaths and collection devices can contain urinary incontinence in men. Many older men suffer from retraction of the penis though few writers mention this problem. It can be almost impossible to fix a urinary sheath onto a retracted penis. Using a pubic pressure device can correct retraction and make it possible to fit a urinary sheath. Pubic pressure devices must be correctly fitted. They can be obtained if the GP sends a referral letter to the surgical appliances department (usually at the local hospital). The resident is seen, assessed to determine suitability and if suitable a pubic pressure device is ordered.

Complications of using urinary sheaths

Allergy and tissue damage – Most urinary sheaths are made from latex (though pure silicone sheaths are now available) and research indicates that many men can suffer from a skin rash and an allergic reaction to latex. Sheaths are normally held in place with adhesive or a strap fixed around the shaft of the penis that the sheath fits over. One researcher found that 40% of men using urinary sheaths had experienced allergic reactions to either the sheath material or the adhesive used to fix sheaths[16]. Sheaths are rolled on to the penis and if the sheath is not the correct size a ring of sheath material can compress the shaft of the penis. This can cause tissue damage and in extreme cases pressure necrosis[17].

Outflow obstruction – It is important that sheaths are the correct size and are made of materials that do not twist too easily. Sheaths that are too large can easily twist at the tip of the penis and can cause outflow obstruction. Older men are particularly at risk of outflow obstruction as the prostate enlarges with age. Outflow obstruction predisposes to infection and can lead to ureteric reflux and in some cases to pyelonephritis and renal damage that can cause renal failure[18].

Infection – Wearing a urinary sheath increases the risk of developing a urinary tract infection. One study found that 87% of older men who wore urinary sheaths developed infection over a five month period[19].

Preventing complications

You can prevent complications by taking the following action.

Ensure that you assess the person's suitability for a sheath
A male resident who has a large residual urine (over 150 ml) may be suffering from outflow obstruction and a urinary sheath would be inadvisable.

Patients with compromised immune status are at high risk of developing infection.

Patients with allergies may react to adhesive or material – test by cutting a piece of sheath off and strapping to inner aspect of arm for 48 hours, then inspect.

Patients who are circumcised are more at risk of tissue damage because urine comes in direct contact with tip of penis.

Choose the right material

Latex allergy is increasingly common

Consider silicone sheaths

Choose the right size

Check the length – to avoid the risk of twisting and outflow obstruction

Check the width – to avoid the risk of pressure necrosis and tissue damage

Give enough fluid

Ensure fluid intake is adequate – concentrated urine will cause skin damage

Provide good hygiene

Remove sheath and wash at least once daily. Ensure that foreskin is retracted and tip of penis is cleaned. Failure to ensure this is done can lead to infection, phimosis and stricture.

Preventing skin problems in incontinence

Individuals who suffer from urinary incontinence are at risk of developing infection, macerated skin and even sores[20]. Using soap to wash the person after each incontinent episode normally presents no problems. Soap though is alkaline (pH 9) and can strip the skin of essential oils. Stripping the skin of oils can render it more likely to become dry and crack; any break in skin integrity predisposes a person to infection and increases the risk of pressure sores. Some practitioners now recommend that the skin should only be washed with plain water; others recommend that the skin should not be washed after incontinent episodes. Personally I feel that the skin should be washed after each episode of incontinence to remove traces of urine that can damage skin; pH balanced soap, skin washes, soap with moisturisers (available in unperfumed versions), Simple Soap, pH balanced cleansing lotions and emulsifying ointment can all be used to clean skin, retain the acid mantle of the skin at pH 5.5 and maintain skin health. If the skin is sore, plain water should be used. Many continence advisers do not recommend the use of barrier creams. Overuse of barrier creams can clog up incontinence pads and lead to leakage.

Conclusion

Using research-based care enables you to:

- Choose the right type of product to contain incontinence
- Choose the right size of product to contain incontinence
- Contain incontinence effectively
- Reduce nursing workload
- Avoid the complications of poorly managed incontinence
- Enable the person to maintain dignity.

There is no one 'correct method' to achieve these aims. You need to offer continence management strategies that are as individual as the people you care for.

References

[1] Fader, M.J., Barnes, K.E., Malone Lee, J.G. & Cottenden, A.M. (1986) Incontinence garments; results of a DHSS study. *Health Equipment Information*, 159.

[2] Journet, C. (1981) *DHSS Aids Assessment Programme: Incontinence Aids for Handicapped Children*. The Stationery Office, London.

[3] Cottenden, A.M. (1986) Incontinence pads; clinical performance, design, technical properties. *Journal of Biomedical Engineering*, **10**, 506–514.

[4] Malone Lee, J.G., McCreery, M. & Exon Smith, A.N. (1982) *A Community Study for the Performance of Incontinence Garments*. DHSS Aids Assessment Programme. The Stationery Office, London.

[5] Bridle, K. (1999) *Nappies and the environment*. Hampshire County Council website: www: hants.og.uk

[6] Cottenden, A.M. (1992) Aids and Appliances for Incontinence. In: *Clinical Nursing Practice*. Roe B (ed.). Prentice Hall, Hemel Hempstead.

[7] Noonan, E. (1990) Disposing of the disposables. *Nonwovens Industry*, July, 20–26.

[8] Haeker, S. (1985) Disposable Vs reusable incontinence products. *Geriatric Nursing*, **6**, 345–347.

[9] Hu, T., Kaltreider, D.L. & Igou, J. (1990) The cost effectiveness of disposable versus reusable diapers. *Journal of Gerontological Nursing*, **16**(2), 19–24.

[10] Grant, R. (1982) Washable pads or disposable diapers. *Geriatric Nursing*, July/August, 248–251.

[11] Palmer, M.H. *et al.* (1991) Risk factors for urinary incontinence one year after nursing home admission. *Research in Nursing & Health*, **14**(6), 4054–4062.

[12] Silberg, J. (1977) A hospital study of a new absorbent bed pad for incontinent patients. *Medical Journal of Australia*, 14 April, 512–516.

[13] Pottle, B. (1986) When the sheets were changed. *Nursing Times*, 26 November, 64–66.

[14] Smith, B. (1985) A comparative trial of urinary incontinence aids. *British Journal of Clinical Practice*, **39**(8), 311–319.

[15] Clancy, B. (1989) Bed protectors; no easy choice. *Nursing Times*, **85**(33), 70–75.

[16] Bransbury, A.J. (1979) Allergy to rubber condom urinals and medical adhesives in male spinal injured patients. *Contact Dermatitis*, **5**, 317–323.

[17] Golji, H. (1981) Complications of external catheter drainage. *Paraplegia*, **19**, 189–197.

[18] Jayachandran, S., Mooppan, U.M.M. & Kim, H. (1985) Complications from external (condom) urinary drainage devices. *Urology*, **xxv**(1), 31–34.

[19] Ouslander, J.G., Greengold, B. & Chen, S. (1987) External catheter use and urinary tract infections among incontinent nursing home patients. *Journal American Geriatrics Society*, **35**(12), 1063–1070.

[20] Palmer, M.H., German, P.S. & Ouslander, J.G. (1991) Risk factors for urinary incontinence one year after nursing home admission. *Research in Nursing and Health*, **14**(6), 405–412.

Chapter 9

Risk Management

Introduction

In the past nurses, especially those caring for older people, tried to keep people safe. In 1986 I remember the registration officer requiring that every resident's bed had bed rails 'to prevent falls'. The culture that we worked in was a blame culture and nurses covered their backs and took no risks. Now that has changed and nurses are encouraged to empower and enable residents and to manage risk rather than seek to eliminate it.

Risk has been defined as:

'The possibility of incurring misfortune or loss'
'To be exposed to danger or loss'
'To be vulnerable'

Life is full of risks. We take risks every time we get out of bed, every time we step in the car, every time we cross the road. If we decide to cower under the duvet, we merely exchange one set of risks for another. We cannot avoid risks entirely but what we can do is reduce the probability that major problems will occur. In order to do that, we need information. Our decisions are only as good as the information on which they are based.

This chapter aims to:

- Enable you to identify risk
- Enable you to classify the degree of risk and seriousness of outcome
- Provide information about relevant legislation
- Help you to obtain further information about risk management

---

Why identify and classify risk?

Managers of registered homes and nurses in charge of a shift must be able to identify and manage risk. There are three reasons why nurses must manage risk: to protect residents, to protect staff and to manage well. Recently the UKCC stated: 'The ultimate aim of risk management is the promotion of quality'[1].

In 1997, according to Health and Safety Executive figures, 67 people were blinded, 1006 lost limbs and 303 people were poisoned at work. In 1998, 261 people were killed in workplace accidents[2].

While we would all agree that life is about risk and without risks life would be dull and impoverished[3], it is clear that risk must be managed. Life is about responsible risk-taking about weighing up costs and benefits. If professionals are to manage risk, they must be able to identify it and measure it. If you cannot measure something then you cannot manage it.

Can we manage risk?

It is important to recognise that no home can ever hope to offer a totally safe environment. No home should be expected to offer a totally safe environment[4,5]. Instead, the home should develop policies that identify potential risks and should work with residents and families to determine the acceptable level of risk[6].

No home can ever hope to offer staff a totally safe environment. Homes cannot hope to eliminate the chance combination of circumstances that lead to accident. People with responsibility for health and safety within homes have to strike a balance between offering an enabling environment and a safe environment. In order to do this, managers and staff must develop policies that identify potential risks and they must work together to determine acceptable levels of risk.

Hazards

A hazard is the potential to cause harm or damage:

> 'Hazard identification is the systematic consideration of all the equipment, processes, activities etc. associated with your work and that of others in the home, that may cause anyone personal injury or ill health or that may cause damage to property.'[7]

Hazards can potentially harm residents, staff, relatives and other visitors. Table 9.1 gives details of possible hazards that residents may face. As you can see from Table 9.1, residents are at risk not only from staff practice but also from the actions of other residents and relatives. One resident may wet on the toilet floor, exposing other residents to the risk of falls or injuries. A relative may bring in medication for her mother's pain, and give it to her exposing the resident to many risks. The home is also hazardous to staff. Table 9.2 outlines some of the risks that staff are exposed to in the workplace.

As you can see from these tables, if a home is not safe for staff, it is not safe for residents. Residents can be put at risk by other residents as well as by staff. Staff can be put at risk by thoughtless or overworked colleagues who fail to report hazards. Staff can be put at risk by managers who fail to take health and safety seriously. Managers can be placed in impossible situations by staff who think health and safety is solely a management responsibility. Health and safety in the workplace must be a team effort.

Risk evaluation

When you have identified hazards the next step is to determine the level of risk. Is the level of risk high, medium, or low? The risk assessment process is:

Table 9.1   Some potential hazards to residents.

Hazard	Cause	Consequence
Abuse	Staff, relatives, residents	Physical and psychological harm
Alteration of room layout	Staff, relatives, residents	Physical and psychological harm
Changes in floor level	Design of home	Falls, injury
Chemicals left out	Staff	Skin damage, ingestion
Fire	Equipment, staff, residents, relatives	Physical and psychological harm
Floors strewn obstacles	Staff, residents, relatives	Falls, loss of mobility
Inappropriate care	Staff, relatives	Loss of independence, neglect
Inadequate, absent lights	Poor maintenance, design	Falls, injury
Manual handling techniques	Staff, relatives	Falls, dislocations, injury
Medication	Staff, GPs, relatives	Adverse reactions, illness
Poorly maintained furniture	Staff, management	Falls, injuries
Poorly maintained equipment, e.g. wheelchairs with flat tyres, broken brakes	Staff, management, outside agencies	Falls, injuries
Stairs	Design, management, inspectors	Falls, injuries
Wet floors	Staff, residents, relatives	Falls, injuries

Step one: Identify hazards
Step two: Who is likely to be exposed to these hazards?
Step three: Evaluate risk associated with each hazard
Step four: Implement specific measures to eliminate or reduce hazards
Step five: Check if these measures have been effective

Managers carrying out risk assessment can feel overwhelmed. You may identify 20 or 30 potential hazards in one area, such as the kitchen. Where do you start? How do you begin to prioritise?

Risk ratings

Assessing the level of risk as high, medium or low enables you to begin to prioritise. Is the chef likely to burn his hand on a saucepan? The difficulty with this approach is that although something might be very likely to happen, the consequences might not be very serious. Assessing the risk and the severity makes it easier for you to determine priorities. Table 9.3 shows how this works.

Table 9.2 Some potential hazards to staff.

Hazard	Cause	Consequence
Abuse	Residents, relatives, manager, staff	Physical and psychological harm
Alteration of room layout	Residents, relatives, staff	Physical
Biological hazards	Contact body fluids, infected material	Hepatitis and blood borne infection
Changes in floor level	Design of home	Falls, injury
Chemicals	Working practice, poor ventilation	Skin damage, inhalation
Fire	Equipment, staff, residents, relatives	Physical and psychological harm
Floors strewn with obstacles	Staff, residents, relatives	Falls, loss of mobility
Inappropriate staff care	Manager, inspectors	Stress, illness
Inadequate, absent lights	Poor maintenance, design	Falls, accident, injury
Manual handling techniques	Inadequate equipment, space, training or staffing	Injury, stress, burnout
Needle-stick injury	Poor practice, inadequate facilities	Infection, illness, injury
Poorly maintained furniture	Staff, management	Injuries
Poorly maintained equipment, e.g. wheelchairs with flat tyres, broken brakes	Staff, management, outside agencies	Injuries
Stairs	Design, management, inspectors	Falls, injuries
Wet floors	Staff, residents, relatives	Falls, injuries

Table 9.3 Risk rating.

Risk likelihood	Consequence severity	Risk rating
High = 3	Death/major injury = 3	$3 \times 3 = 9$
Medium = 2	Minor injury = 2	$2 \times 2 = 4$
Low = 1	No injury = 1	$1 \times 1 = 1$

Using this method enables you to draw up a risk scale. Table 9.4 illustrates this. Using a risk scale gives you the ability to determine what you need to sort out today and how to prioritise all the other risks within the home. You can then draw up a table to enable you go through the home identifying risks and determining priorities. A sample form that you may wish to use is given at the end of this chapter.

Table 9.4 Risk scale.

Risk rating	Potential consequences	Priority
3 × 3 = 9	Highest risk, most serious consequence	Urgent, highest possible priority
3 × 2 = 6	High risk, serious consequence	High priority
2 × 2 = 4	Medium risk, less serious consequence	Medium priority
1 × 3 = 3	Low risk, most serious consequences	Medium priority because of the severity of consequences
2 × 1 = 2	Medium risk, less serious consequences	Medium priority
1 × 1 = 1	Low risk, less serious consequences	Low priority, but do not ignore

Control measures

Identifying and measuring risk gives you the ability to begin to manage that risk. You must deal with high risk, severe consequence risk urgently. Control measures aim, wherever possible, to eliminate risk. If elimination is not possible then introduce measures to control risk.

Evaluation

How do you know if your policies are working? Unless you evaluate, you do not know. Evaluation is crucially important. Sometimes we do not notice changes in the workplace; reviewing risk assessments enables you to pick up those subtle changes that might otherwise be missed. The following sections look at other relevant legislation.

Legal aspects

There are several laws governing health and safety in the workplace. These are:

- Common law
- The Health and Safety at Work Act 1974
- Management of Health and Safety at Work Regulations 1992, amended 1994
- Control of Substances Hazardous to Health 1988 – known as COSHH
- Reporting of Injury, Disease and Dangerous Occurrences Regulations 1995 known as Riddor
- Manual Handling Operations Regulations 1992
- Fire Safety Regulations 1997

Common law

Common law has evolved over the last 1000 years and is unwritten. Under common law, each of us has a 'duty of care'. Employers, statutory bodies and professionals who breach this duty may be sued for negligence. In negligence claims the person suing must prove:

- That the company/person had a general duty of care to prevent fore-seeable injuries
- That the failure to prevent injury was negligent
- That this failure caused the injury.

The case history below illustrates how negligence claims can work.

Case history

In 1996, a resident's bath oil was spilt on a vinyl 'nonslip' floor. The care assistant bathing the resident accompanied the resident to her room. She did not mop up the bath oil, as she was busy. Anyhow, it was the last bath of the morning. Soon the domestic would come to clean the bathroom. Unfortunately, the domestic didn't come soon enough. The resident's elderly visitor, noting that the bath oil had not been brought back from the bathroom went to fetch it. She slipped on the floor and fractured her femur. She sued the home for negligence. Her solicitor argued that the home was negligent in failing to prevent a foreseeable accident. The nursing home settled out of court on legal advice.

People whose actions have contributed to their injury may be found 'contributory negligent' and any damages awarded may be reduced. This will be discussed in more detail later in this chapter under manual handling.

The Health and Safety at Work Act 1974

The Health and Safety at Work Act was introduced in 1974[8]. The Act is the main piece of legislation and outlines broad principles concerning health and safety. Other more recent legislation is more specific. The Act is a piece of criminal law and people who fail to comply with the Act can be prosecuted and fined or jailed if found guilty.

Employer responsibilities are:

- Those who employ more than five people must prepare, review and revise a written health and safety policy. This should acknowledge and comply with legislation.
- Employers must ensure the health and safety of employees at work and other people on the premises.
- Employers must display a certificate of employer's liability insurance
- Employers must display the poster *Health and Safety Law – what you should know* or distribute leaflets giving this information.
- Employers must ensure that employees receive adequate and appropriate information, instruction and training to carry out their work safely.

Employee responsibilities are:

- Employees must comply with legislation and ensure that their actions do not adversely affect others
- Employees are entitled to sue their employers if they have been injured in the course of their work.

Self-employed people (such as the window cleaner) must comply with legislation and ensure that their actions do not adversely affect others. Manufacturers and suppliers must ensure that their products are safe when used properly. They must provide health and safety information about their products.

Management of Health and Safety at Work Regulations

The Management of Health and Safety at Work Regulations 1992 were amended in 1994 by the Management of Health and Safety at Work (Amendment) Regulations. It is these regulations that require employers to carry out risk assessments. The key points of the regulations are as follows.

Employers are required to:

- Assess risks associated with the business to determine how to eliminate or minimise those risks
- Take action to eliminate or minimise risks
- Appoint 'competent persons' to help meet the requirements. This can be the manager or a member of staff. If no one within the home has the skills, then consultants can be used.
- Ensure that temporary staff (including agency staff) are informed of any health and safety information and/or the skills necessary to do their job.
- Consider the capabilities of each individual to do their work safely.

Employees are required to:

- Adhere to the instructions, policies and procedures laid down by their employer
- Report any shortcomings in the employer's arrangements – for example, if there are instructions that Mrs X is to be moved using the hoist but the hoist is broken.

New and expectant mothers

The workplace can damage the health of mothers and that of their unborn children[9]. Research shows that working long hours, working shifts, heavy physical labour and stress can affect pregnancy[10]. The 1994 amendment regulations recognise that new and expectant mothers are particularly vulnerable in the workplace. Employers must carry out specific risk assessment that includes the risks to expectant, new mothers and mothers who are breast-feeding. The Health and Safety Executive produce guidance[11]. RCN members can obtain a free guide from their local RCN office.

Control of Substances Hazardous to Health 1988 (COSHH)

COSHH regulations distinguish between the hazards and risks of substances commonly used in the home. The manager's responsibilities under COSHH are to:

- *Identify hazardous items.* Some common kitchen hazards are bleach, disinfectant, descaler and dishwasher powder.

- *Identify how these items could affect health.* Ensure that potentially harmful substances such as bleach are labelled. Maintain a file of chemicals used and action to be taken in case of splashing or swallowing. Your suppliers can provide this information.
- *Devise secure storage systems.* Ensure that potentially hazardous substances are stored under lock and key. Beware the bottle of bleach under the sink or staff leaving cleaning trolleys where they are easily accessible.
- *Train staff.* New national minimum standards recommend induction courses and three study days for all staff, including ancillary staff.

Reporting of Injury, Disease and Dangerous Occurrences Regulations 1995 (Riddor)

Riddor legislation is not specific to care environments. It was in fact drafted with the building industry in mind. Under Riddor, employers or designated managers must report the following occurrences to their local Health & Safety Executive (HSE)[12].

Death or major injury
In the case of death, or major injury requiring hospitalisation, to a member of staff, the public or a subcontractor, the manager must telephone the HSE and details will be taken. This should be followed up with a completed accident report on form F2508 within ten days of the occurrence. Relevant reportable injuries are:

- Fracture other than to the fingers, thumbs or toes
- Amputation
- Dislocation of the shoulder, hips, knee or spine
- Acute illness requiring medical treatment where there is reason to believe that this resulted from exposure to a biological agent or its toxins or infected material.

Over three-day injury
If an accident occurs, including an assault, connected with work and the employee or contractor is unable to work for three days or more, then a completed accident report form must be sent to the HSE. This three-day period includes non-working days. If a member of staff injures her back and has one day off, unless she reports that she is taking her days off as usual you should report the incident to the HSE.

Disease
If a doctor informs you that an employee is suffering from a reportable work-related disease, you must send a completed disease report form (F2508A) to the HSE. Relevant examples are:

- Skin diseases such as occupational dermatitis. Current HSE opinion is that this includes latex allergy and hand dermatitis.
- Infections such as hepatitis, tuberculosis, legionellosis and MRSA.

Dangerous occurrences

This near-miss clause compels mangers to report occurrences that could have but did not cause serious injury. If a wall collapsed and narrowly missed hitting someone, this should be reported. The HSE should be telephoned and a completed form (F2508B) sent within ten days. Relevant examples are:

- Unintended collapse of a wall or floor in a place of work
- A chandelier falling from the ceiling
- Explosion or fire causing suspension of normal work for over 24 hours
- Collapse of load-bearing parts of lifts.

Records

Employers must keep records of any injury, reportable disease or dangerous occurrence. You can comply with legislation by keeping copies of the report forms in a file, recording details on computer or maintaining a written log.

Fire Precautions (Workplace) Regulations 1997

In the past, fire safety regulations were determined by the local fire officer. The fire officer visited and decided which particular measures were necessary to comply with fire safety regulations. On 1 December 1997, the new regulations came into force. These implemented part of the general fire safety provisions of the European Framework and Workplace Directive. The regulations specify minimum fire safety standards in places where people work. In situations where the employer does not have control over part of the workplace, this is the responsibility of the person who has control. If an employer leases an office in a block, the landlord or letting agent would have responsibility for common areas outside the employer's control, such as stairs and hallways. In nursing homes employers' responsibilities are:

- Risk assessment
- Fire detection and warnings
- Means of escape
- Provision of fire fighting equipment
- Planning for an emergency and training staff.

Risk assessment

Managers are already required to assess health and safety risks. Fire safety can either be incorporated into this or carried out separately. You need to keep a formal record and determine if your current arrangements are satisfactory. If you need to change anything, record any proposed changes. You need to inform staff of any changes. Ensure that staff have access to this in case they need to refer to it.

Nursing homes should already be complying with the other aspects of legislation.

Documentation

The UKCC recently commented that it considered that professionals had both a legal and professional duty of care. They emphasised the importance of record keeping: 'The approach to record keeping which courts of law adopt tends to be "if it is not recorded it has not been done".'[13]

Summary

Employers, managers and professionals have a legal responsibility to ensure that the workplace is as safe as possible. This can be achieved by proactive work, such as risk assessment, and reactive work, such as acting after accidents have occurred. Risk assessment involves identifying hazards and determining the level of risk posed by these hazards. Risk management involves eliminating hazards, wherever possible, and acting to reduce risks when this is not possible. Auditing enables you to discover how effective your health and safety policy is.

Conclusion

Risk assessment is becoming increasingly important. Homes that fail to assess and document risk are wide open to claims of negligence and malpractice. The national minimum standards will increase the emphasis on risk assessment.

Moving and handling

Only one group of workers, those working in the building industry, are more likely than nurses to be injured at work. Most nursing staff are at high risk of back injury. Employers, managers and staff have legal responsibilities to ensure that residents and staff are not injured during moving and handling. Legislation requires assessment of all moving and handling tasks. New guidance states that 'other than in an emergency' nurses should no longer manually handle patients.

This section aims to:

- Update you on the latest expert opinion regarding moving and handling
- Refresh your knowledge of legal responsibilities
- Enable you to assess manual handling risks in your workplace
- Discuss how to assess an individual's manual handling risk
- Discuss how to educate staff and promote safe practice

Legal aspects

Research carried out in an elderly care ward indicated that two nurses lifted an average of $2\frac{1}{2}$ tons an hour. Another research project surveying more than 3000 nurses found that one nurse in six suffered low back pain as a result of handling patients. Legislation aims to prevent workers becoming injured at work. The relevant legislation is the Health & Safety at Work Act 1974[14] and the Manual Handling Regulations 1992. The Manual Handling Regulations aim to prevent back injury by evaluating handling tasks and reducing or eliminating the need for manual handling. Employers have legal duties to: 'so far as reasonably practical, avoid the need for employees to undertake any manual handling operations at work which involve the risk of their being injured.'

Manual Handling Regulations

The regulations are supplemented by guidance from the Health & Safety Executive[15] and the Health and Safety Commission[16]. The key points are as follows.

Weight limits
Neither the regulations nor the guidance contain any weight limits. These documents state that there is no threshold below which handling must be regarded as safe.

Assessment
All manual handling operations must be assessed. In a home, this means that every operation that involves lifting must be assessed. Do you know how much a full laundry bag full of damp towels, etc. weighs? What is the weight of the soap powder or detergent drums? How will they be moved? How much do the boxes of incontinence pads weigh? Where are staff expected to store things like incontinence pads? Lifting upwards is dangerous. The guidance produces numerical guidance to simplify assessment of minor tasks.

Every individual who requires manual handling should be assessed. This manual handling assessment should include weight, factors affecting handling and methods to be used to handle the resident. Ideally, the home should have a designated manual handling co-ordinator responsible for assessing manual handling. Manual handling of residents is discussed in detail later in this chapter.

Training
Employers have a legal duty to provide training to enable staff to move residents and avoid injury. The latest recommendations are that all staff receive classroom-based training on induction. Training required will depend on previous level of training but should be between two and five days. Regular refresher training is required with one day a year in-house or classroom-based[17]. Written records of staff training should be kept. These should include details of handouts and information supplied to staff, including what is not acceptable within the home, for example manual handling or certain types of manual handling.

Equipment
The employer is required to provide a range of equipment to enable staff to handle residents and other loads safely. The range of equipment available within a nursing home may include hoists, standing hoists, transfer boards, monkey poles and sliding sheets. Under legislation, the employer could argue that provision of equipment is not necessary because the cost of supplying equipment *greatly* outweighs the risk of injury. This stance is

unlikely to cut much ice with the employer's insurer. Increasingly insurers demand evidence of risk assessment before agreeing to insure. In 1996, the RCN legal department won more than £8.5 million in compensation for members who suffered back injuries.

Recording accidents

The employer is required to introduce procedures for recording accidents, investigating causes and, when possible, setting up systems to prevent their recurrence.

Staff responsibilities

Staff have responsibilities under the code. They must enable employers to develop and implement a code of practice on the handling of residents, and they must inform the employer of any situation that might present 'a serious and imminent danger' and any shortcomings in the arrangements for manual handling. These include lack of staff, lack of equipment, faulty machinery, injuries or accidents, illness or disability affecting handling capacity. Pregnancy is neither an illness nor disability but pregnant women are more vulnerable to back injury than other workers. Staff must comply with employer's policies on moving and handling, and nurses must have access to and follow the written individual handling assessments.

Nurses are responsible for updating assessment of resident handling needs, recording any accidents that occur and helping to investigate and set up systems to prevent recurrence.

To lift or not to lift?

For many years, the Royal College of Nursing has pressed for a no lifting policy. In 1992, the RCN and the National Back Pain Association produced a code of practice that included statements about weight limits. The code stated that, under ideal conditions, no nurse should take the full weight of any resident weighing more than 30 kg, i.e. about five stones. The weight limit for two nurses was 50 kg, i.e. 7 st 12 lb. The guide was updated in 1993 and stated that in practice very few residents could be lifted manually. The guidance condemned four lifting techniques as unsafe. These were the drag lift, the orthodox lift, lifting with the resident's arms around the nurse's neck and the use of poles or canvasses.

The latest guidance[18] states: 'You must not lift people because:

- They weigh too much and are unpredictable
- It is difficult or impossible for people to get into a safe position to lift
- Nurses are at risk of injury in all manual handling techniques
- Most lifts include a risk of injuring the resident
- Manual lifts are not therapeutic; they do not improve the resident's mobility.'

The 1998 guide states that: 'There is no such thing as an emergency. It is the manager's responsibility to ensure that all eventualities have been planned for in advance.' The guidance distinguishes between foreseeable emergencies and real emergencies. Managers are responsible for creating plans for foreseeable emergencies. Foreseeable emergencies include:

- Cardiac or respiratory arrest
- Collapsed residents and staff in a range of situations
- Handling residents in the accident and emergency area
- Fire, bomb and other evacuations.

Lifting manually is only permitted in what the guide defines as four real emergencies. These are situations where the victim must be moved to safety immediately. There is no time to get equipment or plan the move. Risks may have to be taken when the person is:

- In water and in danger of drowning
- In an area that is on fire or filling with smoke
- In danger from bomb or bullet
- In danger from a collapsing building or other structure.

Status of the guide

The guide does not affect primary legislation. It is an advisory document and the techniques it condemns are not banned. Many physiotherapists have expressed concern that this advice will adversely affect resident rehabilitation. New guidance from the Chartered Society of Physiotherapists recommends that if a particular technique is the only one possible, the physiotherapist must now justify its use and carry it out safely. They stress the importance of assessing and documenting manual handling techniques. Physiotherapists should not, the guidance concludes, assume that others who lack physiotherapy backgrounds can be taught such techniques[19].

Managers cannot afford to ignore this guide. In legal cases, the previous edition has been used as a guide. If you are using manual handling techniques in your home, every person lifting must be trained. Every person being moved must be assessed. Documentation must be impeccable, otherwise the home is open to being sued for negligence or fined for breach of health and safety legislation.

Nurses refusing to lift

In 1989, Nurse Grant was reported to the UKCC professional conduct committee for gross professional misconduct because she refused to lift a patient. She was found not guilty. In 1996, the UKCC stated that it would look at such cases on an individual basis. In the UKCC's view, although the most important consideration is the safety and well-being of the resident, it must not be at the expense of the nurse's health and safety. It stresses the importance of the nurse documenting reasons for refusal. The UKCC has yet to comment on how the latest guidance affects their position.

Agency nurses

The agency nurse is not directly employed by the home but recent court cases have found the employer responsible in such cases. The courts consider that the employer must take reasonable steps to ensure that contractors such as agency nurses have been trained and assessed as competent in lifting and handling residents. At the time of writing, one nursing home is being sued because a registered nurse from the agency was asked to help lift a resident. The nurse developed back pain the next day and is suing.

Managers and employers should ensure that they have a written assurance from the agency they use that staff are fully trained in the moving and handling of residents.

Vicarious liability

Vicarious liability means that the employer is responsible for the actions of employees. Even if an employee breaches the employer's guidance, the employer is liable. In one case, where two nurses were lifting on the count of three and one failed to lift, the employer was found liable. In another case, where two staff lifted a resident and one injured her back, the employer was found liable. The manual handling assessment and care plan stated the resident was to be hoisted.

Contributory negligence

When nurses breach employer's guidance, injure themselves and sue, the question of contributory negligence arises. If the nurse used a prohibited lift, or lifted when she should not have done, she may be 'contributory negligent'. If she is considered 25% at fault then damages will be reduced by this amount. In some cases, the employer is held to account because policies are unworkable. One employer's guidance stated that hoists must be used to toilet residents but the hoists would not go through the toilet doors.

Assessing workplace manual handling risks

Figure 9.1 outlines responsibilities under the Act, showing the questions that must be asked. When you have completed your assessment you must document your findings and the measures you have taken to reduce risk. Guidance recommends that you date your assessment and carry out another assessment every year. If you have evidence to suggest that your policies are not working, you will need to reassess as soon as you are aware of this.

Assessing an individual's risk

Every resident should have a moving and handling assessment. It is good practice to complete a short assessment even on residents who do not require assistance. The assessment should indicate when the person requires help and what help is required, and should detail any aids that will be used. This assessment should be documented and referred to in the care plan. The assessment should be updated every six months, or sooner if the individual's needs change.

Educating staff and promoting safe practice

In the NHS the costs of staff back pain are £480 million a year[20]. Although the Manual Handling Regulations were introduced in 1992, the level of back injury has not fallen[21]. Why? Is it because hospitals and homes do not assess people although they are required to do so? Is it because staff do not always

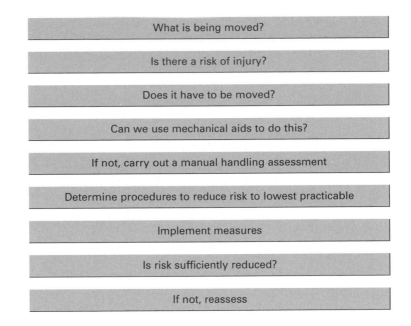

Fig. 9.1   Guide to manual handling responsibilities.

move people in the ways that the assessments identify? Is it because our new ways of moving people have introduced a new set of risks? The reasons are not yet clear. What is clear is that we need to educate staff and reinforce good practice. We need to stop moving people around so much and encourage those who can move to move themselves.

Documentation

Nurses are not good at documenting what they have done. This is not surprising because the amount of paperwork nurses are required to complete has risen by 39% in the last five years. The time nurses spend with residents has fallen proportionally. Unfortunately, if you do not have the documentation to support your claims, inspectors and the courts will consider, 'if it isn't documented, it isn't done'. It is difficult to balance the need to document with the need to spend time with increasingly frail and vulnerable residents. Some homes are now using computers to plan and manage care and to complete assessments. Nurses report that this does save time once they have become used to the system. Perhaps this will be something we will all be doing when the next edition of this book is published.

Falls

Older people are more likely to fall than any other group. The National Service Framework for Older People identifies the reduction of falls as a major issue. Frail elderly people are at great risk of falling. Falls can be fatal. Some nursing home staff do not yet have the skills to minimise the risk of falls. Research suggests that some staff try to prevent falls by discouraging walking, using wheelchairs and using sedation. These strategies are counterproductive. It is possible to find out who is at risk of falling and to reduce risks[22]. You need to know why older people fall and how to prevent falls.

This section aims to:

- Explain why falls occur
- Discuss ways to reduce falls
- Enable you to assess risk factors
- Discuss how to manage risk

The risk of falls

The risk of falls rises with age; 30% of 65 year olds, 50% of 80 year olds, and every 85-year-old falls once a year[23]. Almost all hip fractures (90%) occur in people aged over 70 and are caused by falls[24]. Seventy percent of deaths caused by falls occur in very elderly people[25]. Nursing home residents are three times more likely to fall than people living in their own homes[26]. A study in Spanish nursing homes found that women were more likely to fall than men. The average female nursing home resident had two falls a year. Three-quarters of male residents fell once a year. A third of residents had two or more falls in six months. A study in a Japanese nursing home found that 37% of residents had at least one fall a year.

Why do falls occur?

If we do not intervene, our residents will fall. Before we can begin to intervene, we need to know why our residents fall. Many factors influence the person's risk factors relating to the individual and to the environment.

Factors relating to the individual

Poor mobility increases the risk of falls. The person who is less mobile loses muscle strength and balance deteriorates[27].

Poor vision increases the risk of falls. Researchers found that 76% of residents admitted to a geriatric unit following a fall had poor vision; 40% needed glasses, 37% had cataracts, 14% senile macular degeneration. Seventy nine percent of individuals with poor vision were treatable[28].

Cardiac disease, especially poorly treated cardiac disease, increases the risk of falls[29]. When the person stands up the pulse rate fails to rise rapidly maintaining blood supply to the brain. The person feels dizzy and may fall or walk less, or walk fearfully.

Parkinson's disease, arthritis, and poor depth perception also increase the risk of falling[30]. Parkinson's affects the gait and makes it difficult to balance and walk. Arthritis leads to pain and joint instability, increasing the risk of falls.

Fear of falling and the anxiety brought on by moving to a new environment increase the risk of falling[31]. One study investigated people who had fallen. People who became fearful after falling gradually became less able to balance, less able to walk easily and became more confused than those who were not afraid[32]. The person who is terrified of falling will probably fall.

Depression increases the risk of falling. Many of our residents are depressed. These residents are becoming less able and more frail[33]. As the level of disability increases, the depression increases[34]. Depression makes people more accident-prone[35] so the risk of falls increases and the person becomes more miserable and fearful.

Medication increases the risk of falling. Older people are more vulnerable to the effects of medication than any other group. Unfortunately, older people are more likely to be prescribed medication than any other group. Older people consume 43% of all prescribed medicines, more than any other group[36]. More than 90% of people aged 75 or over are prescribed regular medicines[37]. Older people are prescribed an average of four medicines[38]. In US nursing homes, the average resident is prescribed an average of eight regular medicines[39].

Antidepressants increase the risk of falling[40] by between 50% and 200%[41]. Tricyclic antidepressants can cause a fall in standing blood pressure and this can lead to dizziness and fainting[42]. Well-informed doctors are aware that tricyclic antidepressants increase the risk of falls. When the newer seratonin reuptake inhibitor antidepressants such as fluoxetine were introduced, doctors thought that they were safer and would not increase the risk of falls[43]. Soon research from nursing homes was disproving this. A study of over 2000 people living in Tennessee nursing homes proved that there was little difference in fall rates in those treated with tricyclics and newer antidepressants. Every person receiving antidepressants had a higher rate of falls than those who were not. The rate of falls increased as the dose of antidepressant rose[44]. Older people receiving antidepressants are more likely to fall and fracture a hip than those who are not[45].

Sedatives and benzodiazepines increase the risk of falling. The risk is dose-related and increases in line with the number of sedatives and anti-depressants taken[46].

Other factors that can increase the risk of falls are poor nutrition, anaemia and infection.

Environmental factors

Environmental factors can cause falls. In Australia, government offered older people free home safety checks and subsidised the cost of modifications required. Modifications included non-slip flooring, improved lighting and grab rails. The total number of falls fell by 63%[47]. In Norway, researchers found that environmental modifications reduced falls by 48% and the number of fractures fell by 26%. There was no reduction in the rate of falls in nursing homes, possibly because the nursing home environment was much safer than older people's homes[48].

Reducing the risk of falls

Small changes can reduce the risk of falls dramatically[49]. Identifying the individual risk factors will enable you to work most effectively. Changes that will reduce the risk of falls include the following.

Encouraging exercise

Exercise programmes and specific exercises to improve balance (Tai Chi) reduce the number of falls[50]. People most at risk of falling benefit most from exercise programmes[51]. People who fall frequently benefit from exercise programmes[52]. Frequent fallers become more confident and less fearful. Muscle strength increases and the risk of falls is reduced.

Improving ability to transfer

Immobile people are less likely to fall than those who walk. Many immobile people who fall do so when transferring. Teaching people how to transfer safely reduces the risk of falls during transfers.

Reviewing medication

Minimise drug treatment. Ensure that residents are only prescribed drugs they need. Every drug has costs and benefits; weigh up the costs of certain drugs as well as the benefits. Ensure drugs are reviewed regularly; write review dates on medicine charts if you can. Eliminate the use of hypnotics; the risks far outweigh any benefits claimed in this group. Reduce sedatives to the lowest possible level, review regularly and use with caution. If a resident requires an antidepressant be aware of the risks. Use in the smallest possible dose for the shortest time. Watch for side effects. Only around 60% of residents with serious medical conditions take medication regularly enough to achieve any benefit[53]. Ensure that residents take prescribed medication.

Enhancing vision

Many residents admitted to nursing homes have not had an eye test in years. Make sure vision is as good as it can be to reduce the risk of falls.

Providing aids

Many older people are more confident and stable if they use a walking aid. Ensure residents who require aids obtain them. People with a history of toppling out of the chair trying to reach something often benefit from a 'Helping hand' aid. People with arthritis in the knees whose knees 'give' may benefit from a knee brace to improve joint stability. People with shortening after repair of fracture often benefit from a raised heel on one shoe to improve stability. People with poor tone following stroke may find a calliper supports the limb and prevents falls.

Improving nutrition

People who are well nourished feel healthier and happier and are less likely to fall than malnourished and anaemic individuals.

Assessing an individual's risk of falling

Assessing the person's risk of falling enables you to identify the risk factors that apply to an individual. A sample risk assessment form is given at the end of the chapter. You can then draw up a care plan and use a problem solving approach. You may find that despite your efforts the person retains a high risk factor. You need to go on and discuss how you manage this risk.

Managing risk

People who fall are more likely to fracture if they have osteoporosis. Older people who have osteoporosis may be prescribed calcium and vitamin D supplements to prevent further bone loss. Some people with osteoporosis will require other treatments that have been proven to increase bone mass. Treating osteoporosis reduces the risk of fracture. People who fall to the side are more likely to fracture. Older people with a history of falls, fractures and joint replacement can reduce their risk of fracture by wearing hip protectors. These absorb the impact of a fall and reduce the risk of fracture[54].

Documenting risk

It is vitally important that you document any risk assessment and write up the actions you have taken in the care plan. If you agree risk taking with the resident or relative, it is important to document this. Increasing numbers of homes are asking residents or relatives to sign risk management documents.

Communication

Some risk management documents are useless because staff have no access to them or are not aware of them. Risk management is a team effort and if it is to work, everyone must know what has been agreed.

Conclusion

Nursing home residents are at risk of falling. General policies can reduce the risk of falls. Individual assessments reduce risk still further. Measures to protect vulnerable individuals reduce the risk of fracture if falls occur.

Record keeping

Not all accidents are recorded. Sometimes we are busy, the person appears uninjured, and we never get round to recording the accident. Some nurses work in cultures where they are expected to keep people safe. In such places, accidents are viewed as failures. Nurses may fear that they will be blamed if accidents occur. In such cultures, there is the temptation not to record minor accidents. This makes it more difficult to prevent accidents because there are ten minor accidents for every major accident. Often we can learn from the minor accidents and prevent serious accidents occurring. Accidents are an important part of the audit trail. They let you know whether management policies are working or not. Sometimes your policies work but throw up a new set of problems. Only when these have been identified can they be dealt with.

This section aims to:

- Enable you to obtain relevant information about accidents
- Enable you to identify the factors leading to accidents
- Enable you to act to reduce risk
- Discuss legal obligations

Recording accidents

Any decision that we take is only as good as the information it is based on. Most accident forms are designed to meet legal requirements, not to help us prevent recurrence. If you aim to use the accident form to help you manage risk, you need a form that is tailored to your workplace or one very similar. Ideally, you should be able to change the form.

Many inspectors insist that nurses record accidents in bound books with sequential numbering. This is to avoid the possibility of forms being destroyed. You can comply with such requests and still get the information you need. Draw up and number your forms using a computer, then have them bound. Any high street printer can bind your forms in a hard cover book for around £5.

Lessons from accidents

Falls are the commonest type of accident. If you are to prevent falls and other accidents occurring you need to obtain certain information. The sort of information you need to have on your accident form includes the following.

What happened?

Most falls occur in the afternoon when the person is alone in the bedroom. Often there is no witness. If you are to prevent accidents, you need to know what happened. What was Doris doing when she fell? Did she fall off the chair? Did she fall while walking?

If you do not find out what happened you have little chance to prevent future occurrences. Doris might have slipped off her chair because staff put her bag out of reach. She might have fallen because the pressure-relieving cushion you have sat her on is making her wobble. You need to know.

What else was going on?

Many accidents occur when staff are busy. Perhaps there is too much going on at once. Perhaps you can consider ways to ensure staff are not split too many ways at the same time.

What time was it?

When you look at the timing, you will find that there are peak times when accidents occur. These peaks are linked to biorhythms and resident and staff activity. If you can identify peak risk times you can reduce, though never eliminate, these peaks.

Was anyone else involved?

One person's actions can sometimes lead to several apparently unrelated accidents. You may identify a problem with residents slipping on a wet floor. The floor could be wet because one domestic consistently leaves the floor wet or one resident splashes the floor.

Was equipment at fault?

One of the most maddening things is that when equipment is at fault and causes an accident, someone *always* knew about the faulty equipment. This is often because a minor unreported accident that caused no harm has already occurred. You need to make sure that when equipment is faulty, faults are reported and equipment is not used.

Any recent changes?

Older people are more vulnerable to accidents in certain circumstances. If the person's medication has been changed, this may affect balance and reaction. If the person has moved from one room to another, this can increase accident risk. Perhaps the person has gone off her food and is feeling weak and faint. You may know these things but will you remember them in six months?

Anything we can do to prevent recurrence?

Asking this question gives staff permission to let you know what they think the solutions are. Often they are right.

Reducing accident risk

Now that you know what is going on you can begin to introduce safeguards. You can use a problem solving approach to reduce the risk of accidents.

Case history

At the Cedars, they had had several major accidents. Registration officers were concerned and visiting frequently. The newly appointed matron did not know where to start so the Cedars employed a specialist gerontology consultant.

The adviser found that accidents, mainly falls, peaked at certain times, usually in the early morning and early afternoon. In the morning, night staff were rushed off their feet. They were expected to prepare and give out breakfasts, give out medication and clear breakfast trays. Night staff were also required to wash and dress certain residents. If it was bath day the day staff undressed the person and bathed her. In the morning call bells rang for a long time before being answered. Many residents who required help tried to get to the toilet unassisted and fell. Almost all of the residents were taking night sedation. By early afternoon, the combination of early waking and the residual effects of night sedation were taking their toll. Some of the residents were so exhausted they could barely see straight or put one foot in front of the other.

The adviser recommended:

- Reorganising the routine so that day staff gave out most medications.
- Changing the culture so that residents had more choice about when they got up
- Improving relations between day and night staff. Both sets of staff felt pressurised to get things done before the other shift came on.
- Physical examination and investigations to determine the causes of falls. This uncovered one case of undiagnosed Parkinson's disease, one individual with postural hypotension, and one anaemic individual suffering from a slow gastrointestinal bleed caused by non-steroidal anti-inflammatory drugs.
- Review of every resident's medication. This led to all hypnotics being phased out over a period of 12 weeks. Sedative use was almost eliminated.
- Introducing individual programmes to improve balance and mobility.

Within 12 weeks, accidents became rare. The inspectors congratulated staff on the improvements made and the daily visits ceased.

Cultural factors

The culture of a home can affect accident rates. In homes where dependency is high and staff feel under pressure, accident rates can rise. Staff rush to get things done and get through the work. Often when staff are rushed and pressurised, accidents can occur. Dependency within our homes is higher than ever before but resources have fallen in real terms. We are all being expected to do more and more with less and less.

Environmental factors

The environment in which residents live can increase the risk of accidents or minimise risks. The Health and Safety Executive identify two major hazards within nursing homes: radiators and lifts.

Radiators are hazardous to residents because of the high surface temperatures. Each year over 200 cases of nursing home residents suffering severe burns are reported to the HSE. Many of these residents have fallen and lain against a radiator until discovered by staff. Others are burnt when their limbs touch radiators and poor sensation, poor movement, communication difficulties and confusion prevent the person moving or calling out. The possibility that residents will be injured by high surface temperature radiators is foreseeable. To fail to act to eliminate this hazard is indefensible.

This risk can be significantly reduced by installing low surface temperature radiators, kick space heaters mounted high on a wall or underfloor heating. These changes can be expensive in most existing homes but are being specified in most new-build homes or extensions. Existing homes can significantly reduce the risk by installing radiator covers. These can be purchased or custom made. Hundreds of homes are prosecuted every year for failure to manage the risk of burns by taking such action. In Cornwall the Health and Safety Executive informed homes that they would be visiting. Many homes failed to carry out risk assessments despite this warning and now face prosecution for breaches of health and safety legislation.

Lift doors cause many accidents in nursing homes. Most lift doors work on a time delay. People have a certain time to enter the lift. After this time, the doors begin to close. Usually the lift door springs open when it meets an obstacle such as a leg. Scores of slow moving nursing home residents have suffered soft tissue injury when the lift door hits delicate, easily damaged skin. This is a predictable risk. Installing an infrared beam prevents such injuries. The lift only closes when the beam from both sides of the doors meets. If there is someone or something in the way, the door will not close. Now Health and Safety Executive officers are issuing notices when such an accident occurs. Failure to comply will result in prosecutions.

Other identified environmental hazards include:

- Poorly maintained wheelchairs. If a wheelchair does not have well-pumped up tyres the brakes will not work effectively and a person may fall on transfer. If faulty breaks are not repaired, a person may fall.
- Poorly maintained aids. A walking aid has rubber grips, known as ferrules, on the ends to prevent the aid sipping. Ferrules that have lost tread can lead to falls. The joints on Zimmer frames may work loose and

require tightening. Loose joints on frames can lead to the frame collapsing and injury occurring.

- Poor lighting, especially on stairs, can lead to falls; this means visitors and staff are most at risk as few if any of our residents are able to walk upstairs.
- Poorly maintained floors can cause falls. In older buildings, the floorboard that springs up can cause a bump. The older person with gait problems may trip. Fraying carpet and damaged vinyl can cause similar problems.

Accident review

All accident reports should be reviewed by the nurse manager, for two reasons: to discover the causes of the accident and how the accident affected the individual. The circumstances surrounding the accident may be new. The brakes may have just failed on the wheelchair but you need to be sure that the wheelchair has been taken out of use and a repair arranged. The person may have just commenced on a new drug but this may need to be reviewed urgently.

The individual may be fearful because of the fall. As fear increases the risk of falls, you may need to develop a plan of care to tackle this fear and prevent further falls. The individual may have fractured. This almost certainly indicates osteoporosis and you may need to discuss treatment with the GP.

Reviewing accidents enables you to identify the factors that have contributed to the accident. You may discover that the safeguards you put in place are not as effective as you hoped. You may find that a measure you introduced has introduced another set of risks. You may decide that the only way to prevent a person injuring themselves falling out of bed is to put a mattress on the floor. Then you find that staff are finding it difficult to get the person up in the morning or sit the person up in bed.

Education and training

Some accidents occur because we ask care assistants to perform tasks that they do not have the skills to perform. The best homes now offer a structured induction programme for care assistants. National minimum standards require that all homes provide care assistants with a comprehensive induction programme. This induction programme combined with increased levels of NVQ qualified care assistants may help to ensure that we have staff who are more able.

Abuse

Older adults are vulnerable to abuse. We know from enquiries into abuse in local authority children's homes that abusers have moved undetected from home to home because managers failed to recognise the warning signs of abuse. In September 1998 the Department of Health convened a multi-professional working group to draw up a code of practice to deal with suspected abuse in vulnerable adults[55]. This was published in 1999. There are plans to register all care workers (see Chapter 1) and to introduce a code of conduct. This will help weed out abusers. A review of accidents will enable managers to pick up the warning signs of abuse and to act promptly.

Legal aspects

The Care Standards Act and health and safety legislation require you to record accidents. Accidents and dangerous occurrences that fall within Riddor must be reported to the local Health and Safety Executive. Records of accidents must be kept until seven years after the last entry. We live in a world where relatives are more likely to sue than they were ten years ago. People seem to expect so much more than they once did. Nurses worry about what will happen if relatives sue. What will happen if Doris' daughter sues me for negligence? In such circumstances, the nurse will not be judged against impossibly high standards but against the standards of a 'professional nurse'. Documentation enables you to demonstrate that you have been aware of risks and have introduced safeguards.

It is important to realise that most complaints arise because of poor communication and poor relationships. One of the best ways to avoid these problems is to work with relatives. Let them know that you are on their side working to provide the best possible care for their loved one.

Conclusion

Reviewing accidents is not simply a case of 'locking the door after the horse has bolted'. Reviewing accidents can enable you to figure out why the horse bolted and to reduce the likelihood of other horses bolting. Reviewing accidents is part of the audit process and can help all staff learn. Good management systems also enable staff to pick up poor practice and suspected cases of abuse. Accident review enables managers to provide high quality care.

Ethical issues

In the long stay, geriatric hospitals conditions were grim. Attitudes were different then. Those of us working in the geriatric hospitals were left to get on with it. Our work was not scrutinised or inspected. Our job was to care for the patient and we got on with it. No one ever checked how well or how badly we performed. We used cotsides to stop people falling out of bed. We used Buxton chairs to prevent people falling out of chairs. We used feeding cups to stop people spilling tea over themselves. No one ever asked us about our philosophy of care or risk management. It is different now. We are expected to have a philosophy of care and policies on risk management. Our policies and accident rates are scrutinised carefully.

Whose life is it anyhow?

When we write our policies, it is easy to lose sight of the people that the policies aim to benefit. It is easy to forget Doris, Annie, Ethel and Charlie. They will not be the ones complaining if they think we have it wrong. The people we have to watch out for are our colleagues, the relative, the inspector and sometimes the boss. Consider the following cases with an ethical dimension and write down what you would do in each case.

Case history

Mrs Davis came to live at the home when her husband died. She improved physically but was bored and depressed until recently. You discovered that Mrs Davis had been a confectioner. Now Mrs Davis spends most of her time in the kitchen decorating cakes. She is making figures for the Christmas cake when the inspector arrives. The inspector says that you are breaking every health and safety rule in the book. Mrs Davis could burn herself on the soup simmering on the stove. The cook could not move fast enough to stop it. Mrs Davis, a resident, is preparing food for other residents. This is exploitation and Mrs Davis does not have a food hygiene certificate. The inspector demands your assurances that residents will in future stay out of the kitchen and other dangerous areas. What do you do? How can you justify your actions?

Case history

Annie Jones loves the garden. Every evening she takes a stroll in the beautiful gardens that surround the home. One evening Annie stumbles and falls. She fractures her wrist. Annie's daughter is furious. She demands that staff prevent her mother walking alone in the garden. 'If mother won't listen to you – call me.' That evening Annie gets up to go into the garden. You offer to accompany her but she declines. 'I just want a little peace and quiet, my dear. There's so little chance to be alone here.' What do you do? How can you justify your actions?

Case history

You are Deputy Matron of the Cedars. You arrive on duty to find that Nelly Shaw's arm is bruised and lacerated. The night sister explains that Nelly caught it on the cot side again. 'She's always doing that.' You check and find that Nelly has caught her arm in the cotside three times in the last year. You remove the cotsides. Nelly sleeps well and there are no problems. Then Matron returns from holiday. She says, 'I can't believe what you've done. What if Nelly falls out of bed? What if she fractures her femur? What if she dies?'. What do you say? How can you justify your actions?

Case history

You are the newly appointed matron of the Cedars. At the Cedars, almost everybody has cotsides; residents are tucked up in bed by 6 P.M. Night staff give everyone night sedation when they come on duty. Residents are wheeled everywhere. Most residents wear slippers. You change things. The cotsides go; the night sedation is discontinued. You introduce a more normal day for residents. You encourage mobility and the pressure sores begin to heal.

Then Fred falls, fracturing his femur. Your boss, the group manager, visits. He says, 'I'm really disappointed in you. This would never have happened when the previous matron was here'. What do you say? How can you justify your actions?

Case history

You are the new regional manager of Evergreen nursing homes. You have arranged a coach to take residents to Brighton for the day. When you arrive at the Cedars, you meet the registration officer. She demands details of how you will deal with any cardiac arrests on the trip. She suggests that you pack oxygen, airways, a portable suction machine and other equipment. Is this reasonable? How do you react?

Balancing choice and safety

When we talk about risk management, we need to be clear about who the risk belongs to. Is it Annie's risk? Do we aim to protect Annie from hurting herself? Is the risk our risk? Do we aim to protect ourselves from censure and blame? Do we aim to cover ourselves? Is the risk the organisation's risk? Do we aim to protect the organisation from being sued?

It is easy for professionals to use risk assessment to protect themselves or their organisations. It is important though to remember that the right to choose how to live our lives is one of the most fundamental of human rights. Everyone has the right to make choices and to take risks. None of us are forced to act logically and if we are honest, we will admit that sometimes we act illogically and take risks. Older people, like other citizens, have the right to take risks. Our role is to set in place safeguards to minimise the risks that people take in leading their lives. If Doris wants to walk along the corridor, we should ensure that she is wearing suitable footwear and her glasses and has her frame. We should ensure that the corridor is not littered with obstacles and that it is well lit. If Doris wants to walk along the middle of the A23, we have a duty of care to prevent this. There are limits to the risks we can enable people in our care to take.

Consent

Consent means the preferences a person makes in their life and how they indicate those preferences. The existence of a wider network of friends, family and advocates enables the person's decision making to be supported by a wider group. This network provides safeguards for the individual. When people do not have a wider network of friends and family, independent advocates can be used[56].

The ability to consent
Individuals are presumed to be competent unless they have been proven not to be so[57]. Confusion does not remove the individual's right to choose. Legal opinion is that capacity should be decided on a decision by decision basis. The person may be unable to handle her financial affairs but perfectly able to decide what to wear or what to eat[58].

Supported decision making
We can learn a great deal from the field of learning disability. In learning disability settings nurses work with individuals, enabling them and supporting them in making decisions within their capability.

The right to take risks
A certain amount of risk taking is healthy and normal, regardless of age. The Queen Mother had a history of falls and fracture. She chose to wear fairly high square heels, not the sensible lace-ups we would suggest to improve

stability. She chose to walk along racecourses using two canes rather than use more stable tripods. Obviously she chose to sacrifice a certain amount of stability for style. This involves an element of risk.

Do professionals know best?

Justin Clark spent 18 years in an institution. Psychiatrists pronounced him 'mentally incompetent'. Justin's parents went to court and a judge released Justin to their care. Justin is unable to speak. A few months after his release he used a Blisssymbol board to speak at a conference:

> 'If people think of you as a person who has many possibilities, then they will create the space for you to grow. If people think of you as a person with limits they usually don't give you so much space and you grow less. All living things are like that. A plant in good earth with water and sun will bear much fruit. A person in healthy surroundings will grow fully. Who makes the decisions? Making decisions helps you grow. You can learn from good decisions and you can learn from your mistakes. Some people believe that because we have a disability we can't make decisions. They start making choices for us. They take our lives into their hands. Then we become vulnerable.'[59]

Our aim in managing risk should always be to enable, not to disable, the people we care for – the people who really matter and the people who are so easily disempowered if we are not sensitive to their needs.

References

[1] United Kingdom Central Council (1998) *Guidelines for Records and Record Keeping.* UKCC, London.

[2] Bergman, D. (1998) Bosses get away with murder. *New Statesman*, 6 November, 29–30.

[3] Counsel and Care (1993) *The Right to Take Risks.* Counsel and Care, London.

[4] Counsel and Care (1992) *What if they hurt themselves?* Counsel and Care, London.

[5] Counsel and Care (2002) *Showing Restraint.* Counsel and Care, London.

[6] Counsel and Care (2002) *Residents taking risks.* Counsel and Care, London.

[7] Tullett, S. (1996) *Health & Safety in Care Homes. A practical guide.* Age Concern, London.

[8] Health and Safety Executive (1974) *A Guide to the Health and Safety at Work Act 1974.* HSE Books, Suffolk.

[9] Salvage, J., Rogers, R. & Cowell, R. (1998) Nurses and children at risk. *Nursing Times*, **94**(43), 34–35.

[10] Williams, N. (1996) Hazards to pregnant women at work. *Modern Midwife*, **3**, 28–30.

[11] Health and Safety Executive (1997) *New and Expectant Mothers at Work; a Guide for Employers.* HS (G) 122. Health and Safety Executive. Sheffield.

[12] Health & Safety Executive (1996) *Everyone's Guide to RIDDOR 95.* Single copies are available free from HSE Books, PO Box 1999, Sudbury, Suffolk CO10 6FS. Tel. 01787 313955.

[13] United Kingdom Central Council (1998) *Guidelines for Records and Record Keeping.* UKCC, London.

14 Management of Health & Safety at Work Regulations and Approved Code of Practice (1992) Stationery Office, London.

15 Health & Safety Executive (1992) *Manual Handling. Guidance on Regulations. Manual Handling Operations Regulations 1992.* HSE Books, Sheffield.

16 Health & Safety Commission (1992) *Guidance on Manual Handling of Loads in the Health Service.* Health & Safety Commission, Sheffield.

17 National Back Pain Association & Royal College of Nursing (1998). *The Guide to the Handling of Residents. Introducing a Safer Handling Policy*, revised 4th edn, p. 69. National Back Pain Association & Royal College of Nursing, Teddington, Middlesex.

18 National Back Pain Association & Royal College of Nursing (1998) *The Guide to the Handling of Residents. Introducing a Safer Handling Policy*, revised 4th edn, p. 238. NBPA & RCN, Teddington, Middlesex.

19 Chartered Society of Physiotherapy (1998) *Moving and Handling for Chartered Physiotherapists.* Chartered Society Physiotherapy, London.

20 Clinical Standards Advisory Group (1994) *Report of a Clinical Standards Advisory Group on Back Pain.* Stationery Office. London.

21 Royal College of Nursing (1996) *Hazards of Nursing. A study commissioned by the RCN conducted by the Institute of Employment Studies using data from a national survey of 6,000 registered nurses in RCN membership.* Royal College of Nursing, London.

22 Rawsky, E. (1998) Review of the literature on falls among the elderly. *Image Journal of Nursing Scholars*, **30**(1), 47–52.

23 Steinway, K.K. (1997) Falls, causes and consequences. *American Family Physician*, **56**(7), 1815–1823.

24 Runge, M. (1997) Multifactorial pathenogenesis of gait disorders and hip fractures in the elderly. *Z Gerato Geriatric*, **30**(4), 267–275.

25 Commodore, D.I. (1995) Falls in the elderly population: a look at incidence, risks, healthcare and costs. *Rehabilitation Nursing*, **20**(2), 84–89.

26 Thapa, P.B., Brockman, K.G., Gideon, I., Fough, B.L. & Ray, W.A. (1996) Injurious falls in non-ambulatory nursing home residents, a comparative study of circumstances, incidence, and risk factors. *Journal American Geriatric Society*, **44**, 273–278.

27 Gialloreit, L.E. & Marazzi, M.C. (1996) Risk for falls in the elderly. Role of activities of daily living and of subjective assessment of health status. A case controlled study. *Recenti Prog Med*, **87**(9), 405–411.

28 Jack, C.I., Smith, T., Neoh, C., Lye, M. & McGalliard, J.N. (1995) Prevalence of low vision in elderly residents admitted to an acute geriatric unit in Liverpool; elderly people who fall are more likely to have low vision. *Gerontology*, **41**(5), 280–285.

29 Shaw, F.E. & Kenny, R.A. (1997) The overlap between syncope and falls in the elderly. *Postgrad Med J.* **73**(864), 635–639.

30 Northridge, M.E., Nevitt, M.C. & Kelsey, J.L. (1996) Non syncopal falls in the elderly in relation to home environments. *Osteoporosis International*, **6**(3), 249–255.

31 Luukinen, H., Koski, K., Kivela, S.L. & Laippala, P. (1996) Social status, life changes housing condition, functional abilities, and lifestyle as risk factors for recurrent falls among the home dwelling elderly. *Public Health*, **110**(2), 115–118.

32 Vellas, B.J., Wayne, S.J., Romero, L.J., Baumgarten, R.N. & Garry, P.J. (1997) Fear of falling and restriction of mobility in elderly fallers. *Age, Ageing*, **26**(3), 189–193.

33 Parmalee, P.A., Katz, J.R. & Lawton, M.P. (1992) Depression and mortality among the institutionalised aged. *Journal Gerontology*, **47**, 3010.

[34] Katz, J.R., Miller, D. & Oslin, D. (1998) Diagnosis of late life depression. In: Salzman, C. (ed.) *Clinical Geriatric Psychopharmacology*, 3rd edn, pp. 133. Williams and Williams, Baltimore.

[35] Katz, J.R., Curlick, S. & Lesher, E.I. (1988) Use of antidepressants in the frail elderly, when, why and how. *Clinics Geriatric Medicine*, **4**, 203–222.

[36] Audit Commission (1994) *A Prescription for Improvement. Towards more Rational Prescribing in General Practice*. Audit Commission, Stationery Office, London.

[37] Harris, C.M. & Darjda, R. (1996) The scale of repeat prescribing. *British Journal of General Practitioners*, **46**(412), 649–653.

[38] Purves, I. & Kennedy, J. (1994) *The Quality of General Practice Repeat Prescribing*. Department of Primary Health Care, University of Newcastle upon Tyne, Newcastle upon Tyne.

[39] Broderick, E. (1997) Prescribing patterns for nursing home residents in the US. The reality and the vision. *Drugs, Aging*, **11**(4), 255–260.

[40] Myers, A.H., Baker, S.P., Van Natta, M., Abbey, H. & Robinson, E.G. (1991) Risk factors associated with falls and injuries among elderly institutionalised persons. *American Journal Epidemiology*, **133**, 1179–1190.

[41] Ray, W.A., Griffin, M.R. & Malcolm, E. (1991) Cyclic antidepressants and the risk of hip fracture. *Archives of Internal Medicine*, **151**, 754–756.

[42] Roose, S.P., Glassman, A.H., Giardina, E.G.V., Walsh, B.T., Woodring, S. & Bigger, J.T. (1987) Tricyclic antidepressants in depressed residents with cardiac disease. *Archives General Psychiatry*, **44**, 273–275.

[43] Li, X., Hamdy, R., Sandborn, W., Chi, D. & Dyer, A. (1996) Long term effects of antidepressants on balance, equilibrium, and postural reflexes. *Psychiatry Res*, **63**, 191–196.

[44] Parashottam, B. Thapa, Patricia Gideon, Amanda B. Milam & Wayne A. Ray (1998) Antidepressants and the risk of falls among nursing home residents. *New England Journal of Medicine*, **339**, 857–882.

[45] Liu, B., Anderson, G., Mittman, N., To, T., Axcell, T. & Shear, N. (1998) Use of selective seratonin reuptake inhibitors of tricyclic antidepressants and the risk of hip fractures in elderly people. *Lancet*, **351**, 1303–1307.

[46] Weiner, D.K., Hanlon, J.T. & Studenski, S.A. (1998) Effects of central nervous system polypharmacy on falls liability in community dwelling elderly. *Gerontology*, **44**(4), 217–221.

[47] Thompson, P.G. (1996) Preventing falls in the elderly at home; a community based approach. *Med J Australia*, **164**, 520–523.

[48] Ytterstad, B. (1999) The Harstad injury prevention study; a community based prevention of fall fractures in the elderly evaluated by means of a hospital based injury recording system in Norway. *Int J Circumpolar Health*, **58**(2), 84–95.

[49] Myers, A.H., Young, Y., Langlois, J.A. (1996) Prevention of falls in the elderly. *Bone*, **18**, (suppl. 1) 875–1015.

[50] Province, M.A., Hadley, E.C., Hornbrook, M.C., Lipsitz, L.A., Miller, J.P., Mulrow, C.D., Ory, M.G., Sattin, R.W., Tinnetti, M.E. & Wolf, S.L. (1995) The effects of exercise in falls in elderly residents. A preplanned meta-analysis of the FICSIT Trails. Frailty and Injuries Co-operative Studies of Intervention Techniques. *Journal American Medical Association*, **273**(17), 1341–1347.

[51] Rizzo, J.A., Baker, D.I., McAvoy, G. & Tinetti, M.E. (1996) The cost effectiveness of a multifactoral targeted prevention program for falls among community elderly persons. *Medical Care*, **34**(9), 954–969.

[52] Graffmans, W.C., Ooms, M.E., Hofstec, H.M., Bezemer, P.D., Bouter, L.M. & Lips, B. (1996) Falls in the elderly a prospective study of risk factors and risk profiles. *American Journal of Epidemiology*, **143**(11), 1129–1136.

53 McGavock, H. (1997) *A review of the literature on drug adherence*. Royal Pharmaceutical Society of Great Britain. London.

54 Greenspan, S., Myers, E.R., Kiel, D.P., Parker, R.A., Ayes, W.C. & Resnick, N.M. (1998) Fall direction, bone mineral density and function; risk factors for hip fracture in frail elderly nursing home residents. *American Journal Medicine*, **104**(6), 539–545.

55 Department of Health (1999) *No Secrets. Guidance on Prevention of Abuse*. Department of Health, London.

56 Ryan, T. & Holman, A. (1998) Pointers to control. People with learning difficulties getting direct payments. VIA, London.

57 British Medical Association and the Law Society (1995) *Assessment of Mental Capacity. Guidance for Doctors and Lawyers*. BMA, London.

58 British Association of Social Workers (1998) Mental incapacity and decision making; professional implications for social workers. BASW, Birmingham.

59 Clarke, J. (1991) Where you live can make you vulnerable. *Entourage*, **6**(4), 11.

Risk Assessment Form

Name of home_____

Person completing form_____

Date_____

Hazard Identified	Possibility Score	Consequence score	Risk rating	Action

Comments

Key to risk rating

Risk rating	Potential consequences	Priority
3x3=9	Highest risk, most serious consequence	Urgent, highest possible priority
3x2= 6	High risk, serious consequence	High priority
2x2=4	Medium risk, less serious consequence	Medium priority
1x3= 3	Low risk, most serious consequences	Medium priority because of the severity of consequences
2x1= 2	Medium risk, less serious consequent	Medium priority
1x1=1	Low risk, less serious consequences	Low priority, but don't ignore

Fall Risk Assessment Form

Name_____
Age_____
Gender_____

Step one: identify risk factors

Risk factors: Tick box if present.

☐ Visual problems   ☐ Polypharmacy
☐ Peripheral neuropathy   ☐ Sedative use
☐ Arterial disease   ☐ Antidepressant use
☐ Postural hypotension   ☐ Use of sedatives & antidepressants
☐ Cardiac disease   ☐ Environmental hazards identified
☐ Arthritis of knees and hips   ☐ Any other risks identified
☐ Parkinson's disease   ☐ Incontinence
☐ History previous falls   ☐ Cognitive impairment
☐ Fear of falling

Step two complete POMS scale

Performance Orientated Mobility Screen (POMS)

Adapted from Tinnetti ME (1996). *Performance orientated assessment of mobility problems in elderly patients.*
Journal American Geriatric Society, 34; 119–126

Ask patient to:	Normal	Abnormal	Possible causes abnormality
Sit down in chair, 16–18″ seat height	Able to sit down in one controlled movement without using arm rests.	Sitting is not a smooth movement. Falls into chair or needs armrest to guide	Myopathy, arthritis, Parkinson's, deconditioning
Rise from chair	Able to get up in one smooth movement without using armrests.	Uses armrests and/or moves forward in chair to propel self up. Requires several attempts to get up.	Myopathy, arthritis, Parkinson's, deconditioning
Stand, for about 30 seconds, after rising from chair.	Steady, able to stand without support.	Unsteady, loses balance.	Postural hypotension, vestibular or proprioceptive dysfunction, adverse drug effects.
Stand with eyes closed for about 15 seconds	Steady, able to stand without support	Unsteady, loses balance without aide	Postural hypotension, vestibular or proprioceptive dysfunction, adverse drug effects
Stand with eyes open. Nurse nudges on sternum three times using light pressure	Steady, needs to move feet but able to withstand pressure and maintain balance.	Unsteady, begins to fall	Postural hypotension, vestibular or proprioceptive dysfunction, adverse drug effects.
Walk in a straight line approximately 15 feet at the person's usual pace and then back again.	Gait continuous, no hesitation; walk in a straight line, feet clear floor.	Gait is non-continuous with deviation from straight path, feet scrape, or shuffle on floor.	Visual, vestibular, proprioceptive, foot disorders, adverse drug effects, improper walking device, or shoes.
Walk a distance of five feet and turn around.	No staggering, steps are smooth and continuous.	Staggering, steps are unsteady and discontinuous.	Visual, vestibular, proprioceptive, foot disorders, adverse drug effects, improper walking device, or shoes.

Step three: Referral
Refer patient to GP if you have identified problems that require medical treatment.
Refer to orthotist if specialist footwear required
Refer to physiotherapist if required

Step four: Plan care
Plan and implement care to reduce risk factors.

Step five: Evaluate
Reassess if patient condition changes or strategies ineffective.
Additional comments:

Form completed by: _____
Date: _____

Chapter 10

Preventing Pressure Sores

Introduction

There is little research into the incidence of pressure sores in nursing homes. Research carried out in 1999 in nursing and residential homes indicates a prevalence of over 6%[1]. Research indicates that the incidence of pressure sores in UK hospitals is 15%, and in NHS elderly care units it varies from 4% to 34%. The majority of people in NHS hospitals who have pressure sores have developed them in hospital. The NHS spends an estimated £200 million each year on treating pressure sores[2].

Sometimes if a person develops a pressure sore in a home, staff say 'There was nothing we could do'. But if we are honest we must admit it is not exactly a badge of honour. Although people living in nursing and residential homes are at high risk of developing pressure sores, most pressure sores can be prevented. The risk of residents developing pressure sores has risen as dependency has risen. The number of pressure sores will rise unless we act to reduce risk[3]. In some homes staff provide specialist mattresses and overlays for most residents, and routinely change residents' positions two hourly. This scattergun approach fails residents and staff. There are only so many resources and only so much time. Inevitably some residents are overtreated while others are undertreated. Understanding why pressure sores develop and assessing risk accurately enables nurses to target resources effectively. The goal of skilled professional care is to assess risk and rectify, wherever possible, factors that predispose to pressure sores. Care should be planned to prevent the development of pressure sores.

This chapter aims to:

- Enable you to understand why pressure sores develop
- Enable you to assess pressure sores risk
- Enable you to document risk
- Enable you to act to reduce risks

What is a pressure sore?

'A pressure sore is an area of localised damage to the skin and tissue and usually occurs over bony prominences such as the base of the spine, hips and heels. They are caused by a range of internal and external factors but the primary factor is unrelieved pressure that occludes microcirculation.'[4]

A pressure sore is caused by unrelieved pressure on the skin, or shearing forces. Shearing forces can occur when an individual is lifted or moved. Blood supply is interrupted and tissue death occurs. Anyone of any age will develop pressure sores if the skin is subject to unrelieved pressure, but it is recognised that certain groups of people are at greater risk.

Why pressure sores develop

Three major factors contribute to pressure sores developing: pressure, shear and friction.

Pressure is the single most important factor in the development of pressure sores. Capillaries supply oxygen-rich blood to the skin and drain away deoxygenated blood. The pressure in a capillary is 32 mmhg at the arterial end and 12 mmhg at the venous end. Unrelieved pressure reduces the capillary pressure and prevents the skin receiving oxygen and nutrients. Tissues deprived of oxygen and nutrients die and pressure sores develop.

Shear affects the deep tissues. The tissues attached to the bone are pulled in one direction and the skin surface sticks to bed linen or clothing causing the tissue to distort. Shearing forces may be caused by a person slipping down the bed or chair or by poor handling techniques. The person who keeps sliding down the chair is subjecting her sacrum to shearing forces. Staff who pull the person back up (because it takes too long to use a hoist) are also subjecting the person's tissues to shearing forces. If you put a film or hydrocolloid dressing on a person's sacrum and find that it curls up at the edges, this is an indication of shear caused either by the person sliding down in the chair or poor handling techniques. Shearing and pressure are inter-linked.

Friction occurs when two surfaces rub against each other. This friction strips the epidermis away and can produce shallow ulcers and blisters.

Risk factors

Ageing increases the risk of developing pressure sores; 70% of people who develop pressure sores are over 70 years old[5]. Ageing is associated with changes to the skin. The skin becomes dryer and the amount of collagen fibres are reduced. Collagen acts as scaffolding in the skin and loss of collagen makes the skin more vulnerable to damage. Some older people have skin that is more prone to damage than others. Individuals on long-term steroid therapy, and others who have thin papery skin, are more prone to develop tissue damage.

Reduced mobility increases pressure risk. Normally, even when we think we are sitting still we make micro adjustments to our position. Reduced mobility stops us fidgeting and adjusting our posture. If the person is unable to change position unaided or to walk unaided, he or she depends on nursing staff for position changes.

Chronic illness makes the individual more likely to develop pressure sores. Chronic illness such as diabetes can affect circulation and make the person more vulnerable to pressure damage. Anaemia is common in people living in nursing homes and reduces the ability of blood to oxygenate tissues – this increases the risk of pressure damage.

Sensory impairment is common in stroke survivors who live in nursing homes. Some people with diabetes develop peripheral neuropathy. People who have sensory impairment are often unaware of discomfort caused by pressure.

People with cardiac and circulatory problems have reduced blood flow to the tissues and are more vulnerable to skin damage.

Nutrition is a very important factor in the development of pressure sores[6,7]. Obesity can predispose an individual to pressure sores as adipose tissue has a poorer blood supply than normal tissue. Obese people can be hot and sticky, and moist clammy skin is vulnerable to infection and tissue breakdown. Very thin older people lack a protective layer of fat – they have bony prominences and are at extremely high risk of developing pressure sores.

Urinary incontinence if poorly managed can cause skin damage and lead to pressure sores. Urine can cause dermatitis, maceration and excoriation of the skin. Any skin damage increases the risk of pressure sores.

Poor handling and positioning increase the risk of skin damage. Clothing made of nylon or synthetic fibres can cause tissue damage. Nylon can make the person more likely to slide down the bed. Synthetic fibres do not absorb perspiration and can lead to moist sticky skin that is easily damaged. Other factors that increase risk are infection, pain, stress and lack of sleep.

Chronic illness and its physical effects make an individual more likely to develop pressure sores. Individuals with cardiac and arterial problems suffer from compromised circulation. Blood flow to tissues is reduced and damage can occur more readily than in individuals with a healthy circulation.

Individuals who are not lucid, or who are drowsy, often because of the effects of medication, are less aware of pressure on skin. They are less likely to complain of discomfort and are often dependent on nursing staff to relieve pressure. Individuals who have sensory loss, perhaps as the result of diabetic induced peripheral neuropathy, or other neurological problems, are often unaware of pressure and discomfort and are dependent on nursing staff to relieve pressure.

Medication can increase the risk of pressure sores developing. Hypnotics and psychotropic drugs can lead to drowsiness. The person who is drowsy is less likely to move and may develop a pressure sore because of this. Non-steroidal anti-inflammatory drugs (NSAID) can lead to slow blood loss and anaemia. This can increase pressure sore risk. NSAID can also impair healing because they impair the inflammatory response required to enable wounds to heal.

Older people who live in nursing homes are among the most disabled of their generation. They are more likely to suffer from chronic illness, more likely to have impaired levels of consciousness, more likely to suffer from neurological disease and more likely to be admitted in a malnourished state.

The older person admitted to a nursing home may be admitted with a sore. Research carried out in Liverpool indicated that 28% of people with pressure sores were admitted with them[8]. The nursing home resident is extremely vulnerable and at high risk of developing pressure sores. The goal of skilled professional nursing care is to prevent pressure sores developing and to heal any pressure sores present on admission.

Assessing and reducing risks

An ounce of prevention is worth a ton of cure. The best way to prevent pressure sores developing is to assess the person's risk and use a problem solving approach to reduce risk.

It is vital that you use a risk assessment scale to determine the person's level of risk. Assessment should be carried out when the person is admitted and whenever there are any significant changes to the person's health. There are a number of risk assessment scales. Each scale scores risk factors and the scores indicate the individual's risk of developing a pressure sore. Assessment scales enable you to assess risk and to plan care to prevent pressure sores occurring. The assessment scale should take into account all the risk factors and accurately predict the risk of damage occurring.

Doreen Norton developed the Norton scale in 1962[9]. The Norton score assesses five risk factors. By the 1980s health care changes, such as surgery being carried out on the very old and increasing longevity, led many nurses to question its accuracy.

Many other risk assessment scales were developed but the one that was commonly adopted was the Waterlow scale. The Waterlow scale was developed by Judy Waterlow in 1985 and was made available commercially[10]. The Waterlow scale includes additional factors such as age, nutritional status, skin type and diseases, including those that affect circulation. It was designed to assess the risk status of all patients from the cradle to the grave. Waterlow evaluated the scale three years after its introduction, on a geriatric unit for four weeks. The wards used were one acute admissions ward and one rehabilitation ward. The Waterlow scale is subjective. Two nurses assessing the Waterlow scale on the same patient on the same day may get different scores. This means that the scale may overpredict the risk of a person developing a pressure sore, and time and resources may be spent wastefully. The scale may also underpredict the risk and the person may not, despite the best of nursing intentions, receive the level of care required to prevent pressure sores developing[11].

The Braden scale was developed in the US in the 1980s. It was developed to take account of increased knowledge about the factors that lead to pressure sores. It is an objective scale and eliminates the problem of different nurses assessing an individual's risk differently. The Braden scale has been extensively researched with large numbers of elderly people. Research suggests that the Braden scale is more accurate than any other risk assessment scale[12].

It is important that nursing staff at the home decide which scoring system will be used. The score should be determined on admission, but it must be stressed that scoring is an ongoing process and should be carried out whenever there is a major change in an individual's condition. It is also a good idea to periodically check a person's score; sometimes residents' risk factors change so slowly that we do not register them.

The benefits of assessment scales

Accurate research-based assessment scales enable you to predict more accurately an individual's risk of developing a pressure sore. This is invaluable. The individual at low risk can sleep on a foam or hollow fibre overlay or replacement mattress rather than a specialist overlay or mattress replacement. Most older people would prefer this to an unnecessary specialist product. The individual at low risk can sleep undisturbed. The individual at high risk of developing pressure sores will benefit from increased staff interventions to reduce risk and prevent pressure sores developing. Nursing workload is reduced when risk is accurately assessed and equipment and care can be targeted accurately.

The benefits of nursing expertise and observation

Assessment tools are 'tools'. They are designed to complement the experienced nurse's professional judgement, not to replace it. Assessment tools can never replace good nursing observation and experience[13]. Norton, Waterlow and Braden are not at the resident's bedside – you are. Nurses know that although two individuals may have the same risk factors and receive the same treatment, one person may still develop the early signs of tissue damage. It is important to look at pressure areas and to ensure that care assistant colleagues are aware of the importance of reporting immediately any signs of tissue damage.

Adopting a problem-solving approach

It is vital that that you follow through the results of your assessment with appropriate nursing interventions. Often when nurses identify that a person is at high risk of developing pressure sores, they rush to provide pressure-relieving equipment. This is an important part of the solution but it is not *the* solution. A holistic approach benefits the nurse and the person cared for. Mobility is a key factor in the development of pressure sores. If the person is immobile, can you enable them to improve mobility? Ensuring that the individual has suitable shoes and aids, organising physiotherapy, and helping the individual to exercise and regain mobility, reduce the risk of pressure sores. If the person is unable to turn over in bed unaided, can you help? If not, can you refer the person to an occupational therapist who may be able to suggest aids to help the person regain ability? Could a physiotherapist help? Would a review of medication to improve pain control help?

If the person is malnourished, can you encourage them to eat a healthy balanced diet with sufficient nutrients, calories and protein? If not, can you ensure that the person sees a dietician? This will reduce the risk of tissue breakdown. If the person is a poorly controlled diabetic, can you work with medical staff to help the person gain better control? If the person is anaemic can the anaemia be treated? Anaemia increases the risk of pressure sores developing; treating anaemia not only reduces risk, it also makes the person feel much better.

If the individual is incontinent can the incontinence be treated? A continence promotion programme may help the individual regain continence. If the incontinence cannot be treated, can it be managed effectively? Poorly managed urinary incontinence predisposes an older person to tissue breakdown. Many nurses feel an indwelling urinary catheter reduces the risk of an individual developing pressure sores and is an essential part of treatment if the individual is incontinent and has a pressure sore. Many individuals are admitted to nursing homes with urinary catheters in situ and some nurses fear that if they remove the catheter they will increase the risk of an individual developing a pressure sore. Urinary catheterisation increases the risk of infection and is associated with increased mortality rates. Urinary catheters should only be used if clinically indicated (see Chapter 7). Some older people are so distressed by the fact that they have a urinary catheter that they do not wish to get better. Many can, with the help of skilled professional nursing, regain quality of life.

Case history

Margaret Mitchell was admitted to a nursing home following repair of a fractured femur. She was immobile, had a urinary catheter in situ, was suffering from a large deep pressure sore to her sacrum and had lost all will to live. She was malnourished, in pain and curled into a foetal position. Her glasses had been lost and she could see little without them. Analgesia was given, the wound swabbed and redressed and admission procedures completed. Margaret was at her lowest ebb and felt that she had come to the nursing home to die. The admitting nurse worked with Margaret to identify her needs and ensure that these were met. Margaret's catheter, which made her feel 'dirty and smelly', was removed and she regained continence using continence promotion strategies as detailed in Chapter 7. She regained mobility when provided with suitable shoes, a frame, glasses and physiotherapy. Nutritional needs were met, her wound was dressed and pressure relieving devices were used. Margaret regained not only mobility and continence but also her self-respect and zest for life.

If the person has cardiovascular disease can this be managed more effectively? If the person is drowsy because of hypnotics or sedatives can these be discontinued? Can nursing measures be used to promote healthy natural sleep? Encouraging exercise and leisure activities will make older people feel more alert. It is unlikely that such individuals will require hypnotics to help them sleep; their days will be full and active and they should sleep well. The risk of the individual developing pressure sores is further reduced.

Pressure relieving aids

Individuals at low risk of developing pressure sores – those who do not suffer from chronic illness, who are not malnourished, who have no sensory loss and who are not incontinent – are still at risk of developing pressure sores if their skin is subject to unrelieved pressure for more than a few hours. Older people who are at risk of developing pressure sores may suffer from tissue damage even if their position is changed every two hours.

The areas of the body most at risk of ischaemic damage are the sacrum, heels, buttocks and greater trochanters. Almost half of all pressure sores develop on the sacrum and almost 20% develop on the heels[14]. The aim of pressure-relieving aids is to relieve and redistribute pressure to avoid tissue damage. The features of the ideal pressure-relieving mattress replacement or overlay are:

- Redistributes pressure evenly
- Is impermeable
- Allows the skin to breathe
- Is easily cleaned
- Is comfortable at all times
- Enables nurses to care without restriction
- Is reliable and does not break down
- Is competitively priced.

Unfortunately the ideal mattress does not exist. A range of pressure-relieving overlays and mattress replacements exist. Foam overlays, alternating-pressure overlays and mattresses replacements, static systems and low air loss beds are all available. Assessment of risk enables you to choose the appropriate pressure-relieving equipment to prevent the development of, or treat existing, pressure sores.

What sort of equipment do I need?

If the person you are caring for is slipping down the chair and is at risk of shear, your first priority must be to obtain a comfortable chair that will provide support and prevent the person slipping down. You may have a suitable chair in the home or you may have to consider purchasing a special chair. If you can stop the person slipping out of the chair you will have reduced shearing forces and the risk of pressure sores.

If you are buying chairs for the home it is worth considering chairs with integral pressure-relieving cushions. The seat cushion of the chair is made of a pressure-redistributing foam that reduces pressure sore risk. When you place a pressure-redistributing cushion on top of a chair you increase the height of the chair and this can make it more difficult for a person to get up. Placing a cushion on top of a chair also makes the seating arrangement less stable.

If the person is at risk of developing a pressure sore or indeed has a pressure sore, it is important to consider cushions as well as pressure-redistributing mattresses, replacements and overlays. Cushions are available in a range of materials including foam, memory foam, gel and powered alternating-pressure cushions.

If the person is at risk you need to provide a pressure-relieving mattress or overlay. Standard 'hospital' foam mattresses are not suitable surfaces for people at risk of developing pressure sores. The old hospital foam mattresses have been superseded by a new generation of foam mattresses. These new foam mattresses are better at redistributing pressure and reduce pressure sore risk. Powered alternating-pressure mattress replacements and overlays also reduce pressure sore risk[15].

It is important that you do not use donuts or water filled gloves in an attempt to reduce pressure on sore heels, as these devices actually increase pressure on the heels and make them more likely to develop pressure sores.

How do I choose the 'right' equipment?

In the past, decisions on what support surface to use were based on the results of risk assessments. If the Waterlow scale was at a certain point, a certain support surface was recommended. In 1999 McGough examined this issue and concluded that there was insufficient evidence to recommend using risk assessment scores as a basis for pressure-relieving equipment[16].

It is possible to measure the interface pressure using an interface pressure monitor; however, this is not a reliable indicator of how a support surface will perform. A more holistic approach is now recommended. The latest guidance states that decisions on support surfaces should be based on the following factors:

- Is the person comfortable?
- Is the person able to move?
- Does it prevent the person from getting up?
- Is it relieving pressure?
- Is the skin improving?

Buying equipment

People who are admitted to nursing homes are usually immobile and at high risk of developing pressure sores. The standard foam mattress offers no protection and is no longer recommended for people at risk of developing pressure sores. You can purchase foam overlays and place these on top of foam mattresses to reduce pressure risk. The problem with overlays is that they raise the height of the bed. This can make it difficult for people to get up, even with help. Raising the height of the bed also increases risk of injury if the person falls out of bed.

If you are purchasing new mattresses it makes sense to use foam-based, low pressure mattresses. These are more expensive than standard foam mattresses but work out cheaper than buying a foam mattress and an overlay.

Alternating-pressure mattresses are available either as mattress replacements or as overlays. The mattress replacement system is by far the best option because it does not raise the height of the bed or create an unstable surface; however replacement systems are much more expensive than overlays. If you are buying a powered alternating-pressure system, consider one that provides a cushion and an overlay. Some systems are designed so that you can remove the pump and use it to power a cushion when the person is sitting in a chair.

Most suppliers will send a representative to visit the home. The representative will provide technical details and copies of research reports and papers relating to the product and its use in preventing or treating pressure sores. Nursing staff will be shown how to use the product. Most companies will lend you a piece of equipment for evaluation purposes – equipment is now loaned for approximately two weeks. You can then compare and evaluate products before purchase. A product that appears less expensive but is unreliable or less effective may well be the most expensive in the long term. The budget conscious nurse should always ask for a discount if more than one item is being purchased.

Changing position

Aids are intended to serve as a supplement to, and not a substitute for, nursing care. It is important to help the person change position frequently. The frequency of position changes will be determined by the condition of the skin and the person's comfort. Details of how often position should be changed should be documented in the care plan.

Assessing wounds

Pressure sores are preventable in the vast majority of cases if individuals receive high quality individualised care that meets their needs. Caring for individuals who are at extremely high risk of developing pressure sores, and preventing the sores occurring, is a mark of high quality professional care. The incidence of pressure sores is an important indicator of care. Many individuals are admitted to nursing homes with pressure sores acquired either in hospital or in the community. It is not always possible to determine either the presence of or the extent of a pressure sore during an assessment visit.

All individuals admitted to a nursing home should have their risk assessed on admission. This is important as the individual's condition (and risk factors) may have changed since the initial assessment. Individuals who have pressure sores should have a full assessment. This should include the site of the wound and its size. A record of the wound size and depth should be made. A grid can be used to trace the wound and the depth can be measured with a probe. You can take a photograph – using digital and Polaroid cameras avoids developing delays.

There are two widely used methods of classifying pressure sores. One classifies wounds in five categories[17] while another uses four categories. Senior nursing staff within the home should decide which classification system they will use. The classification should be recorded. Table 10.1 gives details of the Torrance classification.

Senior nursing staff within the home should determine which classification system they will use, and the classification should be recorded. It is important to note that blanching hyperaemia is an ineffective test on individuals with dark skins. In stages 1 and 2 you need to be alert for colour changes in the person's skin and for warmth.

A wound assessment chart can be used to provide a baseline measure of the wound. This can be updated at each dressing change.

Treatment of pressure sores

The principles of wound care are given in Chapter 6. Individuals who have pressure sores are at risk of developing infection; details of infection control strategies are outlined in Chapter 5.

Table 10.1 Torrance classification of pressure sores.

Stage	Description
1	Reddening is present. Light finger pressure causes the skin to whiten. This is referred to as 'blanching hyperaemia'. The whitening indicates that capillary circulation is intact and undamaged
2	Reddening remains when light finger pressure is applied. This is referred to as 'non-blanching hyperaemia' and indicates that capillary circulation is damaged. The skin may be broken
3	The skin is ulcerated and subcutaneous tissue is ulcerated
4	The ulcer extends into subcutaneous fat. Underlying muscle is inflamed and swollen
5	The ulcer extends into muscle or bone

Documentation

Assessment of individuals who have acquired or who are at risk of developing pressure sores should be ongoing. The care plan should indicate this continuing process and should record changes in risk factors. You must document findings, intention, action and outcome when delivering care. Documentation safeguards the nurse from accusations of failing to provide appropriate care. We live in a changing world and individuals and their relatives are more likely to consider legal action if they feel care has been inadequate. In such situations, if care is not documented there is no proof that it has been provided. Many nurses give care but fail to document that care. Some mean to write it up later but get interrupted and never get around to documenting it. Practising in such a way is unsafe and puts the nurse and the resident at risk. Table 10.2 gives an example of part of a care plan.

Staff education

As nurses we have a professional duty to remain clinically up to date and to provide research-based care. We also have a duty to ensure that the resident receives research-based care, even when we are not directly providing that care. Our role includes the education and supervision of our care assistant colleagues and ensuring that the resident receives quality care at all times.

National minimum standards require homes to ensure that increasing numbers of care assistants are qualified to NVQ level 2. However, the current NVQ level 2 syllabus has very little information about preventing pressure sores. Most care assistants are unaware of the factors that contribute to the development of pressure sores. They may be unaware of the importance of relieving pressure and of the damage friction can cause to skin. They may have been taught to give reddened skin a good rub; such action can further damage a compromised circulation and contribute to tissue damage.

As a registered nurse you are responsible for educating care assistants and explaining not only what care must be given but why it must be given. It is important that you emphasise the need to report any changes in skin colour

Table 10.2 Sample of first two sections of a care plan.

Problem	Aim	Action	Review
1. Risk of pressure sores – Braden = 12	• To prevent pressure damage • To maintain healthy skin	• Use dynamic pressure-relieving mattress • Use dynamic pressure-relieving cushion • Assist to change position two-hourly • Improve nutritional status (see 2) • Improve continence (see 3) • Report changes in skin	
2. Malnourished – BMI = 19, weight = 42 kg	• To enable Mrs Jones to gain weight • To reduce pressure sore risk	• Provide high calorie diet • Provide snacks • Encourage to eat meals and snacks	

or any signs of skin damage. Staff who understand the reasons why care is carried out in a certain way are more motivated and able to work with nurses to provide high quality care.

Pressure sores cause pain and suffering, and can lead to infection and even death. Individuals who develop pressure sores, especially extensive cavity wounds, require high levels of skilled nursing care. It is important that care is holistic and person centred and meets the individual's needs. The vast majority of pressure sores are preventable. Our goal as skilled professionals is to act to prevent the development of pressure sores, rather than react to their occurrence.

References

[1] Sheils, C. & Roe, B. (1999) Pressure sore care. *Nursing Standard*, **14**(6), 41–44.

[2] Department of Health (1993) *Pressure Sores. A Guide for NHS Purchasers and Providers*. Department of Health, London.

[3] European Pressure Ulcer Advisory Panel (1999) Pressure ulcer prevention guidelines. *EPUAP Review*, **1**(1), 7–8. Available on www.epuap.com. or Tel. 01865 228264.

[4] Reed, S. & Hambridge, K. (2001) Implementing best practice in pressure ulcer prevention. *Nursing Times NT Plus supplement*, **97**(24), 69–71.

[5] Bergstrom, N., Braden, B. & Kemp, M. *et al.* (1996) Multi-site study of the incidence of pressure ulcers and the relationship between risk level, demographic characteristics, diagnosis and prescription of preventative interventions. *Journal of the American Geriatric Society*, **44**, 2–30.

[6] Allman, R.M. (1997) Pressure ulcer prevalence, incidence, risk factors and impact. *Clinics Geriatric Medicine*, **13**(3), 421–436.

[7] Lewis, B.K. (1998) Nutritional intake and the risk of pressure sore development in older patients. *Journal of Wound Care*, **17**(1), 31–35.

[8] Sheils, C. & Roe, B. (1999) Pressure sore care. *Nursing Standard*, **14**(6), 41–44.

[9] Norton, D. *et al.* (1962) *An Investigation of Geriatric Nursing Problems in Hospital*. National Corporation for the Care of Old People, London.

[10] Waterlow, J. (1988) The Waterlow card for prevention and management of pressure sores: towards a pocket policy. *Care, Science and Practice*, **6**(1), 8–12.

[11] Waterlow, J. (1997) Practical use of the Waterlow Scale. *British Journal of Community Health Nursing*, **2**(2), 83–86.

[12] Bergstrom, N. & Braden, B. (1992) A prospective study of pressure sore risk among the institutionalised elderly. *Journal American Geriatric Society*, **40**(8), 747–758.

[13] Rycroft Malone, J. & McInness, E. (2000) *Pressure ulcer risk assessment and prevention*. Technical report. RCN, London. This can be downloaded from www.rcn.org.uk

[14] Dealy, C. (1991) The size of the pressure sore problem. *Journal of Advanced Nursing*, **16**, 663–670.

[15] Cullum, N., Deeks, J., Song, F. & Fletcher, A.W. (2000) Beds, mattresses and cushions for preventing and treating pressure sores. (Cochrane Review) Website: www. update-software.com/cochrane/login.htm

[16] McGough, A.J. (1999) A systematic review of the effectiveness of risk assessment scales used in the prevention and management of pressure sores. MSc thesis, University of York. Cited in Rycroft Malone, J. & McInness, E. (2000) *Pressure ulcer risk assessment and prevention*. Technical report. RCN, London. This can be downloaded from www.rcn.org.uk

[17] Torrance, C. (1983) *Pressure Sores Aetiology Treatment and Prevention*. Croom Helm, Beckenham.

Chapter 11

Nutrition

Introduction

Nutrition is an issue that has been receiving increased attention since the publication of *Hungry in Hospital*[1]. The report was critical of the attention nurses paid to the nutrition of older people in hospital and prompted the UKCC to issue a statement saying that it was the nurse's responsibility to ensure that patients were adequately fed[2].

This chapter aims to enable you to:
- Understand how ageing affects nutritional needs
- Understand how illness affects appetite and nutritional needs
- Understand how medication affects appetite
- Measure nutritional status
- Provide a healthy diet for frail older people

The nutritional needs of older people

In the early twentieth century when old age pensions were introduced, few people lived long enough to collect them. Now, ever increasing numbers of people are surviving into their eighties and nineties and every year 5000 people celebrate their one hundredth birthday. Unfortunately we still know very little about the nutritional needs of very old people. In 1992 when the Committee on Medical Aspects of Food Policy published their report on nutrition, they made recommendations for further research and commented on the lack of data available[3]. In the absence of appropriate research we have to rely on information obtained from studies of younger adults[4]. This means that we do not know if nutritional requirements change in extreme old age. We do not know if older people have the same intakes of nutrients as younger people. We do not know how prevalent nutritional deficiencies are in older people. We do not know if health promotion strategies such as losing weight or cutting down on dietary fat are effective or even appropriate to older people. Researchers in the US consider that people over the age of 70 have special nutritional needs and they have developed special dietary guidance for people aged 70 or over[5].

The incidence and consequences of malnutrition

Older people are at risk of becoming malnourished and the risk increases with age[6]. Malnourished people can be obese, of normal weight or thin.

Malnutrition affects the immune system in the following ways (based on Chandra's 1993 work[7]):

- Reduces the rate of wound healing
- Increases the risk of infection
- Reduces the secretion of IgA antibody that protects mucosal surfaces
- Reduces the effectiveness of mucosal barriers to infection, so infections such as thrush and urinary tract, chest and eye infections are more common
- Reduces immune response even in moderate malnutrition, so infections are more likely
- Reduces the ability of phagocytes to ingest bacteria, so infections are more severe
- Reduces the response to immunisation, so vaccinations such as the Flu Vac are less effective.

Research indicates that many healthy older people living in their own homes suffer from vitamin deficiencies. Medication can impair absorption of vitamins and minerals. Low levels of vitamins and minerals can reduce the ability of the immune system to fight infection[8]. Older people are most likely to suffer from deficiencies of iron, zinc and vitamin C. Vitamin supplements that correct these deficiencies lead to a reduced rate of infection[9].

Many older people are admitted to hospital malnourished – unfortunately many become even more malnourished in hospital[10]. Cook-chill plated systems used in hospitals reduce vitamin C content by between 45 and 76%[11]. Immobility reduces the appetite and increases the risk of malnutrition.

Malnutrition increases the risk of infection. It also leads to loss of respiratory muscle and increases the risks of chest infection. Immobility increases the risks of constipation. Constipation can lead to poor appetite and urinary retention and increased risk of urinary tract infection[12].

Malnutrition inhibits mobility and delays recovery[13]. Weight loss leads to muscle loss, which affects respiratory muscles and leads to reduced respiratory function. This makes it more difficult for individuals to cough and expectorate and increases the risk of chest infection[14]. Research suggests that 36% of older people living in continuing care and nursing home settings are malnourished[15].

Malnutrition sets up or is part of a cycle of exhaustion, poor mobility, poor appetite and depression. Providing a nutritious diet and enabling people to eat it breaks this circle and improves health.

Meeting nutritional needs

In order to meet an individual's nutritional needs you have to provide sufficient calories, vitamins and nutrients. We eat not only to provide fuel for our bodies but also for comfort and enjoyment, so food provided must be acceptable to the person receiving it.

In 1995 the Caroline Walker Trust established an expert group to study the dietary requirements of people living in continuing care settings. The group studied local authority homes, residential homes and nursing homes. They found that in 1994 every home should have been spending £15 per resident per week to ensure that the person received an adequate diet. Some homes spent 35% less than this on food[16].

Many frail older people rarely go outdoors. Half an hour's winter sunlight on the hands and face enables the body to make Vitamin D and this helps maintain strong bones. In 1991 researchers found that 40% of people living in long-stay hospitals, residential and nursing homes suffered from vitamin D and calcium deficiency due to inadequate exposure to sunshine[17]. People with dark skins require greater exposure to sunlight to manufacture vitamin D. Inadequate intake of calcium, and vitamin D deficiency, increase the risk of osteoporosis and fracture. Box 11:1 outlines ways to reduce vitamin D deficiency and fracture risk.

Box 11.1   **Ways to prevent calcium and vitamin D deficiency.**

- Serve full cream milk as removing the fat from milk also removes the vitamin D.
- Encourage and enable individuals to sit in the sunshine. Patios and windbreaks can reduce the risk of chills
- Ask GPs to consider prescribing calcium and vitamin D supplements to housebound people. This significantly reduces the risk of hip and other fracture[1]
- Serve cream cakes, full fat cheese, butter and margarine, as these are rich sources of vitamin D

It is important to be aware that not all residents living in a home have the same nutritional needs. Individuals living in nursing homes can have very different dietary requirements. Providing all individuals with the same diet will lead to some individuals becoming malnourished, resulting in poor health. One research study carried out in an NHS long stay unit investigated the reasons why some individuals lost weight while receiving what *appeared* to be an adequate diet. This study revealed that the individuals concerned ate all the food provided and were not suffering from malabsorption or metabolic disorders, but they were all slow or clumsy eaters or were dependent on nursing staff to feed them. All had difficulty in communication and were unable to tell nursing staff that they were hungry. None of them had access to snacks. The reason for their weight loss was that they were simply not getting enough food to meet their requirements. This has been termed 'institutional starvation'[18]. Individuals living in nursing homes are particularly at risk of malnutrition for the following reasons:

- Some residents will have difficulty feeding themselves and will be dependent on nursing staff for feeding, many will be receiving medication which may impair appetite or interfere with the absorption of nutrients, and individuals are dependent on the home to provide meals
- Some individuals do not have relatives or friends to provide the snacks with which all patients in all care settings traditionally supplement their diets
- Most individuals are suffering from physical or mental disabilities that resulted in their coming to live in a nursing home.

How illness affects the ability to eat a balanced diet

Illness can make it difficult for older people to eat. Loss of the use of a limb, neurological problems, arthritis or weakness can cause older people to experience problems cutting up food and transferring it from plate to mouth. Illness can lead to problems with chewing and swallowing. Understanding the problems that older people face and using a problem solving approach can help them enjoy a balanced diet.

Parkinson's disease can cause intention tremor, resulting in food slipping off the fork or spoon, which can be very embarrassing to older people. Prescribed antiparkinsonian medication given an hour before meals often reduces intention tremor and enables individuals to enjoy a meal in company without the fear of dropping food. The individual's doctor is often able to adjust the times that prescribed medication is given if informed of eating problems.

Individuals with neurological problems as a result of conditions such as strokes, multiple sclerosis or motor neurone disease can have problems with fine muscle control. Food may slide across the plate when the individual is attempting to eat, or the plate may slip or move. The use of plate guards or plates with an upturned rim can prevent food sliding off plates; small pizza plates look more 'normal' than plate guards. Special anti-slip mats can be placed under plates and bowls to prevent them moving.

Individuals who are hemiplegic experience great difficulty in cutting up food and may have to rely on nursing staff to do this. Providing cutlery specially designed for people who can only use one hand can enable individuals to retain independence. This cutlery has a knife edge on one side and fork prongs on the other. A plate guard or a rimmed plate should be provided, at least until the individual has become used to cutting and spearing food one handedly.

Arthritic individuals can find it difficult to grip cutlery. Providing special cutlery with hand grips can enable older people to retain independence. Arthritic individuals can sometimes find commercially produced cutlery with grips too heavy to use. Foam insulation designed to keep pipes from freezing can be bought from DIY shops. This is sold by the metre and costs less than a pound. A sleeve of this foam, designed for 15 mm pipes, fits neatly around normal cutlery, providing very light but easy to grip cutlery. The foam slips off easily so that the cutlery can be washed. When the foam becomes grubby it is thrown away.

Pottery cups and mugs full of tea can be too heavy for arthritic and frail older people. Nurses often offer lightweight plastic feeding cups in these circumstances. Melamine cups and mugs are lightweight and look just like ordinary cups, so are a more dignified alternative in many cases. These can be obtained from supermarkets and hardware shops. They are normally used for picnics, and budget conscious nurses will stock up on them in autumn when shops reduce prices.

Some older people have extremely poor eyesight or are partially sighted. Individuals who have suffered from visual loss because of glaucoma tend to lose peripheral vision. Food at the edges of the plate may remain uneaten because it cannot be seen. Using a large plate and placing all the food in the centre of it can enable some partially sighted people to see their meal.

Individuals who suffer from macular degeneration and peripheral neuropathy can distinguish red, black and yellow more readily than other colours. Mashed potato, fish and cauliflower presented on a white plate may be invisible to some partially sighted individuals. Black, red or yellow plates provide a contrast and enable individuals to see the food on the plate. Such plates can be difficult to obtain and extremely expensive, but are available in melamine in shops and hardware stores, where they are sold for picnics.

Individuals can develop hemianopsia after strokes and may only be able to see half of the food on the plate. The individual should be encouraged to look around and should be shown the uneaten portion of food. If this is ineffective, placing all the food on the half of the plate the individual can see will usually help. If the plate is to small for this you may have to rotate the plate halfway thorough the meal.

Older people often complain that 'food doesn't have any taste any more'. Taste buds atrophy with age and older people often use more sugar and salt than before to add taste to food. Yet it is often assumed that older people prefer bland food. Many nursing homes offer mild cheddar when extra mature may well taste like mild to an older person. A bland diet can be boring and unappetising. Nurses should encourage the home's chef to offer tasty alternatives to the traditional nursing home diet. Chilli con carne, pizza or jellied eels may tempt jaded appetites, and variety is the spice of life.

The amount of saliva produced declines with age. Older people may find some food too dry to eat easily. The nurse can ensure that water and drinks are provided with the meal so that individuals can wash their food down. Oesophageal peristalsis declines with age and some older people can find swallowing difficult. Advising such individuals to take smaller mouthfuls, to chew food thoroughly and to wash food down with a drink, will help.

Strokes can affect fine muscle control of the tongue, jaw and lips. This can make chewing difficult and dentures can slip during eating. Fastidious older people can be mortified when they develop these problems and may prefer to go hungry rather than 'show themselves up' in public. This situation requires careful handling. Food always tastes better when eaten in company but if an individual is embarrassed by eating difficulties, meals can be served in the person's room. It is important to emphasise to the person that this is at their request and not because nursing staff or residents find their eating difficulties offensive.

Many people regain fine muscle control of the lips, jaw and tongue spontaneously after a stroke, but speech therapists can teach people exercises that help speed up this process. As control improves the individual should be encouraged to join other residents and enjoy a meal in company. Eating alone is rarely as pleasurable as eating with others.

Many older people wear dentures. Many older people have had their dentures for many years and some dentures no longer fit as well as they once did. Poorly fitting dentures reduce an older person's ability to eat a wide range of foods and can cause gums to become painful. Many older people benefit from having new dentures; others can benefit from having dentures adjusted or relined to ensure a more comfortable fit. Very frail individuals can have temporary soft liners fitted to their dentures to relieve pain and discomfort. Information on obtaining dental services is given in Chapter 13.

Medication and nutrition

Many prescribed medications affect appetite.

Antidepressants increase appetite and lead to weight gain. Often a person who is depressed begins eating properly because she is feeling better. Improved nutrition leads to increased well-being. Sedatives *can sometimes* help the agitated person feel more settled and this can lead to a person eating a proper meal instead of picking at food. If the person is sedated unnecessarily or receives inappropriately high doses of a sedative, this can hinder the person's ability to eat. Drugs used to treat non-insulin dependent diabetes can increase or decrease appetite. One group of oral hypoglaecemics, known as biguanides, e.g. metformin, depress appetite. These can help overweight diabetics lose weight. Another group of oral hypoglaecemics, the sulphonlureas e.g. glibenclamide, glycaside, increase appetite and can help underweight diabetics gain weight. Anticholinergic drugs given to treat bowel spasm or urge incontinence can cause a dry mouth and this can reduce appetite.

Some medications can impair the absorption of vitamins and nutrients; others can lead to nutritional deficiencies. Antacids reduce the absorption of dietary iron and iron tablets. Vitamin C increases the absorption of iron. Giving a glass of orange juice with an iron tablet increases absorption by 40%. Non-steroidal anti-inflammatory drugs given to control pain and inflammation can lead to gastric ulceration and slow steady loss of iron. Corticosteroids given long term increase the excretion of vitamin C. Corticosteroids also lead to reduced protein absorption and loss of muscle and bone. Phenytoin reduces the absorption of vitamin D and folic acid. People on long-term phenytoin benefit from calcium and vitamin D supplements to prevent bone loss, and folic acid to prevent pernicious anaemia.

Sedatives and night sedation, if given in inappropriate doses, lead to daytime drowsiness and reduced food intake.

Individuals with special dietary needs

Older people who have wounds or pressure sores or who have undergone a recent operation require additional protein, vitamins and calories to enable healing to take place. Active people require larger helpings of food than the inactive. Some older people are very active and can have very high calorie requirements. Older people suffering from dementia who walk around the home constantly may be unable to tell nursing staff that they are hungry, and if they are not offered sufficient food to meet their requirements they can rapidly lose weight.

Some older people are unable to chew food as a result of illness; other older people, including people with end stage dementia, tend to spit out meat and lumpy food. Some can manage to swallow a soft diet but in many cases food must be puréed. It is easy to underfeed individuals who are having a puréed diet as liquid added makes portions appear larger than they actually are. Meat and vegetables should be puréed separately and not mixed together. The person can then choose to eat preferred foods and can leave food that is not liked. If food is mixed together it appears unappetising and a person has no choice but to eat it all or refuse it all. Individual puréed foods can melt into each other on a plate and look unappetising. Pottery or stainless steel serving dishes with three compartments, designed for serving vegetables, can be used to keep meat, potato and vegetable purées separate.

Principles of diabetic diet

Detailed information about diabetes and diabetic diet can be found in Chapter 15.

The incidence of diabetes rises with age. The pancreas becomes less efficient at producing insulin as adults age. Some older people are thought to become less sensitive to the effects of insulin as a result of age. Many older people suffer from maturity onset or type II diabetes. This is usually controlled either by diet or a combination of diet and oral hypoglaecemic drugs.

The treatment of diabetes has changed dramatically. Twenty years ago diabetics were advised to weigh food and the aim of diabetic treatment was to avoid blood sugars that were higher than 4–6 mmols, the normal range in non-diabetics. This was replaced by a more liberal approach to diet and people with diabetes were taught to measure units of 10 g of carbohydrate, known as portions. A typical diabetic diet might consist of three portions of carbohydrate for breakfast, a one portion snack mid morning, a three portion lunch, a one portion tea, a three portion dinner, and a one portion bedtime snack. People with diabetes were advised to eat foods high in fat but low in carbohydrate, such as cheese and eggs, if the diet failed to satisfy appetite. Now people with diabetes of normal weight are advised to eat a diet high in fibre and low in fat, with sufficient carbohydrate allowed to satisfy hunger. Older people who are overweight and diabetic are usually advised to lose weight. This, together with avoiding sugar and sweet foods, often controls diabetes.

Normally the aim in diabetic management is to maintain blood sugar at levels which avoid the risk of hypoglycaemia and avoid the long term risks of hyperglycaemia. Hyperglycaemia can, in the long term, lead to renal failure, peripheral neuropathy and diabetic retinopathy. These changes take decades to occur.

Older people with maturity onset diabetes who are living in nursing homes are usually in their eighties and nineties and their diabetes is usually of recent onset. Most physicians specialising in diabetes do not consider older people who develop maturity onset diabetes to be at serious risk of the long-term effects of hyperglycaemia. They tend to adopt a more liberal approach to diabetic control in such patients. It is generally agreed that older people who are non-insulin dependent and are not suffering any ill effects from their diabetes, such as drowsiness or thirst, can safely maintain blood sugars of around 10 mmol. Maintaining blood sugars that are higher than normal is thought to be preferable to exposing older people to the risks of hypoglycaemia.

Oral hypoglaecemic drugs act by stimulating the islets of Langerhans in the pancreas to produce more insulin and by decreasing insulin resistance, and they are prescribed if diabetes is not controlled by diet. Advice on diabetic diets can be obtained from community-based dieticians who can provide dietary advice for nurses and residents.

Insulin dependent diabetes is less common in older people. Community-based diabetic nurse specialists will visit older people with diabetes and provide advice on treatment and diet.

Vegetarians

Increasing numbers of people have become vegetarian. Some people eliminate meat from their diet but continue to eat fish, eggs and dairy products. Other people consume no animal products and are known as vegans. Particular care must be taken to ensure that a vegan diet is varied and balanced and supplies trace elements and nutrients. Vegans can be at risk of iron deficiency anaemia but a diet rich in fruit (especially apricots), cereals, nuts, beans and lentils avoids deficiency. Green leafy vegetables (especially broccoli) reduce the risk of folate deficiency.

Individuals who have had a vegan diet for many years may develop vitamin B_{12} deficiency if they are not careful to include yeast extract in their diets. Soya milk fortified with calcium or sesame paste (tahini) provides calcium normally obtained from cow's milk. Vitamin D normally found in diary products is a fat-soluble vitamin. It can be manufactured by the body and half an hour's exposure of the hands and face to the sun daily is sufficient, even in winter, to enable the body to manufacture vitamin D. Older people consuming a vegan diet, who do not go out of doors, are at risk of vitamin D deficiency. All margarine has vitamin D added and eating three slices of bread spread with margarine each day will supply an individual with sufficient vitamin D.

Caring for people from ethnic minority communities

Government statistics indicate that only 2% of older people come from minority ethnic communities. Older people from these backgrounds are less likely to enter nursing homes than older people from the host population. This may be because few services are tailored to their needs. Older people from all backgrounds should be offered a diet similar to that which they would choose to eat at home. This diet should reflect religious and ethnic background.

Jewish people do not eat pork or shellfish. Some Jewish people maintain a strict kosher diet and have separate areas within their kitchen for preparing dairy foods and meat. Separate crockery and utensils are also used for dairy foods and meat. Animals are killed in a specific way to ensure that meat is kosher. There are a number of nursing and residential homes throughout the UK that care specifically for people of the Jewish faith. These homes are able to prepare kosher food. Most nursing homes lack the facilities to prepare kosher food; in many cases the individual's family wish to bring it in. Ready-prepared kosher meals are available through the kosher meals service in many areas of the UK. The local hospital dietician can provide details as hospitals obtain kosher meals in this way. Older people of the Jewish faith who do not observe a strict kosher diet usually do not eat pork or shellfish and do not consume meat and dairy products at one sitting. In practice this may mean that the individual eats roast beef, roast potatoes and vegetables followed by apple pie, but does not have custard because it contains milk, and has a cup of tea without milk.

Older people of the Muslim faith do not eat pork. Strict Muslims eat meat that has been killed in a special way so that all blood is drained from it; this is known as halal meat. It is possible to obtain halal meat from halal butchers, and it can be prepared for eating normally. If it is not possible to obtain halal meat, strict Muslims may wish to avoid meat.

Individuals who follow the Hindu faith do not eat beef. Some Hindus are vegetarian and do not eat any animal products. They follow a vegan diet as outlined earlier.

Assessing nutritional status

Weight and height are reliable indicators of nutritional status in younger adults, but these are less reliable in older people. You can work out a person's body mass index (BMI) by using the following formula:

$$BMI = \frac{body\ weight\ in\ kilograms}{(Height\ in\ metres)^2}$$

In theory the BMI classification gives you the following results:

BMI	Weight
Less than 20	Underweight
20–25	Ideal weight
25–30	Overweight
30+	Obese

There are a few problems with using BMI in very old people. Oedema may mask weight loss so although a person's BMI appears satisfactory it is concealing undernutrition. Low protein levels lead to a low serum albumen. When serum albumen levels are low, fluid leaches into the tissues causing oedema. Increasing protein intake leads to improved nutrition but if you use BMI as the sole indicator of nutritional status it can appear that nutritional status is worsening.

It can be difficult to obtain an accurate height measurement with some older people. Osteoporosis can lead to collapse of vertebrae and if you measure the person they appear shorter than they actually are. People with osteoporosis can develop spinal curvatures and this makes it difficult to measure height accurately. In order to calculate BMI you have to measure height and that involves standing up. Two-thirds of nursing home residents are unable to stand unaided.

Mindex

Measuring the distance from the web of the fingers to the sternal notch when the arm is held horizontally gives you a demi-span measurement. You can then use the demi-span to work out the person's height[19].

Height for men = 1.2 × demi-span +71

Height for women = 1.2 × demi-span +67

You can then use these measurements to obtain a BMI. You can also use the measurement to work out the mindex. This is calculated as:

$$\text{Mindex} = \frac{\text{Weight in kg}}{\text{Demi-span in metres}}$$

Demi-span and Mindex measurements overcome the problems of measuring height but can remain inaccurate when oedema is present. People with cardiac and liver disease may retain fluid in the abdominal cavity and this is not visible.

Upper arm circumference

Upper arm circumference measurements, known as mid arm circumference (MAC) measurements, can provide information about nutritional status. A single measurement is of little use but ongoing measurements enable you to determine if the person's nutritional status is improving or worsening. MAC measurements are useful for people who are too frail to be weighed.

Biochemical tests

Serum albumen is reduced in renal and liver diseases and some cancers lead to reduced serum albumen. Generally though it is a good indicator of chronic malnutrition. Tests are also available to test for deficiency of specific nutrients such as vitamin C or zinc.

General measures to reduce malnutrition

Nurses working in nursing homes can introduce general measures that reduce the risk of malnutrition, including:

- Providing snacks. Researchers studying the difference in diet between well nourished and poorly nourished older people living in nursing homes found that the poorly nourished people did not have snacks. Generally the poorly nourished people were confused or required assistance to eat. Staff conscientiously gave these residents their meals but the meals had insufficient nutrients to prevent malnutrition. This presented no problem to the well nourished residents who were able to eat independently and raid their biscuit tins and eat cake in the afternoon, but the dependent and confused residents rarely got the snacks.
- Encouraging and enabling older people to eat independently. Providing appropriate aids such as plates with deep rims and non-slip mats to prevent slippage, enables many people to eat independently. People who eat independently eat more than those who are fed.
- Watching wastage. If a meal is moved from kitchen to table to bin, it is not doing the person any good. Watching wastage enables you to identify problems and to take action to prevent malnutrition.
- Providing supplements if a meal is declined or appetite is poor. The

research shows that nutritional supplements given at appropriate times do not reduce appetite, and improve health.

- Organise the home to prevent unnecessary interruptions at mealtimes. Make sure that medications are given out before or after the meal (as appropriate). This allows people to enjoy the meal without disturbance. Ensure that the dressings are completed before or after mealtimes. Beginning your meal when everyone else is finishing spoils the pleasure of a meal and reduces intake.
- Ensure that all staff are available to help residents who require help to eat.
- Ensure staff take time and make sure mealtimes are pleasurable and unrushed.

Specific measures to reduce malnutrition

If a person is malnourished you need to develop a problem solving approach. Table 11.1 outlines common problems and solutions.

Table 11.1   Common nutritional problems.

Problem	Possible solutions
Dental problems, e.g. dental cavities[20]	Refer to dental surgeon for treatment
Ill-fitting dentures	Refer to dental surgeon for treatment
Medication reducing appetite	Ask GP to review medication
Reduced appetite	Offer enriched diet
Swallowing difficulties	Refer to GP and speech and language therapist to improve swallowing Refer to dietician for dietary advice Provide soft, thickened or puréed diet as tolerated

It is important to present food attractively so that it will appeal to people with poor appetites. Food should be freshly cooked and appeal to the eyes as well as the appetite. Only a very hungry person would relish cauliflower, mashed potatoes and white fish! An enriched diet will help correct nutritional deficiencies. Ageing affects appetite and providing meals rich in nutrients and energy reduces the risk of malnutrition. The challenge for chefs is to pack as many nutrients and calories as possible into small portions of food[21]. The way food is served is very important. Dining rooms should be welcoming and staff should encourage residents to linger over their meals. It is important to avoid developing a culture where meals are viewed by staff as a chore to be gotten over as quickly as possible – they should be a pleasure.

The role of dietary supplements

Older people who are malnourished should be offered large helpings of normal food, and should also be offered nutritious snacks. Some older people are unable to eat enough to meet their dietary needs, and dietary supplements should be considered. You should ask the individual's doctor to contact the community dietician; they cannot accept referrals from nurses. The dietician will visit the individual to assess the diet eaten and discuss dietary preferences with the individual. Dieticians usually bring samples of supplements so the person can taste them. The dietician will then recommend a range of dietary supplements that can be prescribed by the individual's doctor.

There are ranges of flavoured drinks that are high in calories and have added vitamins and minerals. Some are fruit flavoured and can be given through the day instead of water or squash. Other drinks are milk based and available in a variety of flavours. High protein puddings are also available and can be given as snacks. A number of dietary supplements are available as tasteless white powders and these can be mixed into food to provide additional calories.

Dietary supplements can be prescribed for individuals suffering from dysphagia and a range of other conditions. Details can be obtained from the latest issue of the British National Formulary. It is important to be aware that dietary supplements are intended to supplement meals not substitute meals. Sometimes supplements can be self-defeating. If you give a resident a supplement and she is then too full up to eat her meal, you need to think again. It is important that you get the message across to care assistant colleagues that a small carton of a dietary supplement is not a substitute for dinner.

High fibre diets and their role in preventing constipation

Constipation becomes more common as adults age. Disorders of the gastro-intestinal tract, such as irritable colon syndrome, haemorrhoids and anal fissure, can lead to constipation. Neurological problems, such as dementia, stroke, Parkinson's disease and disseminated sclerosis, can also lead to constipation. Endocrine disorders and prescribed medications, such as iron, antacids and analgesics, can contribute to constipation. Factors such as lack of exercise, immobility, inadequate fluid intake and pain can also cause it.

Nursing practice can contribute to constipation. Nurses must examine practice within their workplace and ensure that older people have sufficient time and privacy to open their bowels. Some practitioners suggest that constipation in older people should not be treated with an increase in dietary fibre[22]. Laxatives and suppositories or enemas are recommended because it is thought that a high fibre diet can cause the rectum to become loaded with soft faeces[23]. The dosage of laxatives, however, can be extremely difficult to calculate. Osmotic softeners that are often used to treat constipation in older people can cause the rectum to become loaded with soft faeces and individuals can leak soft faeces. Irritant laxatives can cause abdominal pain, cramp and diarrhoea, and can lead to faecal incontinence.

Introducing high fibre foods gradually into an older person's diet can eliminate the need for laxatives in many older people and contribute to general well-being. It is often thought that a diet is magically transformed into a high fibre diet by adding tablespoons of bran to porridge or soup. Any sensible older person will refuse food which has had bran stirred in. High fibre foods, such as bran flakes, Weetabix, Shredded Wheat and muesli, can be offered as alternatives to cornflakes. Prunes, apricots and fruit compote provide additional fibre, vitamins and nutrients. Wholemeal bread high in fibre and B vitamins is a tasty alternative to sliced white bread. Cakes, crumbles and pastries can be made with 50% wholemeal flour. Many cakes such as banana cake and date loaf provide additional fibre and taste delicious. Digestive biscuits, wholemeal shortbread and wholemeal cookies with added nuts and raisins can be offered instead of custard creams. Lentils, barley and pulses can be added to soups and casseroles.

Eating a diet rich in fibre can be enjoyable and in many cases cures constipation and reduces the need for laxatives. Some older people do not wish to eat wholemeal bread or cereals high in fibre but benefit from other fibre-rich foods introduced subtly into their diet[24]. It is essential that individuals who are consuming a diet rich in natural fibre drink at least two litres of fluid each day. Offering extra cups of tea, water, squash and fruit juice helps ensure that fluid intake is adequate.

Reduced fibre diets and their role in managing bowel problems

Some older people who suffer from diarrhoea benefit from a high fibre diet. The fibre absorbs excess water and the stool is more formed than before. In others this is ineffective. Some older people who are profoundly disabled, perhaps because of neurological disease, develop faecal incontinence. Helping the individual to the toilet after breakfast, when the gastro-colic reflex is at its strongest, often results in a bowel action. Such nursing interventions can prevent faecal incontinence in many extremely disabled, cognitively impaired older people. Some older people, though, remain faecally incontinent. In these individuals a high fibre diet can result in the bowel becoming loaded with soft faeces, and continual leakage can occur. A low residue diet normally results in constipation and this can be treated with suppositories or a mini-enema.

Conclusion

Frail older people are at risk of malnutrition. Nurses can enable older people to eat a healthy diet that enhances the older person's quality of life and protects against illness and disease.

References

1 Association Community Health Councils in England and Wales (ACHEW) (1997) *Hungry in Hospital*. ACHEW, London.
2 United Kingdom Central Council (1997) Responsibility for the feeding of patients. *Registrars Letter*. UKCC, London.
3 Committee on Medical Aspects of Food Policy (COMA) (1992) *The Nutrition of Elderly People*. Report on Health and Social Subjects no. 43. The Stationery Office, London.
4 Webb, Geoffrey, P. & Copeman, June (1996) *The Nutrition of Older Adults*. Arnold, London.

5 Drewnowski, A. & Warren-Mears, V.A. (2001) Does aging change nutrition requirements? *J. Nutr. Health Aging*, 5(2), 70–74.

6 Department of Health (1992) *The Nutrition of Elderly People*. Report on Health and Social Subjects no. 43. The Stationery Office, London.

7 Chandra, R.K. (1993) Nutrition and the Immune System. *Proceedings of the Nutrition Society*, **52**, 77–84.

8 Goode, H.P., Penne, N.D., Kelleher, J. & Walker, B.E. (1991) Evidence of cellular zinc depletion in hospitalised but not in healthy elderly subjects. *Age & Ageing*, **20**, 345–348.

9 Chandra, R.K. (1992) Effect of vitamin and trace element supplementation on immune response in elderly subjects. *Lancet*, **340**, 1124–1127.

10 McWhirter, J.P. & Pennington, C.R. (1994) Incidence and recognition of malnutrition in hospitals. *British Medical Journal*, **306**, 945–948.

11 McErlain, L., Marson, H., Ainsworth, P. & Burnett, S.A. (2001) Ascorbic acid loss in vegetables: adequacy of a hospital cook-chill system. *Int. J. Food Sci. Nutr.*, **52**(3), 205–211.

12 Chandra, R.K. (1991) McCollum Award Lecture 1990. Nutrition and Immunity. Lessons from the past and new insights into the future. *American Journal of Clinical Nutrition*, **53**, 1087–1102.

13 Bastow, M.D., Rawlings, J. & Allison, S.P. (1982) Benefits of supplementary tube feeding after fractured neck of femur: a randomised control trial. *British Medical Journal*, **287**, 1589–1592.

14 Bistrian, B.R., Sherman, M. & Blackburn, G.L. (1977) Cellular immunity in adult marasmus. *Archives of Internal Medicine*, **137**, 1408–1411.

15 Friedman, R. & Kalant, N. (1998) Comparison of long-term care in an acute institution and in a long term care institution. *CMAJ*, **159**(9), 1107–1113.

16 The Caroline Walker Trust (1995) *Eating Well for Older People*. The Caroline Walker Trust, London.

17 Committee on Medical Aspects of Food Policy (1991) *Dietary Reference Values for Food Energy and Nutrients for the United Kingdom*. Report on health and social subjects no. 41. The Stationery Office, London.

18 Prentice, A.M. (1988) Is severe wasting in elderly mental patients caused by excessive energy requirement? *Age & Ageing*, **18**, 158–167.

19 White, A. *et al.* (1993) *Health Survey for England*. The Stationery Office, London.

20 Sheiham, A. & Steele, J. (2001) Does the condition of the mouth and teeth affect the ability to eat certain foods, nutrient and dietary intake and nutritional status amongst older people? *Public Health Nutr.*, **4**(3), 797–803.

21 Drewnowski, A.M. (2001) Impact of Aging on Eating Behaviors, Food Choices, Nutrition, and Health Status. *J. Nutr. Health Aging*, 5(2), 75–79.

22 Ardron, M.E. & Main, A.N.H. (1990) Management of constipation. *British Medical Journal*, **300**, 1400.

23 Roe, B. & Williams, K. (1994) *Clinical Handbook for Continence Care*. Scutari Press, Harrow.

24 Nazarko, L. (1993) Preventing Constipation. *Elderly Care*, 5(2), 32–33.

Chapter 12

Stroke

Introduction

Over half of all people admitted to nursing homes have suffered a stroke. These individuals are very disabled; more than three-quarters are unable to transfer from bed to chair unaided[1]. When stroke survivors are admitted, we can offer care that enables or care that disables. If we are to offer enabling care we need to be aware of the causes and consequences of stroke. Stroke is responsible for 10–12% of deaths in industrialised countries. Most people who suffer stroke are elderly. The risk of stroke doubles every decade after the age of 55, and 88% of people who die as a result of stroke are aged 85 or more.

In industrialised societies the incidence of stroke fell by an average of 5% every decade until the mid 1980s[2]. Now the incidence of stroke in industrialised societies is again rising because people are living longer. The incidence of stroke is rising in line with the increase in people aged 85 and over. Every year 120 000 people living in the UK suffer a stroke. Within a month 24 000 of the people who suffered stroke will have died. Within six months 30 000 people will have fully recovered from the effects of stroke. The remaining 66 000 people will have some degree of disability[3]. The most disabled stroke survivors require continuing care and are referred to nursing homes. Research indicates that 25% of all people who have first strokes are admitted to nursing homes. Almost 50% of stroke survivors are severely affected and more than half of them are cared for in nursing homes 90 days after stroke. A year after stroke almost 70% of the most disabled stroke survivors will require a period of nursing home care[4].

This chapter consists of six sections: causes and consequences of stroke, rehabilitation, fluids and diet, communication, bladder and bowel problems, and ethical issues.

Causes and consequences of stroke

This section aims to:

- Discuss normal brain function
- Discuss the causes of strokes
- Explore current treatment of stroke
- Explain how stroke affects mobility, comprehension, the ability to eat and the ability to control bladder function

Normal brain function

The adult human brain accounts for 2% of body mass but requires 20% of cardiac output. The brain receives its blood supply from two vertebral arteries and two carotid arteries. These arteries join up in the brain to form the 'circle of Willis'. The brain requires an average of 50 ml of blood per 100 g of body tissue per minute. Some areas of the brain, such as the cortex and the basal ganglia, require higher levels of blood flow; other areas, such as the white matter, have lower blood flows[5]. The brain metabolises over five times more oxygen than glucose. In a healthy well-nourished adult the brain receives a constant supply of well-oxygenated blood and functions to capacity.

Stroke is an interruption to the blood supply to the brain. The World Health Organisation definition of stroke is[6]: 'Rapidly developing clinical signs of focal (or global) disturbance of cerebral function with symptoms lasting 24 hours or longer or leading to death with no apparent cause other than of vascular origin.'

Causes of stroke

Cerebral ischaemia and cerebral haemorrhage lead to stroke.

Cerebral ischaemia

Cerebral ischaemia, lack of blood perfusing the brain, is the commonest cause of stroke. Research demonstrates that 80–90% of strokes are caused by cerebral ischaemia[7]. An embolus or multiple emboli blocking part of the cerebral circulation cause the ischaemia. The most common emboli are blood clots but fat cells, gases and malignant cells can also cause emboli. Emboli can originate in the heart, aorta, carotid or vertebral vessels; most originate in the heart.

Causes of cardiac emboli

- Mitral valve stenosis
- Mitral valve prolapse
- Bacterial endocarditis
- Cardiac myopathy
- Rheumatic heart disease
- Cardiac arthymias, especially atrial fibrillation.

Cerebral haemorrhage

Bleeding into the brain is responsible for 10–20% of all strokes. There are two causes of brain bleedings: haemorrhage and aneurysm. Spontaneous haemorrhage into the brain has a high mortality rate; between 13% and 56% of patients die within a month of stroke.

A weakening of the walls of the arterial muscles causes aneurysm. The artery dilates and either ruptures or leaks, releasing blood into the brain. Scientists do not yet know the reason aneurysms develop but there are two theories. The congenital theory is that arterial weakness is genetic; supporters of the genetic theory point out that there is often a strong family history of aneurysm. The degenerative theory is that certain factors, including age, hypertension, smoking, lean body mass and arteriosclerosis, lead to roughening and damage of the arterial walls. This damage reduces the strength of the arterial walls and leads to aneurysms. Aneurysm causes 6–10% of strokes; between 22% and 25% of all patients die within a month of stroke. Aneurysm is most common in people in their fifties and sixties.

Consequences of stroke

Whatever the cause of stroke, the result is that blood supply to the brain is interrupted or totally obstructed. All living tissue requires oxygen and glucose to survive. When the blood flow to tissue is cut off, tissue dies. The damage sustained is dependent on the length of time the blood supply is interrupted and the metabolic rate, which affects oxygen requirements. At the periphery of the ischaemic tissue, circulation is also impaired. The surrounding tissue is dependent on collateral or peripheral circulation for survival.

The extent of disability a person suffers following stroke depends on the site and extent of damage. The areas of the brain that stroke can damage are the cerebral cortex, the thalmus, the limbic system, the cerebellum, the brainstem and the medulla.

The cerebral cortex

The cerebral cortex is a thin covering of grey matter. It is 3–5 mm thick and contains an estimated 15 billion brain cells. It covers both cerebral hemispheres. The cortex is thought to be responsible for voluntary control of many body activities including language, memory, logical thought and self-perception. Damage to the cortex affects language, memory, the ability to work things out and voluntary activity.

The thalamus

The thalamus operates as a switchboard and routes messages from sensory organs to the appropriate part of the brain. The thalamus is linked to speech and is responsible for controlling sleep and wakefulness. Damage to the thalamus affects all aspects of function. Thalamic damage can prevent a message from the bladder getting through to the cortex and preventing reflex bladder emptying. Thalamic damage can prevent a message from the arm that it is getting burnt or crushed reaching motor centres responsible for moving the arm to safety.

The limbic system

The limbic system is the most primitive part of the brain and is concerned with instinctive behaviour and control of instinctive behaviour. The limbic system is interconnected with the hippocampus. The hippocampus is responsible for storing new memories of recent events for later recall. When you return home tonight your hippocampus will release this morning's memories about the way to the train station or where you've parked your car. The hippocampus enables us to recognise faces and to put a name to a face. It is one of the first structures affected by dementia[8]. Damage to the limbic system affects short-term memory.

The cerebellum

The cerebellum stores all information about learnt motor functions. When you learnt to ride a bicycle or do the breast stroke the information about how to co-ordinate these activities was stored in your cerebellum. You'll never forget how to ride a bike unless you have cerebellar damage. The cerebellum receives information from your sensory systems and your cortex; you know at all times where your leg is because your cerebellum is co-ordinating that information. The cerebellum affects muscle tone and is responsible for posture, balance, walking, movement and non-automatic movements. Alcohol causes mild cerebellar disruption and tests carried out by police to find out if a person is drunk test cerebellar function. These include walking in a straight line and closing your eyes and touching the tip of your nose. The ultimate test of cerebellar function is probably standing on one leg pulling on your tights. Damage to the cerebellum affects balance, knowing where your limbs are, and being able to carry out learnt motor functions such as typing or dancing. People with cerebellar damage have difficulty getting started in activities such as walking but get in their stride when automatic motor function takes over.

The brainstem

The brainstem is responsible for hearing and eye movement systems. The pons connects the cortex of a cerebral hemisphere with the opposite area of the cerebellum. This connection enables us to move efficiently and co-ordinates fine motor activity such as threading a needle. Damage to the brainstem affects hearing and eye movements and co-ordination of motor activity.

The medulla

The medulla connects with the pons above and the spinal cord below. It communicates with the brain and spinal cord. Just above the area where the medulla connects with the spinal cord, the nerve pathways cross over. Medullary damage can affect both sides of the body.

How stroke treatment affects outcome

When a stroke occurs some neurones die rapidly but many are simply injured and if the correct treatment was available many of these neurones could be salvaged and damage limited. Our knowledge of how to limit damage after stroke is limited. What we do know is that stroke care in the UK is a lottery. We know that treatment in a specialist stroke unit reduces the risk of dying or requiring continuing care but access to specialist stroke units varies around the UK. Figure 12.1 illustrates access to stroke units.

Research carried out by the Stroke Association in 1999 showed that

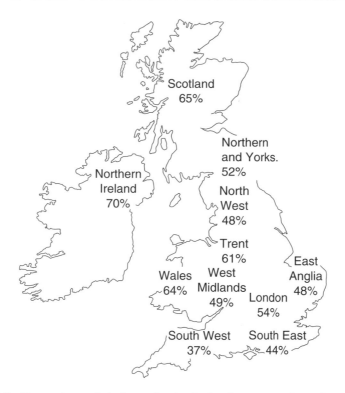

Fig. 12.1 Percentage of stroke patients admitted to or transferred to a stroke unit.

consultants who specialise in stroke medicine look after only 3% of stroke patients. An estimated 7000 people die or require continuing care because of poor care and treatment[9]. Specialist stroke units treat stroke differently from general medical and acute geriatric admission wards. The main differences are that specialist stroke units use oxygen more frequently. This aims to salvage damaged neurones. They use heparin in the case of ischaemic stroke to prevent further strokes. Antipyretics are used to prevent pyrexia as this is thought to increase damage to salvageable neurones. Diastolic blood pressure is stabilised rapidly and maintained at physiologically normal limits while avoiding the trauma and damage caused by hypotension. Patients are stabilised rapidly and mobilised early. People cared for in specialist stroke units are less disabled and have higher levels of functioning than those cared for in general units[10].

Swedish research suggests that the most disabled stroke survivors are discharged early – to nursing homes[11]. Evidence presented to the Royal Commission on long-term care suggested that the most disabled stroke survivors, those destined for nursing homes, receive little physiotherapy because of their age, level of impairment and destination.

How stroke affects mobility

The ability to move is dependent on body systems working together. Turning on a tap requires co-ordination of speed, strength and smoothness of action. You decide to turn on the tap. A message is relayed to your brain and you move your arm and begin to turn on the tap. The tap is stiff – sensory messages are sent from your hand to your brain. Messages from your brain are relayed back to your hand and you increase the force. Any interruption of motor or sensory nerve pathways would prevent you being able to carry out this simple action.

Cerebral control of movement

The primary motor area or motor strip in the frontal lobe controls movement. There are thought to be 17 different areas in the motor strip, each area controlling a part of the body. The left motor strip controls the right hand side of the body. The right motor strip controls the left-hand side of the body. Nerve cells connect the motor strips to the spinal cord.

Ability and quality of movement

Stroke affects the ability to move and the quality of movement. The level of lost ability varies according to the location of the stroke and the size of the damaged area. A mild stroke affecting the motor strip will cause weakness. A severe stroke affecting the motor strip will cause dense hemiplegia. A mild stroke affecting the medulla will cause weakness in both arms or both legs or in all limbs. A severe stroke affecting the medulla will lead to a dense quadriplegia. A stroke affecting the cerebellum will produce difficulty walking. The person will stagger and will have difficulty performing co-ordinated movements. Muscle tone is reduced and the person appears floppy. A stroke affecting the basal ganglia causes tremor.

How much recovery can we expect?

Stroke causes tissue death, tissue damage and tissue swelling. Some of the tissue damaged by low oxygen levels during stroke will recover. The oedema that follows stroke will gradually resolve. Eventually other areas of the brain will take over some of the functions of the damaged tissue. The ability to move, speak and swallow will slowly improve. Despite technological advances such as CAT and MRI scanning it is still very difficult to predict the possible level of recovery. In one study 88% of survivors suffered hemiplegia and hemiparesis but within six months 76% had fully recovered the use of their affected limbs. It can take up to two years for older people to fully recover after stroke. Analysis of research does give an indication of which categories of patients will make good progress[12] and which categories will make poorer progress (Table 12.1).

Conclusion

Older adults are more likely to suffer stroke. Older adults take longer to recover from any illness and few are likely to recover rapidly. The most severely disabled stroke survivors are those admitted to nursing homes. These individuals are normally immobile and incontinent and many have profound difficulties in communicating. Good nursing care can enable many of these individuals to regain skills and enjoy the highest possible quality of life. The next section discusses how to help stroke survivors regain mobility.

Table 12.1   Stroke progress indicators.

Good prospect of recovery	Poorer prospect of recovery
Young – less than 70	Old – more than 70
No severe loss function	Severe loss function
No major communication problems	Major communication problems
Continent	Incontinent
No infection	Spatial defects
No bedsores	Visual defects
First stroke	Previous strokes

Key points

- Stroke is responsible for 10–12% of all deaths
- 88% of people who die from stroke are aged 85 and over
- 80–90% of strokes are caused by ischaemia
- 10–20% of strokes are caused by haemorrhage
- Damage sustained depends on site of damage and duration of ischaemia
- The most disabled stroke survivors, those with the poorest prognosis, are admitted to nursing homes.

Rehabilitation

Every person who suffers a stroke will improve. We do not know how much the person will improve or how quickly. Our role as nurses is crucial in enabling people to function to capacity after stroke. All of us have worked with stroke patients helping them to regain skills only to see everything lost when another stroke occurs. This section aims to help you understand how to reduce the risk of stroke and to enable people to regain skills.

This section aims to enable you to understand:

- Stroke risk factors
- How to reduce stroke risk factors
- Stroke assessment
- Maintaining limb function
- Ways to improve mobility
- Future stroke treatments

Stroke risk factors

People who have suffered stroke are at risk of further stroke. In strokes caused by aneurysm, half will suffer a rebleed within six months. Half the people who rebleed will not survive. Most strokes in older adults are caused by ischaemia. Strokes only occur when there are established cardiovascular problems.

Risk factors that we cannot change
Age – The risk of stroke increases with age; one study shows that the risk increases by 10% every decade.

Sex – Stroke is gender related; men are more likely to suffer stroke but because women live longer there are more female stroke victims[13].

Genetic inheritance – A study of identical and non-identical twins proved the genetic link between stroke[14]. In 1998 researchers found gene mutations that led to abnormalities in cerebral blood vessels and stroke[15]. In 1999 researchers discovered several genetic factors that led to cardiovascular disease and stroke. They found that stroke is a result of interaction between several genetic and environmental factors[16].

Race – Some races have higher stroke risk than others. Japanese people have twice the rate of intracerebral haemorrhage than any other race. In the US researchers have found that black people are twice as at risk of subarachnoid haemorrhage than white people[17]. Another US study found that black stroke survivors had greater levels of disability than white stroke survivors did[18]. A British study found that stroke incidence and severity was race related. Caribbeans had the highest risk factor, then Africans, then Indians and finally whites[19]. Stroke is class related – the higher your social class the less likely you are to have a stroke. Research from the US shows that stroke is the third leading cause of death in black women and the sixth leading cause in black men. Black people have higher levels of hypertension and diabetes than Caucasians[20]. Research being carried out in Kinasha in the Congo suggests that black people metabolise salt more efficiently than Caucasians and that this leads to hypertension and increased stroke risk.

Location – The risk of having a stroke depends on where you live; if you live in Italy you are less likely to have a stroke than a similar person is in Sweden or Scunthorpe. The incidence of stroke increases progressively from the Mediterranean area to Scandinavia. In Northern Europe stroke mortality is 70% higher in winter than in summer. Temperature causes a variation in blood pressure. In the UK the average person's blood pressure rises by 5 mmhg in winter. Cold increases cardiac workload and increases the need for oxygen; this may reduce coronary blood flow. Cold causes peripheral vasoconstriction and this can cause acute pulmonary oedema. Cold increases the concentration of fibrinogen in blood and makes blood more likely to clot[21].

Risk factors that can be altered
Many risk factors can be altered and the risk of stroke is then reduced.

Hypertension is the most important risk factor in stroke. Men with a systolic blood pressure of above 180 mmhg have six times the risk of stroke than normotensive men. Men with a systolic blood pressure of 160–180 mmhg have four times the risk of stroke of normotensive men. Hypertension is of greater significance in black people whose risk factor is even higher at the same levels[22]. Some GPs still consider that high systolic blood pressure is 'normal' in elderly people and do not treat.

Treating hypertension reduces the risk of stroke. One study found that reducing systolic blood pressure to 140 mmhg reduced the incidence of stroke in elderly people by 36%[23]. Hypertension can be treated in three ways: medication to reduce blood pressure, diet to reduce weight and reducing salt. One study involving 975 men aged 60 to 80 examined the effectiveness of these strategies. Patients were divided into two groups – overweight and normal weight. Some men were asked to reduce their salt intake, others to lose weight, others to reduce salt and lose weight, and there was a control group. Blood pressure fell significantly in all intervention groups over a three-month period; 39% of overweight men who lost an average of 3.5–4 kg and reduced salt intake no longer required medication. Reducing salt intake helped lower the blood pressure of men who were of normal weight. Monitoring blood pressure and treating hypertension will reduce the risk of further stroke by 35–40%[24]. If the research in Kinasha is verified, salt reduction may help reduce the stroke mortality and disability in black people.

Cardiac disease increases the risk of stroke. A large study found that people with atrial fibrillation are five times more likely to have a stroke than those in sinus rhythm[25]. People with left ventricular failure and left ventricular hypertrophy are at increased risk of stroke[26]. American research indicates that 45% of older women living in nursing homes suffer from atrial fibrillation[27].

Treating atrial fibrillation and using antiplatelet drugs to reduce clot formation reduces the risk of stroke. The Royal College of Physicians recommend 300 mg of aspirin daily to prevent further stroke when atrial fibrillation is present.

Preventing further strokes

There are several treatment options, which each have costs and benefits. One large study of 19 435 patients found that treating patients with aspirin, 25 mg b.d., reduced the risk of stroke by 18%; treating patients with dipyridamole (an antiplatelet agent) reduced the risk of stroke by 37%. Patients treated with aspirin and dipyridamole reduced the risk of stroke by 37%[28]. Warfarin can be used to prevent stroke but there is a risk of intracerebral bleed. Some doctors consider that, other than in cases when the patients have diseased heart valves, the risks of warfarin use in this group of patients are unacceptably high. Other doctors disagree and think that anticoagulant therapy should be used more in older people[29,30].

Smoking increases the risk of stroke. The level of risk is related to the number of cigarettes smoked. The risk of ischaemic stroke disappears two years after smoking cessation[31]. Exposure to other people's cigarette smoke also increases stroke risk[32].

Alcohol can increase the risk of stroke. Drinking heavily doubles the risk of stroke[33]; however a study of registered nurses found that moderate alcohol consumption reduces the risk of stroke by 30%.

Diabetes increases the risk of stroke. Although many doctors and nurse specialists consider higher blood sugars acceptable in elderly people, good diabetic control reduces the risk of stroke[34,35].

Diet has an important and unrecognised role in stroke prevention. Research indicates that older adults who have a diet low in vitamin C are more at risk of stroke than those with a good intake[36]. A study of registered nurses over fourteen years found that those with a low calcium intake were at greater risk of stroke[37].

Stroke assessment

Before you rush in and begin work on improving the person's mobility – stop and think:

- What are the problems here?
- What needs to be done to help this person regain mobility?
- Who has the skills to do this?

If you do not ask these questions it is unlikely that anyone else will. Your role is to co-ordinate and manage stroke rehabilitation. An example of an assessment form is given at the end of this chapter.

Solutions to common problems

Before you can begin rehabilitation you need to gain the person's trust and co-operation. Ensure that the person is not too tired, in pain or anxious. Do not build yourself and your resident up for failure. If the person requires analgesia, give it well before you begin so that it has time to work. Choose the time of day carefully and build a relationship on honesty and trust. Make sure the person is properly dressed and has clothing that will not inhibit movement. Make sure the person is warm enough; cold can trigger spasticity. Make sure it is not too hot; heat can reduce muscle tone. Make sure the person has suitable footwear with non-slip soles. Begin work in a quiet non-public environment. Noise and distraction make it difficult for the person to concentrate. Inability to do what you ask can be coped with in private but can be humiliating in public.

Positioning

Many nurses think that the priority is to get the person walking, but this is not always true. Begin by making sure that the person is helped to regain muscle control. Often the way staff position stroke patients actually prevents the person regaining muscle control. Sitting the person in a chair with a headrest and fully supporting the back and neck causes muscle weakness. Sitting the person in a chair and elevating the legs on a high footstool, in an effort to reduce oedema, encourages the person to slump and weakens muscles. When you attempt to stand the person up, the person who normally reclines leans backwards because the vestibular system has adjusted to leaning back. When you attempt to stand the person up, who normally slumps forward, she leans forward.

Seat the stroke patient in a short upright-backed chair; the hips should be at right angles and the feet flat on the floor. You should have chairs with differing heights as little legs can dangle! The person's hands and forearms should be positioned on a table. You may be able to encourage the person to read or draw. Make sure that cushions are not too thick or they will cause wobble. Make sure that the chair seat is not too long or the patient will slide out. Make sure that the chair is not too short or it will cause pressure on the back of the upper thighs. Move the person often, hourly if possible. Stand the person up and move them to the toilet; do not bring a commode unless the person requires the toilet urgently. Move the person to the dining room –

do not serve meals at the bedside table. If the person starts to droop take them to bed for a nap. Do not let the person doze off in an abnormal position in the chair, or muscles will adopt abnormal postures that are difficult to correct.

Walking

Do not lift the person into a standing position as this will make it difficult for them to balance. Encourage the person to move forward in the chair, place feet flat on the floor and push up using both arms. Do not expect the individual to walk straight away; give her time to get her balance. If the person cannot get out of the chair unaided, practice this before attempting walking. Use a dining table and chair and get the patient to practice standing up from the chair holding the table for support. Always ask the person to put the good leg first. Do not do too much too soon; little and often is better. This allows the person to build up muscle strength and confidence.

Walking aids

You can obtain suitable aids by asking the physiotherapist or the GP to complete a medical appliances referral form. It is a good idea to have a supply of forms at the home as people forget to fill them in when they return to their office. The resident is then either visited at the home or attends a clinic at the hospital. There the person is assessed and a suitable aid is provided.

Stroke patients should not normally be supplied with Zimmer frames as normal use of both arms and good balance is required to use one. A three-wheeled rollator is more suitable for patients with weakness in one arm. A rollator with forearm supports is more suitable for patients with marked weakness in one arm. Tripods or quadripods (which are more stable) are useful for people with ataxia and/or poor vision.

Spasticity

Clawing of hands is caused by mismanagement of spasticity. Do not give or allow your staff to give the patient a ball, bandage or gamgee pad. This stimulates the grasp reflex and makes things worse. If you have a resident with a clawed hand gently stimulate the wrist and back of the hand. Then put the hand in a bowl of warm water and massage and stretch the hand. Remove the hand when the water cools and dry the hand carefully. Repeat this several times each day. You can use a home-made glove to help reduce spasm; lively splints can also reduce deformity.

Ankle inversion

Sometimes abnormal spastic movements can cause ankle inversion. Exercise helps, especially in a warm bath. If this is ineffective do not attempt to walk the person; refer to the orthotist for possible calliper or lively splint to correct the abnormality first.

Medication to reduce spasm

Spasm and spasticity prevent the person functioning to capacity. Medication can help reduce spasm and help people regain function. There are two available antispasmodics: baclofen (Lioresal) and dantrolene sodium (Dantrium). Baclofen is available in 10 mg tablets and in liquid; it acts by decreasing reflex activity at a spinal level. The normal dosage is 5 mg b.d. increasing to a maximum of 60 mg divided into three doses. The dose can be altered every three days until muscle tone is reduced to the level where the patient can use the affected limbs. Side effects include drowsiness – this usually wears off after a few days, so it is worth watching and waiting – and interaction with antihypertensives. Blood pressure needs monitoring as it can fall and the dose of any prescribed antihypertensives may need adjusting.

Dantrolene sodium acts by reducing the release and uptake of calcium required for muscle contraction. The starting dose is 25 mg daily and it can be increased to 25 mg q.d.s. Side effects include nausea and diarrhoea. Long-term use at high doses can lead to muscle weakness. Baclofen and dantrolene sodium can be used in combination as they work in different ways. Short-term use can be very effective, long-term should be reviewed. It is important to tail off antispasmodics as abrupt withdrawal increases spasticity. Diazepam is also used for spasticity. Its use is not recommended in muscle spasm caused by stroke. It causes a general reduction of muscle tone, does not treat the spasm, reduces concentration, and can affect bladder tone and cause incontinence.

Botulism toxin known as botox can be injected into muscles to weaken certain muscles and treat contractures. A doctor injects the toxin into specific muscles and the toxin acts to paralyse or weaken certain muscle groups. It takes 2–5 days before the effects of the injection become apparent. If the injection has not been effective it can be repeated within 14 days. The injection wears off after 4–6 months and needs to be repeated. Repeated injections weaken certain muscle groups and in theory only eight injections are needed to treat spasticity. In practice doctors find that some people require fewer injections while others require top up injections at 6–12 monthly intervals.

Future therapies

At the moment we know little about how to prevent salvageable neurones from being damaged beyond repair. We know little about how to restore function, but cutting edge research is working on these problems.

Damage limitation therapies

When we looked at what happens during stroke we saw that some cells were damaged but that other cells could be salvaged if only we knew how. One treatment is available to treat acute stroke. Tissue plasminogen activator (TPA) is given within six hours of stroke onset by intravenous injection over an hour. There is a risk of intracerebral bleed. The patient must be scanned to make sure that the stroke was caused by a clot not a bleed before treatment. That means that the patient has to be transported to hospital, seen, scanned and treated within six hours.

In the US, trials of Ancrod are taking place. Ancrod is derived from the venom of snakes known as pit vipers, which are deadly rattlesnakes. The venom of these snakes contains an anticoagulant. Ancrod is given (within six hours of stroke) over a three-day period. A study of 500 stroke patients showed that 42% recovered fully within three hours of Ancrod being commenced[38]. It has a lower risk of intracerebral bleeding than TPA.

Irish or Caribbean coffee may also prevent stroke damage. Researchers have found that one measure of alcohol and two to three cups of coffee taken together offers almost complete protection against stroke damage. They found that alcohol alone made the stroke worse. Coffee alone had no effect. The researchers warned against patients attempting to self-medicate and emphasised the need for further research[39].

Treating existing damage

Stroke leads to muscle wasting. The muscle wasting on the affected side leads to bone loss and osteoporosis[40]. We know that passive movements increase cerebral blood flow and enable brain recovery to take place[41]. Often though it is difficult for nurses on busy understaffed units to give the level of passive movement that stroke patients require. Researchers have developed mini electrodes the size of a grain of rice that are injected into the muscle using a 12 gauge needle. These implants are known as bionic implanted nerve stimulators. They are activated by a radio signal on a patient-worn coil. This controls the frequency and intensity of the stimuli. The doctors then download a set of exercise programmes into the patient-worn coil and the patient's therapy is carried out[42].

Neurologists and engineers have developed a robot arm to help patients carry out arm exercises. The patient is prompted by a video to exercise the arm. If the patient does not move, the robot arm begins the movement; if the patient then begins to carry the movement through, the robot shuts off. Patients who had robot therapy showed improved shoulder and arm movement[43].

Brain cell transplants

Seven stroke patients have had brain cell transplants to replace damaged brain cells. Patients are injected with laboratory grown cells originating in the cancerous tumour teratoma. These are embryonic-like cells and are provided by a company known as Layton Bioscience. They are called LBS neurones. CT scans are used to identify sites to inject cells. Around 2–6 million neurones are injected in and around the stroke-damaged site. This research began in the late 1990s[44].

Conclusion

Stroke patients are at the mercy of the people who care for them. Good stroke management can enable the person to function to capacity; poor management can lead to loss of existing muscle tone and the development of deformity. Assessment of current level of function enables nurses to identify and take action to deal with problems.

Future developments may make all our stroke care skills a thing of the past if doctors can minimise stroke damage.

Key points

- Stroke incidence is related to gender, race, class and country
- Hypertension dramatically increases the risk of stroke
- Treating hypertension significantly reduces the risk of stroke
- Cardiac disease dramatically increases the risk of stroke
- Using antiplatelet drugs dramatically reduces the risk of stroke
- Smoking increases the risk of stroke
- Moderate alcohol consumption reduces the risk of stroke
- Correct positioning is vital to enable good muscle control
- Help the person to stand and balance before walking
- Use exercise and aids to prevent deformity
- Baclofen and dantrolene sodium can help reduce spasticity short term
- Botox may be used more in the future to treat spasticity.

Fluids and diet

Almost half of all stroke survivors have some difficulty swallowing[45,46]. Severe dysphagia is easy to identify but milder cases can be overlooked. Dysphagia can lead to food or drink trickling into the lungs. This can cause aspiration pneumonia and can lead to death[47]. Stroke survivors who suffer further strokes can develop dysphagia. Difficulty swallowing can lead to malnutrition and dehydration. Good nutrition and hydration is vital to health.

This section aims to enable you to:

- Identify signs of dysphagia
- Test swallowing reflex
- Help patients overcome swallowing difficulties
- Provide a suitable diet for people with swallowing difficulties
- Ensure the person with dysphagia receives sufficient fluids

---

Dysphagia

Dysphagia literally means difficulty swallowing. Swallowing is a complex function that involves twenty muscles and five nerves. Dysphagia is more likely to occur if the person has suffered multiple strokes or a brain stem stroke[48]. Although speech and language therapists are the people with specialist knowledge of dysphagia, nurses need to be able to recognise the signs and symptoms[49]:

- Coughing before, during or after swallowing
- Difficult or delayed swallow
- Gurgly voice after swallowing
- Breathlessness or bubbling after swallowing
- Inability to clear food or drink from the mouth
- Inability to hold food or fluid in the mouth.

Assessing for dysphagia

You should assess for dysphagia before offering fluids to a patient who has a stroke or extends a stroke in the home. If you are unsure about the person's ability to swallow and the person does not have any of the symptoms listed above, assess the swallowing ability as follows:

- Make sure the patient is sitting up and the head is bent slightly forward
- Offer a teaspoon of thickened fluid
- If the patient is able to swallow without any symptoms of dysphagia offer a teaspoon of cold water
- If there are no problems offer sips of fluid and observe.

Emergency referral

If the person has signs and symptoms of dysphagia you must withhold fluids and diet and refer the patient urgently. Speech and language therapists are the people with expertise in dysphagia. Speech and language therapists throughout the UK operate an open referral system. This means that you can telephone the speech and language therapist at the local hospital and ask for an urgent assessment. If you explain the problem you should get a visit that day. Speech and language therapists work normal office hours, Monday to Friday. You should also inform the patient's GP of your concerns and request an urgent visit, especially if you suspect that the patient has aspirated food or fluid into the lungs.

Treating dysphagia

The speech and language therapist will visit and advise you about management. If the person has major swallowing problems the dietician will be able to help and advise. Dieticians will only accept referrals from doctors. You can obtain a supply of specialist referral forms from your GP so that the GP can complete the form in the home. Faxing the form and following it up with a call speeds up response time.

Providing suitable diet

People with mild dysphagia have difficulty managing certain types of food. If the person has mild dysphagia avoid:

- Crispy cereals, like cornflakes or Rice Crispies, with cold milk
- Dry crumbly biscuits, e.g. digestives or Hob Nobs
- Sandwiches with loose bits like grated cheese or dry egg
- Soup with hard bits in it
- Dry food
- Crisps, peanuts and cinnamon toast (relatives tend to bring these in).

The person with dysphagia will find it easier to manage:

- Cereals with hot milk, e.g. cornflakes, Rice Crispies, All Bran (with lots of milk), Weetabix
- Cereals with cold milk that have been left standing for half an hour so that they can absorb fluid and soften up
- Soft biscuits, i.e. cookies because these are moist and chewy, not crumbly

- Soup where the bits have been liquidised
- Sandwiches with moist fillings, e.g. egg mayonnaise, cream cheese, tuna mayonnaise
- Food with sauces.

Helping the person to eat

Aim to enable the person to eat rather than feed them. Make sure the patient is in a good position; avoid serving food to the person lying back in bed on pillows – this is the perfect aspiration position. Use plate guards to prevent food slipping off the plate. Use non-slip mats to avoid the plate skidding off the table. If vision is poor, use black or red plates to improve contrast and enable the patient to see the food. Buy or adapt cutlery if necessary. Only give assistance if the person needs help cutting up food; beware care assistants who take over completely and feed the person. This will disable the person. Do not forget to provide, or ask relatives to provide, suitable snacks.

Improving swallowing

Exercise can help strengthen the muscles in the face, mouth and oesophagus. The speech and language therapist will advise. Some helpful strategies include:

- Licking lollipops and ice-lollies. This helps increase tongue movement and reduces the problem of food being 'pocketed' in the cheeks.
- Exercises to practise vowel sounds. These stimulate tone and movement.
- Sucking and blowing through a straw strengthens the soft palate and makes swallowing easier.
- Breathing exercises.

Fluids

People with dysphagia can find it more difficult to drink than to eat. Texture is very important and thickened fluids are easier to manage than liquid. If the dietician recommends thickened fluids you can obtain thickeners on prescription. Avoid feeding cups if the person has dysphagia. In order to drink from a spout the person has to tilt her head back and this opens the airway right up – the odds of aspiration rise dramatically. Use half-full cups – they can be refilled – use straws, use teaspoons but do not use syringes or feeding cups.

Reassessment

Dysphagia improves with time so reassess regularly. The research shows that 29% of people with gastrostomy tubes recover their swallowing ability well enough to have the tubes removed[50].

Case history

Maude, an aphasic stroke victim, was assessed as dysphasic and lived on puréed diet and thickened fluids for some years. When she was admitted to the nursing home she was given a wheelchair to help her improve mobility. Maude scooted around using one leg and one hand to propel herself at breakneck speed around the home. Nursing staff planned to observe Maude eat in the small dining room, but Maude had other ideas. On her second day in the home she whizzed into the large dining room, grabbed a chicken leg from a plate and sank her few remaining teeth into it. Sister moved in to prevent Maude choking to death but Maude scoffed the lot without a problem.

Case history

Betty was admitted with a gastrostomy tube in place. Her swallowing reflex was absent and her prognosis was poor. Two days after admission Betty complained of thirst and asked for a drink. Betty lacked a swallowing reflex but was able to swallow the two pints of saliva we produce daily without problem. Swallowing tests revealed an intact swallowing reflex and no signs of dysphagia. This was confirmed by the speech therapist. Fluids and diet were gradually reintroduced and a fortnight after admission Betty tackled steak, mushrooms and chips.

Maude and Betty got better without anyone noticing! People do recover and defy their diagnosis, so remember to reassess. Some people also suffer small strokes and swallowing can deteriorate, so it is important to reassess if you think swallowing has become more difficult.

Conclusion

Some stroke survivors have severe swallowing difficulties and will require gastrostomy feeding. When gastrostomy feeding is required, health authorities have a duty to provide gastrostomy feeding equipment. Guidance issued by the Department of Health (HSG95/45) makes this clear. Nurses can enable people with moderate difficulty to remain well nourished and well hydrated by using their nursing skills and working with other professionals.

Key points

- Almost half stroke survivors have some difficulty swallowing
- Unrecognised dysphagia can lead to aspiration pneumonia and death
- Do not give diet or fluids if you diagnose dysphagia, seek expert advice
- Offer food that the person can cope with
- Ensure the person sits up properly to eat
- Enable the person to eat
- Offer thickened fluids if advised by the dietician
- Remember to reassess – people improve.

Communication

Communication is not simply about the ability to speak and understand speech. We use all five senses to communicate and receive information. Imagine for a moment that you have had a stroke: you have no feeling in half of your body, you have difficulty understanding what is said and it is difficult to explain what you mean. This is how stroke affects many of our residents. Stroke and the communication problems that often accompany stroke can make people want to curl up and die. Nurses can enable people with communication difficulties to communicate.

This section aims to help you:

- Examine how stroke affects the senses
- Assess communication difficulties
- Overcome barriers to communication
- Understand the principles of sensory integration therapy

Sensory input

We receive input from all five senses. If you walk in the garden your skin will sense temperature, your vestibular system will sense whether the ground is uneven or not, your olfactory system will allow you to enjoy the scent of the flowers and your auditory system will enable you to hear the birds sing. Your brain integrates all these sensory stimuli and you respond. If it is freezing cold, the garden is like a mud bath and the birds are dive-bombing your washing, you will probably retreat indoors. If it is warm and pleasant you will probably remain in the garden. You make these decisions on the basis of information received from a fully functioning sensory system.

How ageing affects sensory input
Ageing affects each of our senses. The eyes are less able to differentiate colour, vision changes, and sense of taste and smell are reduced. To enter the fourth age is to experience a reduction in sensory input (Table 12.2).

Table 12.2   How ageing affects the senses.

Normal	Older person
Sensory stimulation from environment	Sensory stimulation from environment
Normal registration and processing	Abnormal registration because of impaired visual, auditory, olfactory, tactile and gustatory systems
Normal sensory integration and interpretation	Abnormal sensory integration due to impaired sensory, autonomic, proprioceptive and vestibular systems
Appropriate functional adaptive response	Poor and inappropriate adaptive response due to impaired sensory, autonomic, proprioceptive, vestibular systems and age-related mobility impairment or the effects of chronic disease

How stroke affects the senses
We have five senses:

- Visual – seeing
- Auditory – hearing
- Olfactory – smelling
- Kinaesthetic – feeling
- Gustatory – tasting

Stroke can affect each of these senses.

Vision

Our eyes absorb light, and cone cells in the retina distinguish colour and shades. Some nerve cells are sensitive to different types of light, like ripples in water. Electrical impulses travel from the optic nerve to the visual cortex in the occipital lobe[51]. The eye functions as a sophisticated camera and the brain as a computer, enabling us to interpret the signals sent from the eye. In order to see, we require intact and integrated skeletal, visceral, cortical and subcortical systems. We need to be able to fix our gaze on an object, to track a moving object, to focus and to integrate the images from both eyes[52]. Any breakdown in the visual system will cause visual problems. Common visual problems following stroke include:

- *Blurred vision* – caused by damage to the muscles that enable the eyes to focus. Prescription lens may help
- *Visual field loss* – caused by damage to the right or left temporal lobe or the optic nerve or optic chiasm. Training the patient to scan the environment is often effective; if not, you will have to compensate.
- *Nystagmus* (abnormal eye movements causing blurred vision) – caused by damage to the brainstem or cerebellum. Surgery may help in some cases; sensory integration therapy will help.
- *Loss of ability or difficulty in tracking* up, down, left or right – caused by a lesion in either hemisphere, or brainstem damage. Sensory integration therapy may help. In the US researchers are experimenting with the use of computers and video games to help patients relearn tracking skills.
- *Double vision* – caused by reduced control of the eye muscles; in some cases one eye will turn in or out. Patching to alternate eyes helps correct this.

Hearing

Stroke can affect hearing. The usual problems are unilateral hearing loss, muffling of sound or tinnitus. An estimated 20% of people over the age of 80 have impaired hearing and could benefit from a hearing aid. Hearing is lost in the higher frequencies first and female nurses are less easily understood than male colleagues because the frequency of their voices is higher.

Helping people to hear

- Cut down on background noise – close the window, turn off the television and close the door
- Move near to the person
- Get down to the same level as the person
- Face the person
- Do not sit where your face is in shadow
- Do not cover your mouth while speaking. If offered tea do not drink and speak. Do not chew your pen
- Speak directly to the person; do not attempt three-way conversations. Communicating with someone about continence problems is very sen-

sitive; avoid having relatives or students present if at all possible. If someone else *must* be present ask him or her to sit at some distance and to remain silent
- Speak slowly and clearly
- Do not shout; shouting distorts your voice and makes it more difficult to understand. Shouting also alters the tone of your voice and detracts from your efforts to build a therapeutic relationship
- Check that the individual has understood
- If you have not been understood rephrase the sentence
- Use gestures
- Offer to write things down.

Taste and smell

Stroke can affect the person's sense of taste and certain foods taste 'metallic' or 'rotten'. Stroke can affect the sense of smell; it can either be lost, reduced or enhanced.

Touch

Stroke can disturb the sense of touch. The person may experience sensory loss from half of the body. Loss of the ability to feel or be aware of the position of limbs is normally associated with a right-sided lesion (left hemiparesis).

Speech and language

Every year 20 000 people in the UK develop speech difficulties after stroke. There are three types of dysphasia: expressive, receptive and conductive.

Expressive dysphasia, difficulty in expressing yourself through speech, is caused by a lesion in Broca's area. The ability to understand spoken language is intact.
Receptive dysphasia, difficulty in understanding language, is caused by a lesion in Wernicke's area – the temperoparietal region of the cortex[53].
Conductive dysphasia is intact comprehension and ability to express, but an inability to put the two together.

There are three degrees of language impairment – mild, moderate and severe. Some individuals understand every word and gesture but have difficulty in finding the right word. This difficulty in finding words is known as anomia. Communication strategies depend on the degree of dysphasia but include:

- Ensuring that the person is fresh and well rested.
- Reducing distractions.
- Appearing relaxed and unhurried. Watch your body language – people with communication problems are constantly seeking clues to help interpret the environment. They are much more aware of body language and often more skilful at reading it than you are.

- Use charts, pictures and cue cards to help the person communicate.
- Ask the person to show you and encourage the person to use gestures.
- Make sure that the person is wearing her dentures. If they are slipping, a touch of denture fixative can improve speech remarkably.

Difficulty understanding

Dysphasia

People with mild dysphasia understand most of what is said. We can help people with mild dysphasia to understand by:

- Choosing a time of day when the person is alert and not overtired
- Reducing background noise
- Speaking slowly and clearly
- Providing a quiet calm environment and not appearing rushed.

People with moderate dysphasia find it more difficult to understand. They find it difficult to follow long and complicated sentences and some words may only be partly understood. You may 'lose' the person halfway through a sentence. We can help the person to understand by:

- Using simple plain language
- Trying not to use any word with more than seven letters
- Using one idea in each sentence
- Not giving more than one choice in a sentence, as this can be very confusing
- Trying to keep sentences to seven words
- If the person still appears to have difficulties, using five letter words and five word sentences
- Giving the person time to prepare replies.

Remember that this individual is making a great effort to communicate with you. Show that you realise this and appreciate the effort she is making. Do not overtire or stress the person; if the person appears to be tiring then arrange to return and complete the assessment or interview. People with moderate receptive dysphasia rely on tone of voice, gestures and movement to help interpret what is said. Ensure that you can be seen clearly.

People with severe dysphasia can have difficult understanding even single words. Be inventive; use pictures, objects, gestures and cards to help get your message across. Often people with severe expressive dysphasia have difficulty speaking as well and may say yes when they mean no. Devise a foolproof signal such as a 'thumbs up' so that the person can let you know she has understood.

Dysarthria

Dysarthria, difficulty articulating words, is common following stroke and in people with Parkinson's disease. Communication strategies include:

- Making sure the person is fresh and well rested.
- If the person has Parkinson's disease, choosing your time carefully,

normally an hour after anti-parkinsonian medication is best. Do not ask the person to concentrate and make the effort to communicate for long periods when medication is starting to wear off.
- Checking that you have understood by rephrasing the person's words.

Communicating with people who are confused

Multi-infarct dementia (multiple small strokes) cause special problems with communicating. Many people with dementia can be thought of as having been sentenced to solitary confinement. Their only chance of communicating is through the efforts of staff who try to remove as many barriers to communication as possible. If people are not encouraged to use speech and are not stimulated they will deteriorate quickly and unnecessarily[54].

Language breaks down in dementia in stages:

- In the early stages speech becomes empty and vague. Sentences are not completed
- Then word finding becomes a problem. The person has increasing difficulty naming things
- Speech becomes increasingly repetitive
- Speech and conversation is related only to the individual
- Mutism may follow[55].

This inability to communicate can irritate and sometimes overwhelm staff.

Assessing communication difficulties

Stroke patients should be fully assessed after stroke. Vision should be checked by an optician to identify any visual difficulties. If the person has difficulty speaking, reading or writing then refer to a speech therapist. If dentures do not fit, refer the person to a dentist; relining or remodelling of the denture can dramatically improve speech. If the person has sensory or motor problems refer to a physiotherapist and occupational therapist. The nurse's role is to identify problems, and co-ordinate and manage care delivered from the multi-disciplinary team.

Overcoming communication barriers

The strategies outlined throughout this section will enable the stroke patient to communicate more effectively. However, older adults who have strokes face additional sensory difficulties because of age-related changes. Ageing reduces sensory input.

Sensory integration therapy

Sensory integration therapy was developed to stimulate brain function in brain-damaged children. The sensory integration approach is based on neurophysiological and developmental principles. It is based on organising sensation for the benefit of the individual. Integration converts our initial sensations into meaningful perceptions. Spatial awareness is dependent on the integration of visual, auditory and kinaesthetic clues. Sensory motor integration can occur at all levels of the central nervous system from the spinal cord to the cerebral cortex[56]. Sensory integration therapy provides controlled sensory input to the vestibular, olfactory system, muscles, joints and skin[57]. It is now accepted that children's brains are 'plastic' and that the brain has the ability to re-route functions. Stroke patients recover because collateral axons sprout and enable the brain to re-route functions from damaged areas to undamaged areas[58]. Age-related changes can result in sensory loss and reduced ability to interpret stimuli; this sensory deprivation can lead to functional changes that reduce the brain's ability to re-route functions following damage[59]. The use of sensory integration therapy in older adults following stroke is not yet generally accepted and there have been few research studies demonstrating its effects. Some professionals consider that the brain is 'fixed' and not plastic in old age. But the fact that elderly people with massive stroke damage can and do recover function proves that the older brain is plastic[60]. The brain can re-route and recover function.

Many stroke patients within our homes suffer sensory deprivation not because we do not care but because we do not think. Imagine what it is like for the stroke victim unable to move unaided. We put the person in the same chair every day. She sees the same view (if she can see). We put her in easy-to-get-on polyester dresses that her daughter chose. She does not know what the weather is really like because the temperature in the home is constant. Impaired ability to communicate locks her into a tiny world. Sensory deprivation can make grown men weep – it usually takes about three days to break down a trained soldier with sensory deprivation. Is it any wonder that our stroke patients despair? Practising sensory integration therapy in small ways within the home works wonders. Stroking the skin with velvet, tickling with a feather, massaging limbs with aromatherapy oils, taking Mary outside to feel the wind in her hair. Little things to enrich life and stimulate the senses can help people feel that they are alive and not in care.

We still know very little about how the brain works. I believe that one day sensory integration therapy will be part of the mainstream.

Conclusion

To be old is to experience some degree of sensory deprivation. Stroke can increase the degree of sensory deprivation that older adults experience. Insensitive care can further reduce stimuli and lead to depression and despair. Sensitive care can enable the older person to function to capacity and to enjoy the highest possible quality of life.

Key points

- Ageing reduces sensory input
- Stroke can affect all senses
- Communication problems following stroke must be assessed
- Communication strategies can help people communicate
- Sensory stimulation can help people regain abilities.

Bladder and bowel problems

Strokes can cause loss of function, loss of mobility, loss of communication skills, loss of cognitive function and loss of bladder control[61]. Individuals who develop bladder and bowel problems after stroke are usually the people who have been most disabled by stroke[62]. The person is often admitted catheterised with a diagnosis of 'doubly incontinent' written on the discharge letter. Many nurses, and even some continence advisers, think it is futile to consider continence promotion strategies with such individuals. Fortunately they are mistaken; skilled nursing care can enable many people to regain continence after stroke.

This section aims to improve your knowledge of:

- The reasons people develop bladder problems after stroke
- Assessing the reasons for incontinence
- Treatment of different types of incontinence
- The reasons people develop bowel problems after stroke
- Treatment of constipation
- Treatment of faecal incontinence

Why people develop continence problems after stroke

Most people are incontinent immediately after a stroke[63] but within eight weeks most have spontaneously regained continence[64]. However, people who suffer severe strokes tend to have ongoing continence problems. Three factors affect continence after strokes:

- Physiological changes caused by the stroke
- Neurophysiological changes affecting bladder function after stroke
- Factors relating to medical and nursing care and hospitalisation.

Physiological changes
Physiological changes range from the mild to the severe. Short-term memory can be affected. Communication difficulties can include difficulty understanding speech (receptive dysphasia) and problems with speaking (dysphasia and dysarthria). Some individuals lose complete function on one side of the body (hemiplegia); others experience weakness (hemiparesis). Vision is often impaired and visual fields are affected. The individual may lose the ability to move unaided, read or communicate needs. These changes can often lead to depression and feelings of despair.

Neurophysiological changes
Normally bladder control is maintained by the parasympathetic system. We are unaware of any sensation of bladder fullness until the bladder contains around 300 ml of urine. Then we can postpone the need to void until it is convenient. The micturition centre in the brain stem informs us that our bladder is filling up. The micturition centre in the frontal lobe allows us to inhibit urination. The bladder muscle relaxes and capacity is increased. The

urethra remains tightly closed preventing leakage. The autonomic nervous system and both micturition centres must function properly, otherwise we will be unable to maintain continence. Stroke can directly or indirectly cause either the frontal or brain stem micturition centres to malfunction. The level of damage sustained is related to the severity of the stroke. Damage to the frontal lobe causes urge incontinence. Parietal and basal ganglia lesions cause bladder dyssynergia[65].

Urge incontinence

Urge incontinence is also called bladder dysreflexia or detrusor instability. Normally bladder contractions are suppressed while the bladder is filling. The micturition centre in the frontal lobe inhibits bladder contractions. People suffering from an unstable bladder suffer from uncontrolled bladder contractions. Strokes affecting the frontal lobe affect the ability of the micturition centre to inhibit bladder contractions. One research study found that 95% of people who suffered from urinary incontinence after stroke had urge incontinence[66].

Symptoms include:

- Increased frequency of passing urine
- Urgency – having to rush to use the toilet
- Nocturnal enuresis.

Treatment: Investigation of the causes of urgency and adopting a problem solving approach often resolve the problem. Bladder retraining that involves teaching the person to 'hold on' for longer periods often helps. Medication can help to 'dampen down' bladder contractions[67].

Bladder dyssynergia

Normally the bladder contracts and the urethral sphincter relaxes on urination. In individuals with dyssynergia the urethral sphincter fails to relax and complete bladder emptying is not possible. If untreated the bladder becomes overstretched and loses tone (hypotonic bladder), residual urine increases and infection is almost inevitable.

Symptoms include:

- Incomplete bladder emptying
- Passing small frequent amounts of urine
- Leakage on standing
- No leakage in bed
- No nocturnal enuresis.

Treatment: Intermittent catheterisation can, in some cases, help restore normal bladder function. Discontinuing any medication known to affect the autonomic nervous system (such as some antihypertensives) and prescribing medication without such side effects if necessary, can sometimes resolve the problem.

Medication can be prescribed to relax the urethral sphincter. This is sometimes effective, though the side effects – vertigo and postural hypotension – may prevent use because of the risks of falls and fracture. Often individuals with bladder dyssynergia require permanent indwelling urethral catheters. I have found that many alert individuals with dyssynergia prefer to use a catheter valve during the day and a night drainage bag at night.

Contributing factors

Medication can cause incontinence. Diuretics, often prescribed to control leg oedema caused by immobility, can cause incontinence[68]. Muscle relaxants, often prescribed to prevent or treat spasticity, relax the bladder muscle and can cause incontinence[69]. Antihypertensives can disrupt the autonomic nervous system and cause nocturnal enuresis and in some cases urinary retention with overflow incontinence. Insufficient toilets and commodes and lack of privacy can also lead to incontinence.

In the first days or weeks after stroke individuals have little warning of the need to pass urine. It is vitally important that nurses respond promptly to their calls for assistance when the toilet is required. Unfortunately the individual may have difficulty communicating this to nursing staff and incontinence can occur.

Helping people regain continence following a stroke

Awareness of the effects of stroke can enable nurses to plan holistic care that enables the stroke patient to regain abilities.

Catheterisation should be avoided unless the individual is in urinary retention. Most people will regain continence naturally as they recover from strokes; this is not possible if there is a catheter in place. Catheterisation inevitably leads to infection[70]. Infection normally persists for some time after the catheter is removed. Urinary tract infection can cause urinary incontinence[71]. Over three-quarters of people catheterised for three months or more develop inflammatory bladder changes[72]. Catheterisation also makes it more difficult for individuals to regain continence because it rapidly leads to a reduction in bladder capacity[73]. If there are indications for catheterisation, using a catheter to drain the bladder at regular intervals may prevent bladder contraction. There is little research evidence on the use of catheter valves. When the catheter is removed the stroke patient usually has not only to regain bladder control but also to contend with the effects of infection, inflammatory bladder changes and a reduced bladder capacity.

Fluid intake requires careful monitoring; fluid deficits of 10% can cause serious illness. The average person requires 1.5 litres of fluid daily. Fluid requirements rise during illness to two or three litres. Immobility is common after stroke. Immobility increases the risk of urinary tract infection – and the risk of incontinence. An intake of three litres daily prevents urinary tract infection[74]. When Burns conducted a study on a small group of elderly catheterised women, their mean fluid intake was less than 500 ml[75]; so monitor intake carefully – it could be lower than you think.

Communication is vital if we are to meet physical and psychological needs. Be creative. Use cards with large pictures and words. Individuals can waste vital minutes searching for the right sign to indicate that the toilet is required. Making up a special toilet card, with a picture and the word toilet on a sheet of brightly coloured paper or card, can save time and prevent accidents. The person can wait a few moments for tea but not for the toilet! Watch your language. We all speak too quickly and our sentences are too long for many people with communication problems to follow. Try to use five word sentences. Bring up one idea at a time. Offer one choice. Be patient – wait for the person to answer. Enabling the person to communicate with you makes an enormous difference to morale. The person can again develop some control over his or her life.

Mobility – The ability to walk unaided is the most important factor in regaining continence. It is vital that nurses work with the individual and other professionals to enable the person to regain mobility as soon as possible after stroke. The ability to move around unaided or with limited help improves morale, appetite, and bowel and bladder function[76]. Mobilisation, elevation of the feet when sitting out and the use of support stockings can virtually eliminate the use of diuretics to control limb oedema after stroke.

Bowel care receives less attention than previously. The bowel book has been consigned to the nursing history books. Bowel care though is very important. Constipation and faecal impaction can cause or worsen existing urge incontinence. Encourage a diet rich in fibre – if swallowing is difficult puréed fruits and vegetables can be offered. Nursing measures to enable the person to maintain or re-establish normal bowel patterns can virtually eliminate the use of laxatives and enemata[77].

Models of care can influence behaviour. It is easier for everyone to develop caring, trusting relationships with a small number of people. Really using primary nursing (not just going through the motions) can enable individuals to build up trusting relationships. Using an enabling model of care that helps individuals regain dressing skills helps individuals regain continence. Using a custodial model of care that encourages individuals to remain passive while nurses provide care, disables individuals. Delivering care that is tailored to the individual with all their foibles and idiosyncrasies really does make people feel comfortable and safe. In this environment abilities are improved and the amount of psychotropic medication required is greatly reduced.

Specialist treatment

Individuals who have not regained continence within eight weeks of stroke should be investigated. Investigation need not be intrusive or distressing to the patient. Careful history taking and basic investigations can be carried out by appropriately experienced and qualified nursing staff. Most individuals will suffer from urge incontinence. In many instances this can be treated without medication. Some individuals do require drug therapy and must be referred to a medical practitioner. My own experience is that almost three-quarters of individuals can be enabled to regain continence within six weeks. Cognitively impaired individuals and those with severe strokes are less likely to respond to treatment. However, two-thirds of such individuals can remain dry using individual prompted voiding schedules.

Bowel problems after stroke

Constipation is the most common bowel problem after stroke, although some people develop faecal incontinence. This section aims to discuss management of constipation and faecal incontinence. Many stroke patients suffer from constipation; normally a laxative is prescribed. Millions of pounds are spent each year on laxative prescriptions. Constipation and laxative use is highest in older adults; 79% of those in hospitals, 59% in nursing homes and 38% living at home are prescribed laxatives regularly[78]. Constipation is *not* a disease, it is a symptom. Every time a laxative is prescribed without investigating the causes of constipation a health promotion opportunity is lost and the cycle of laxative misuse perpetuated.

Constipation

The causes of constipation are:

- Production of hard stools that are difficult to pass
- Impairment of colonic propulsion
- An insensitive rectum with inability to perceive stool
- A hypersensitive rectum that triggers the urge to defecate when there is very little stool to pass
- Failure of the sphincter to relax during defecation[79].

Ageing does not lead to constipation. A healthy 85-year-old is no more likely to be constipated than a healthy 20-year-old is[80]. Older people are more likely to suffer from ill health than younger people are. Illness, limited mobility, medication and other factors associated with illness can increase the risk of constipation. Offering holistic research-based care can often effectively prevent constipation and promote good health without using laxatives or enemas. Table 12.3 shows factors that can contribute to constipation.

The benefits of bowel management programmes

It is possible to manage bowel care more effectively. The following case history illustrates how one resident benefited from bowel management.

Case history

Mrs Bella Rowland's arthritis had worsened in recent years. Unfortunately the anti-inflammatory drugs she was prescribed had to be discontinued because of gastric bleeding. Mrs Rowland developed cardiac failure following her gastric bleed and suffered a stroke while in hospital. Mrs Rowland was admitted immobile and was taking 20 ml of lactulose twice daily. On alternate days she took two senna tablets. She was prescribed Frumil two tablets each morning, ferrous sulphate 200 mg three times a day and dyhydrocodeine two tablets eight hourly for pain. Her general practitioner reduced her diuretics to one daily. Mrs Rowland's pain was poorly controlled but she was reluctant to take any further tablets because she confessed she felt sick all the time. She agreed to try transcutaneous nerve stimulation to her painful left knee. This was so successful that analgesia was changed to an as-required basis and was seldom used. When she was free of pain and nausea, Mrs Rowland's appetite and fluid intake improved. She began to walk using a frame but her knee tended to 'give'. She was referred to the orthotist who supplied a knee brace to support her knee. Within three weeks Mrs Rowland was able to walk unaided. We offered Mrs Rowland a glass of fresh orange juice with

Table 12.3   Constipation contributing factors.

Gastrointestinal conditions	*Endocrine disorders*
Tumours	Hypothyroidism
Adhesions	Adrenal and pituitary hypofunction
Hernia	
Hypomotility disorders, e.g. idiopathic	*Medication*
slow transit time, idiopathic megacolon	Analgesics
Rectal prolapse	Antacids
Colonic pseudo-obstruction	Iron tablets
Strictures	Hypotensives
Anorectal problems, e.g. haemorrhoids	Diuretics
or anal fissure	Antiparkinsonian agents
Neurological conditions	*Other contributing factors*
Dementia	Lack of privacy
Stroke	Lack of time
Autonomic neuropathy	Lack of dietary fibre
Spinal cord tumour	Immobility
Paraplegia	Pain causing reluctance to defecate
Parkinson's disease	Embarrassment
	Weakness
Gynaecoogical conditions	Cold, dirty, uncomfortable toilets
Endometriosis	
Cystocele	*Psychiatric conditions*
Rectocele	Depression
	Chronic psychosis

each iron tablet, as vitamin C increases iron absorption by 40%. Within six weeks of admission Mrs Rowland's bowel pattern had returned to normal and she no longer required laxatives.

Introducing a bowel management programme

There are four main elements in a bowel management programme:

(1)   Diet, fluids and mobility
(2)   Environmental aspects – nursing practice, privacy, time
(3)   Medical care and medication
(4)   Bowel assessment.

Diet

Fibre increases stool bulk and enables the stool to absorb and retain water. Fibre reduces transit time and produces a soft bulky stool that is easy to pass. People who eat a diet rich in fibre will pass larger, softer stools more frequently. A healthy diet should contain soluble and non-soluble fibre from a variety of sources including wheat, oats, vegetables and fruit[81]. Older people in hospitals and nursing homes may have health problems that make it difficult to eat a high fibre diet. Individuals may have difficulty chewing, masticating and swallowing. However, with a little imagination it is possible to offer even the frailest older person an appetising diet rich in fibre. Fruit can be cut up into small pieces, poached, puréed or juiced. Vegetables can be added to soups, casseroles and stews. Oats, wheat and dried fruit can be added to puddings, cakes and flapjacks. The amount of fibre required varies considerably from person to person. Suggestions for a high fibre diet are given at the end of this chapter.

Fluids

People eating a high fibre diet require a high fluid intake. Older people may have low fluid intakes. Ageing can impair the thirst mechanism and altered renal function impairs the ability to concentrate urine. Some older people cut back on fluids in an effort to prevent incontinence. It is vitally important that nurses ensure people on bowel management programmes have a fluid intake of approximately two litres of fluid daily. Try serving tea and coffee in individual pots so that it stays hot and the person can have a second cup. Serve squashes and cold drinks ice cold. Offer preferred fluids. The older person may enjoy a small gin with lots of tonic, a shandy or a weak beer in the evening and this boosts fluid intake.

Mobility

Walking and moving stimulates peristaltic waves in the colon. Older people can easily become immobile in hospitals and nursing homes because of the effects of illness and nursing practice. Encouraging older people to remain mobile encourages normal bowel function, improves appetite and contributes to well-being[82].

Nursing practice

Nursing practice can directly contribute to constipation. Defecation is an intensely private activity. Most people would prefer to defecate in a locked toilet rather than perched precariously on a bedpan behind screens. Helping frail older people to the toilet and providing a private, unrushed environment enables them to retain normal bowel activity. Some frail older people are at risk of falling off the toilet or commode if left unattended. The Kira commode has been specially designed to support frail older people and to enable them to maintain privacy and dignity, while preventing falls[83]. Removing the commode pan and placing the commode directly over the toilet allows the person to defecate normally in the toilet and gives more privacy.

Medical practice

Many medications can cause constipation and these should be avoided wherever possible. There are often alternatives, for example anti-inflammatory drugs often control pain more effectively than constipating analgesics. Iron preparations can be discontinued when no longer required. Diuretics can lead to dessication of faeces and should be reduced to the lowest possible dose. Regular review of medications not only reduces the risk of constipation but also the risks of polypharmacy in this vulnerable client group. Good medical practice includes the diagnosis and treatment of diseases that contribute to constipation. In nursing homes GPs provide medical care and many rely on the observational skills of the registered nurse to alert them to possible diseases.

Bowel assessment

Individuals who remain constipated despite dietary changes, sufficient fluids, mobilisation and medication review should have a bowel assessment. The purpose of a bowel assessment is to discover the reasons why bowel problems have arisen and to use a problem solving approach. Bowel assessment combines a history and a physical examination. Often the causes of constipation are simple and easily treated. The person with haemorrhoids may experience pain and even prolapse of haemorrhoids on defecation. This can lead to a circle of fear, constipation and pain. Often conservative treatment with suppositories and ointments can not only enable the person to regain normal bowel function but also improve quality of life. A sample bowel assessment chart is given at the end of this chapter.

Faecal incontinence

The commonest causes of faecal incontinence are:

- Constipation with overflow incontinence
- A rectum loaded with soft stool that is difficult to expel
- Loss of sensation and tone in the anal sphincter and lower bowel.

Constipation can be so severe that the patient is faecally impacted. Sometimes nurses perform a manual evacuation in such circumstances and think that they have cleared the bowel. Severe faecal impaction can lead to the entire colon becoming loaded with faeces and it can take days to clear the colon. Only when the bowel has been cleared can you begin to treat constipation in the ways outlined above.

Laxatives such as lactulose, a stool softener, act by drawing fluid into the faeces so that the stool becomes soft. Unfortunately stool softeners do not help propel the stool from the rectum and people with sensory impairment can build up large amounts of very soft stool in the rectum. Clearing the bowel, discontinuing stool softeners and introducing a bowel management programme will often resolve the problem.

Loss of sensation and tone in the anal sphincter and lower bowel is easily diagnosed. On examination the anus gapes and the person is not normally aware of the need to defecate. The rectum and lower bowel is not full of stool. Usually people with this problem are the most severely disabled of stroke survivors. Use a problem solving approach to treat. If the patient is prescribed laxatives have these prescribed PRN and do not give. Aim to help the patient produce a firm stool – you may have to reduce fibre intake. Some older adults, as a result of a life-long diet deficient in fibre, develop diverticular disease and have diarrhoea. Constipating agents such as Lomotil or codeine phosphate (which is also an effective analgesic) can be used in such cases. The alternative, Imodium, is larger and more difficult to swallow, though it is available in liquid form. You can then work to develop a normal bowel pattern by helping the patient to sit on the toilet and try to defecate after breakfast when the gastrocolic reflex is strongest. Using special toilet seats, such as those made by Presalit, make it easier for patients to sit comfortably, and alter the ano-rectal angle to facilitate defecation.

Key points

- 80% of people develop bladder problems after stroke
- If left uncatheterised most people will regain bladder control
- Urinary incontinence is a symptom, not a disease
- The usual causes of urinary incontinence post stroke are urge incontinence and bladder dyssynergia
- Skilled nursing care can enable many people to regain continence following stroke
- Bowel problems are common in the most disabled stroke survivors
- Constipation is the most common bowel problem following stroke
- Bowel management programmes enable you to discover the causes of bowel problems and develop treatment plans.

Conclusion

Bowel and bladder problems following stroke are distressing and embarrassing symptoms. Investigating the causes of bladder and bowel problems and using a problem solving approach improves the individual's health, reduces the use of medication and virtually eliminates the use of laxatives, enemas and suppositories. Introducing a continence management bowel programme enables many older adults to regain function and improves general health and well-being.

Ethical issues

Ethics are collective beliefs or value systems that are held by any social or moral group[84]. As nurses working in continuing care settings we often find ourselves in situations where issues are not clear-cut and there are no easy answers.

This section aims to discuss the dilemmas nurses face in every day practice including:

- To treat or not to treat
- To tell or not to tell
- To resuscitate or not to resuscitate
- Living wills and advanced directives

To treat or not to treat?

Mrs Lister has been resident at the nursing home for five years. She has arterial disease and despite active treatment has suffered small stroke after small stroke. After each stroke Mrs Lister has become more disabled, and for the last six months she has been mute. She shows no signs of awareness and requires total nursing care. Mrs Lister has difficulty swallowing and nursing staff feed her with thickened fluids.

Mrs Lister's family visits every other day though she shows no sign of recognising them. Mrs Lister then suffers another stroke and is unable to swallow. Her GP visits and inserts a nasogastric tube. Mrs Lister's family are devastated and beg you to intervene; they say that they want their mother to be able to die with dignity. What would you do?

What do you think were the GP's reasons for inserting the nasogastric tube? Do you agree with his decision?

To tell or not to tell?

Mrs Lister pulls out the nasogastric tube and the GP agrees to discontinue artificial hydration. Mrs Lister is still unable to swallow and her family come to pay their last respects. Mrs Lister's granddaughter Laura, a university student, is due to arrive this afternoon. Her mother June, Mrs Lister's daughter, comes to see you and asks you not to tell Laura that her grandmother is dying because, 'Laura is so young she's seen nothing of life, she couldn't cope.' What do you say to June?

Laura arrives and after spending some time with her grandmother finds you. She says, 'Granny looks terrible. I've never seen her so ill. Is she going to get better?' What do you say?

Treatment

People enter nursing and medicine because they wish to help people and to 'make them better' but sometimes this is not possible and our goal changes to that of offering a peaceful and dignified death. The difficulty is recognising when patients have entered the 'end stage' when it is appropriate to offer palliative care. Research studies have found that dying patients have all or some of the following signs:

- Profound weakness, usually bedbound, requiring assistance with all care
- Gaunt physical appearance
- Drowsy and cognitively impaired
- Diminished food intake
- Difficulty swallowing medications[85].

Current legal and medical opinion is that doctors should consider the likely outcome of treatment before beginning medical interventions such as nasogastric feeding. Just because we can, does not mean we must. There is a legal distinction between ordinary and extraordinary treatment. Professionals are obliged to give ordinary treatment such as washing the patient and preventing pressure sores. They are not obliged to give extraordinary treatment, e.g. nasogastric feeding to maintain life when there is no hope of recovery[86]. In 1999 the British Medical Association issued a position statement on the ethics of prolonging life by continuing active treatment when there was no hope of recovery. Research indicates that rehydration in the end stage is of no benefit and can cause peripheral and pulmonary oedema if the patient has a low serum albumen[87].

Living wills and advance statements

The British Medical Association ethics committee advises all doctors to take account of the patient's wishes when deciding on treatment. If Mrs Lister had made a living will would she have avoided this indignity? At the moment living wills or 'advanced care directives' have no legal status. Now a government discussion paper is exploring this issue. The paper recommends that people should not be able to refuse 'basic care' to maintain hygiene, oral hydration and nutrition[88].

Telling

At times telling requires great sensitivity and skill. We need to judge when a person is ready and how much he or she really wants to know. We need to have the ability to comfort and support the person we tell. In this situation it is clear that Mrs Lister is dying. It would be easy to go along with June in an attempt to protect Laura, but would we really be protecting her? Would we be depriving her of the opportunity to say goodbye to her grandmother? Every ethical decision we make has consequences.

Ethical principles

The ethical principle of beneficence urges us to choose goodness over badness and in this case nurses should be aware of the potential consequences of their actions.

Conclusion

We think in generalities but live life in detail. As nurses we may have fixed views about what we would do or not do in certain situations, but change our minds when confronted with reality and all its loose ends. The ethical issues raised in this section have not been resolved legally; perhaps issues such as these never will or should be.

References

1 Reardon, M. (1996) Transfers to nursing homes. *Elderly Care*, **8**(5), 16–18.
2 Bonita, R., Stewart, A.V. & Beaglehole, R. (1990) International Trends in Stroke Mortality 1970–1985. *Stroke*, **32**, 989–992.
3 Bonita, R. (1992) Epidemiology of Stroke. *Lancet*, **339**, 342–344.
4 Brown, R.D. Jr, Ransom, J., Hass, S., Petty, G.W., O'Fallon, W.M., Whisnant, J.P. & Leibson, C.L. (1999) Use of nursing home after stroke and dependence on stroke severity a population analysis. *Stroke*, **30**(5), 924–929.
5 Paulson, O.B., Strangard, S. & Edvinsson, L. (1990) Cerebral autoregulation. *Cerebrovascular Brain Metabolic Review*, **2**, 161–192.
6 WHO MONICA Project, Principle Investigation (1988) The World Health Organisation MONICA Project (Monitoring Trends and Determinants in Cardiovascular Disease), a major international study. *Journal Clinical Epidemiology*, **41**, 105–114.
7 Mulley, G.P. (1992) Stroke. In: Brocklehurst, J.C. (ed.) *Textbook of Geriatric Medicine*, 4th edn. Churchill Livingstone, Edinburgh.

[8] Delieu, J. & Keady, J. (1996) The biology of Alzheimer's disease. *British Journal of Nursing*, **2**(1), 162–168.

[9] Professor Shah Ebrahim (1999) *Stroke Care, a Matter of Chance*. The Stroke Association, London.

[10] Indredavik, B., Bakke, F., Sloradahl, S.A., Rosketh, R. & Haheim, L.L. (1999) Treatment in a combined acute and rehabilitation stroke unit: which factors are the most important? *Stroke*, **30**(5), 917–923.

[11] Kumlien, S., Axelsson, K., Ljunggren, G. & Winblad, B. (1999) Stroke patients ready for discharge from acute care – a multidimensional assessment of functions and further care. *Disability, Rehabilitation*, **21**(1), 31–38.

[12] Harada, N., Kominski, G. & Shoshanna, S. (1993) Development of a resource based patient classification scheme for rehabilitation. *Inquiry*, **30**, 4–63.

[13] Sacco, R. & Lipset, C. (1995) Stroke risk factors: identification and modification. In: *Stroke Therapy* Fisher, M. (ed.). Butterworth-Heinman, Oxford.

[14] Bass, L.M., Isaacsohn, J.N., Merikangas, K.R. & Robinette, C.D. (1992) A study of twins and stroke. *Stroke*, **23**, 222–223.

[15] Craig, H.D., Gund, M., Cepeda, O., Johnson, E.N., Ptacek, L., Steinberg, G.K., Ogilvy, C.S., Berg, M.H. & Crawford, S.C. (1998) Multilocus linkage identifies two new loci for a Mendelian form of stroke, cerebral cavernous malformation at 7p 15–13 and 3925 2–27. *Human Molecular Genetics*, **7**(12), 1851–1858.

[16] Rubbattu, S. & Volpe, M. (1999) Genetic basis of cerebrovascular accidents associated with hypertension. *Cardiological*, **44**(5), 433–437.

[17] Broderick, J.P., Brott, T., Tonsick, T., Huster, G. & Miller, R. (1992) The risk of subarachnoid and intracerebra haemorrhage in blacks as compared to whites. *New England Journal of Medicine*, **325**, 733–736.

[18] Horner, R.D., Matcher, D.B., Divine, G.W. & Feussner, J.R. (1991) Racial variations in ischaemic stroke related physical and functional impairments. *Stroke*, **22**, 1497–1501.

[19] Balarajan, R. (1991) Ethnic differences in mortality from ischaemic heart disease and cerebrovascular disease in England and Wales. *British Medical Journal*, **302**, 560–564.

[20] Gillum, R.F. (1999) Stroke mortality in blacks. Disturbing trends. *Stroke*, **30**(8), 1711–1715.

[21] Wimshurst, P. (1994) Temperature and cardiovascular mortality. Deaths from heart disease and stroke are in part due to cold winters. *British Medical Journal*, **309**, 1029–1030.

[22] Shaper, A.G., Phillips, A.N., Pockock, S.J., Walker, M., Macfarlane, P.W. (1991) Risk factors for stroke in middle aged men. *British Medical Journal*, **302**, 1111–1115.

[23] Besdine, R.W. (1993) Stroke prevention in the elderly. *Conn Medicine*, **57**(5), 287–292.

[24] McMahon, S., Peto, R. & Cutleer, J. (1990) Blood pressure, stroke and coronary heart disease. Part 1 prolonged differences in blood pressure; prospective observational studies corrected for the regression dilution bias. *Lancet*, **335**, 827–838.

[25] Wolf, P.A., Abbott, R.D. & Kannel, W.B. (1991) Atrial fibrillation as an independent risk factor for stroke: The Framington study. *Stroke*, **22**, 983–988.

[26] Kannell, W.B. (1991) Left ventricle hypertrophy as a risk factor: The Framington Experience. *Hypertension*, **9**(suppl. 2), 3–9.

[27] Aronow, W.S. (1998) Prevalence of heart disease in older women in a nursing home. *Journal Women's Health*, **7**(9), 1105–1112.

[28] International Stroke Trial Collaborative Group (1997) The international stroke

trial (IST): a randomised trial of aspirin, subcutaneous heparin; both or neither among 19 435 patients with acute ischaemic stroke. *Lancet*, **349**, 1569–1581.

29 Perez, I. *et al.* (199) Use of antithrombotic measures for stroke prevention. *Heart*, **82**(5), 570–574.

30 Deplanque, D. *et al.* (1999) Stroke and atrial fibrillation; was stroke prevention appropriate beforehand? *Heart*, **82**, 563–569.

31 Kawachi, I., Colditz, G. & Stampfer, M. (1993) Smoking cessation and decreased risk of ischaemic stroke in woman. *Journal American Medical Association*, **269**(2), 232–236.

32 Bonita, R., Duncan, J., Truelsen, T., Jackson, R.T. & Beaglehole, R. (1999) Passive smoking as well as active smoking increases the risk of acute stroke. *Tob. Control*, **8**(2), 156–160.

33 Wolf, P.A., D'Agostino, R.D., Odell, P., Belanger, A.J., Hodges, D. & Kannell, W.B. (1988) Alcohol consumption as a risk factor for stroke: The Framington study. *Annals Neurology*, **24**, 177.

34 Wolf, P.A., Cobb, J.L. & D'Agostino, R.D. (1992) Epidemiology of stroke. In: Britt, H.J.M., Mohr, J.P., Stein, B.M. & Yatsu, F.M. (eds.), *Stroke-Pathophysiology, Diagnosis and Treatment*. Churchill-Livingstone, New York.

35 Wannemethee, S.G., Perry, I.J. & Shaper, A.G. (1999) Non-fasting serum glucose and insulin concentrations. *Stroke*, **30**(9), 1780–1786.

36 Gale, C.R. (1995) Vitamin C and the risk of death from stroke and coronary heart disease in elderly people. *British Medical Journal*, **310**, 1565–1566.

37 Iso, H., Stampfer, M.J., Manson, J.E., Rexrode, K., Hennekens, C.H., Coditz, G.A., Spreizer, F.E. & Willet, W.C. (1999) Prospective study of calcium, potassium and magnesium intake and risk of stroke in women. *Stroke*, **30**(9), 1772–1779.

38 Sharman, David (1999) Snake venom could cure stroke. Reported on BBC *Line Health News*, 4 December 1999.

39 Grotta James (1999) Alcohol and caffeine treats stroke. *Presentation at a meeting of the American Neurological Society*, Seattle, October 1999.

40 Ramnemark, A., Nyberg, L., Lorentzon, R., Englund, U. & Gustafson, Y. (1999) Progressive hemi osteoporosis on the paretic side and increased bone mineral density in the non paretic arm the first year after severe stroke. *Osteoporoses International*, **9**(3), 269–275.

41 Nelles, G., Spiekermann, G., Jueptner, M., Leonhardt, G., Muller, S., Gerhard, H. & Deiner, H.C. (1999) Reorganisation of sensory and motor systems in hemiplegic stroke patients. A positron emission study. *Stroke*, **30**(8), 1510–1516.

42 Duncan Graham-Rowe (1999) Mini motivators. Bionic nerves are battling muscle wasting after stroke. *New Scientist*, 11 December 1999.

43 Volpe, B. (2001) Is robot-aided sansorimeter training in stroke rehabilitation a realistic option? *Curr. Opin. Neurol.*, **14**(6) 745–752.

44 Professor Douglas Kandziolka (1999) Brain cell transplants. Stroke and cerebral circulation. Presentation at 24th American Heart Association International Conference.

45 Horner, J. & Masey, W. (1988) Silent aspiration following stroke. *Neurology*, **38**, 317–339.

46 Negus, E. (1994) Stroke induced dysphagia in hospital the nutritional perspective. *British Journal of Nursing*, **6**, 263–269.

47 Park, C. & O'Neill, P. (1993) Swallowing difficulties. The Stroke Association, London.

48 Robins, J.A. & Levine, R.L. (1988) Swallowing after unilateral stroke within the cerebral cortex; preliminary experience. *Dysphagia*, **3**, 11–17.

[49] Sander, R. (1998) Stroke the hidden problems. *Elderly Care*, **10**(1), 27–30.

[50] James, A., Kapur, K. & Hawthorne, A.B. (1998) Long term outcomes of percutaneous endoscopic gastrostomy feeding in patients with dysphagic stroke. *Age, Aging*, **27**(6), 671–676.

[51] Restak, R. (1984) *The Brain*. Bantham Books, New York.

[52] Chusid, J.G. & McDonald, J.J. (1995) *Correlative Neuroanatomy and Functional Neurology*. Lange Medical Publications, Los Altos, California.

[53] Holland, A. (1984) *Language Disorders in Adults; Recent Advances*. College Hill Press, San Diego.

[54] Jones, Gemma (1992) A communication model for dementia. In: *Care giving and Dementia Research and Application*. Tavistock Routledge, London.

[55] Griffiths, H. (1991) The psychiatry of old age: the effects of dementia on communication. In: Gravell, R. & Frances, J. (eds.) *Speech and Communication Problems in Psychiatry*. Chapman Hall, London.

[56] Ayres, A.J. (1980) *Sensory Integration and Learning Disorders*. Western Psychological Services, Los Angeles.

[57] Ayres, A.J. (1980) *Sensory Integration and the Child*. Western Psychological Services, Los Angeles.

[58] Bach, Y. & Rita, P. (1980) *Recovery of Function: Theoretical Considerations for Brain Injury Rehabilitation*. Hans Huber, Bern.

[59] Orly, J.M. & Brizee, K.R. (1979) Sensory coding, sensation perception, information processing and sensory motor integration from maturity to old age. *Ageing 10: Sensory systems and communication*. Raven Press, New York.

[60] Layton, B. (1975) Perceptual noise and ageing. *Psychological bulletin*, **82**, 875–883.

[61] Mulley, G.P. (1982) Stroke. In: Brocklehurst, J.C. (ed.) *Textbook of Geriatric Medicine* 4th edn, ch. 31. Churchill-Livingstone, Edinburgh.

[62] Ouslander, J.G., Morishita, I. & Blaustein, J. (1987) Clinical, functional and psychosocial characteristics of an incontinent nursing home population. *Journal of Gerontology*, **42**(6), 631–637.

[63] Brocklehurst, J.C., Andrews, K., Richards, B. & Laycock, P.J. (1985) Incidence and correlates of incontinence in stroke patients. *Journal of the American Geriatrics Society*, **35**, 540–542.

[64] Borrie, M.J., Campbell, A.J., Caradoc-Davis, T.H. & Spears, F.S. (1986) Urinary incontinence after stroke: A prospective study. *Age & Ageing*, **15**, 177–181.

[65] Rottkamp, B. (1985) A holistic approach to identifying factors associated with an altered pattern of urinary elimination in stroke patients. *Journal of Neurosurgical Nursing*, **17**(1), 37–44.

[66] Khan, Z., Hertman, J., Young, W.C., Melman, A. & Leiter, E. (1981) Positive correlates of urodynamic dysfunction and brain injury after cerebro-vascular accident. *Journal of Urology*, **126**, 86–88.

[67] Nazarko, L. (1996) A matter of urgency. *Nursing Times*, **92**(32), 63–65.

[68] Kirkulata, G.H. (1981) Urinary incontinence secondary to drugs. *Urology*, **18**(2), 243–256.

[69] Nazarko, L. (1994) Drugs, continence, elderly people. *Primary Health Care*, **4**(1), 19–22.

[70] Roe, B.H. (1989) Catheters in the community. *Nursing Times*, **85**(36), 43.

[71] Mollander, U. *et al.* (1990) An epidemiological study of urinary incontinence and related urogenital symptoms in elderly women. *Maturitas*, **12**, 51–60.

[72] Ekelund, P. & Johansson, S. (1979) Polypoid cystitis. *Acta Pathol. Microbiol.*, **87**, 179–184.

[73] Kristiansen, P., Pompiers, R. & Wadtrrom, L.B. (1983) Long term bladder drainage and bladder capacity. *Neurology and Urodynamics*, **2**, 135–143.

74 Pitt, M. (1989) Fluid intake and urinary tract infection. *Nursing Times*, **5**(1), 36–38.

75 Burns (1992) Working up a thirst. *Nursing Times*, **88**(26), 45–47.

76 Nazarko, L. (1996) Power to the people. *Nursing Times*, **92**(41), 48–49.

77 Nazarko, L. (1996) Preventing constipation. *Professional Nurse*, **11**(12), 816–818.

78 Kinnunen, O. (1991) Study of constipation in a geriatric hospital, old people's home and at home. *Age & Ageing*, **3**(2), 161–170.

79 Edwardes, C.A., Tomlin, J. & Reed, N.W. (1988) Fibre and constipation. *British Journal of General Practice*, **11**, 26–31.

80 Heaton, K.W., Radvan, H. & Cripps, H. *et al.* (1992) Defecation frequency and timing and stool form in the general population; a prospective study. *Gut*, **33**, 818–824.

81 Wrick, K.L., Robertson, J.B. & Van Soest, P.J. *et al.* (1983) The effect of dietary fibre source on human intestine transit and stool output. *Journal of Nutrition*, **113**(8), 1464–1479.

82 Nazarko, L. (1996) Power to the people. *Nursing Times*, **92**(41), 48–49.

83 Nazarko, L. (1995) Commode design for frail and disabled people. *Professional Nurse*, **11**(2), 95–97.

84 Thompson, I.E., Melia, K.M. & Boyd, K.M. (1994) *Nursing Ethics*, 3rd edn. Churchill-Livingstone, Edinburgh.

85 Working Party on Clinical Guidelines in Palliative Care (1997) *Changing Gear – Guidelines for Managing the Last Days of Life in Adults*. National Council for Hospice and Specialist Palliative Care Services, London.

86 Glover, J. (1977) *Causing Death and Saving Lives*. Penguin, London.

87 National Council for Hospice and Specialist Palliative Care Services (1997) Ethical decision making in palliative care: artificial hydration for people who are terminally ill. National Council for Hospice and Specialist Palliative Care Services, London.

88 Lord Chancellor's Office (1997) *Who decides? Making decisions on behalf of mentally incapacitated adults*. A consultation paper.

Rehabilitation Assessment Form

Name ....

Patient number ....

Date of assessment ....

Assessment completed by ....

Walking
☐ Chair bound = 1
☐ Walks with help of two staff = 2
☐ Walks with aid = 3
☐ Walks unaided = 4
Score ☐
Reasons/Problems identified

Washing
☐ Totally dependent = 1
☐ Needs major help = 2
☐ Needs some help = 3
☐ Independent = 4
Score ☐
Reasons/Problems identified

Transferring
☐ Totally dependent = 1
☐ Needs assistance one nurse = 2
☐ Needs help two staff = 3
☐ Independent = 4
Score ☐
Reasons/Problems identified

Dressing
☐ Totally dependent = 1
☐ Needs major help = 2
☐ Needs some help = 3
☐ Indepndent = 4
Score ☐
Reasons/Problems identified

Getting out of bed
☐ Totally dependent = 1
☐ Needs assistance one nurse = 2
☐ Needs help two staff = 3
☐ Independent = 4
Score ☐
Reasons/Problems identified

Eating
☐ Totally dependent = 1
☐ Needs major help = 2
☐ Needs some help = 3
☐ Inependent = 4
Score ☐
Reasons/Problems identified

Moving in bed
☐ Totally dependent = 1
☐ Needs assistance one nurse = 2
☐ Needs help two staff = 3
☐ Independent = 4
Score ☐
Reasons/Problems identified

Using the toilet
☐ Totally dependent = 1
☐ Needs major help = 2
☐ Needs some help = 3
☐ Independent = 4
Score ☐
Reasons/Problems identified

Sample menu: examples of high fibre diet

Breakfast

Cereals: All Bran, Bran flakes, Weetabix, Shreddies, Bite Size Shreddies, muesli, porridge. These cereals are easier to swallow if hot milk is added.
Fruit: Compote fruits, soaked dried fruits including apricots, peaches, pears, and prunes. Stewed figs. These fruits can be liquidised if the person has swallowing problems.
Juiced fruits: Whole fresh fruits liquidised and served chilled as a drink.
Bread: High fibre white or wholemeal.
Baked beans on toast.

Lunch

Soup: Made with vegetables, barley, lentils, dried beans served with croutons made from high fibre bread. The soup can be liquidised.
Main courses: Beans, peas, barley and pulses can be added to stews and casseroles. Dumplings made with a mixture of potatoes and white flour* can be served with meat and gravy.
Puddings: Fresh fruit salad, pears poached in redcurrant jelly, water and a little red wine. Whole-wheat crackers butter and cheese.

Afternoon tea

Flap jacks.
Banana tea bread.
Carrot cake.

Supper

Juiced fruits or soup enriched with vegetables, pulses or small whole-wheat pasta shapes.
Jacket potatoes with a selection of toppings.
Baked smoked haddock with cheese sauce, creamed potatoes, peas.
Puddings: Lemon meringue pie with digestive biscuit base.
Rhubarb or gooseberry fool with cream and biscuit topping.
Fresh fruit.

High fibre snacks

Olives.
Peanuts (*Note that these should not be given to people with dysphagia as they fit beautifully into the bronchus*).
Peanut butter on toast or whole-wheat crackers.
Raisins, chocolate covered raisins, chocolate covered peanuts.
Dried fruits (these can be cut up into small pieces).
Banana chips.
Stoned dates.
Yoghurt with puréed fruit.
Fruit spread with bread or crackers.

Bowel assessment form (part 1)

Name:	DOB
Medical diagnosis[1]	Please list all prescribed medications[2]
Nursing diagnosis[3]	
Fluid intake in 24 hours[4]	Mental state[5]
Hearing	Vision
Speech difficulties	Manual dexterity
Difficulty chewing	Difficulty swallowing
Urinalysis[6]	Weight
What is the problem?[7]	How long have you had this problem?
What do you think brought it on?	Does anything make it better?
How does it affect your life?	Does anything make it worse?
How often do you open your bowels?[8]	What is the stool like?
Do you have to strain to open your bowels?	Do you know when you need to open your bowels?
Have you ever had any operations on your bowel or back passage?[9] Tell me about them	Have you ever passed blood when opening your bowels?
Do you have any pain when opening your bowels? Tell me about it	Has your back passage ever fallen down when you were opening your bowels? Tell me about it

[1] The aim is to identify any medical conditions that can contribute to bowel problems.
[2] The aim is to identify any medications causing or contributing to bowel dysfunction.
[3] Please indicate nursing problems.
[4] This can be obtained by unobtrusive observation in lucid individuals. If individual is dependent on nursing staff for fluids maintain a fluid balance chart to obtain information.
[5] Lucid, mild, moderate or severe cognitive impairment.
[6] Pay particular attention to specific gravity as this indicates hydration.
[7] Wherever possible use the person's own words.
[8] Where possible discretely observe to confirm without compromising the individual's dignity.
[9] Individuals sometimes do not tell the GP this one as 'It was years ago'.

Bowel assessment form (part 2)

Physical examination
This is to be carried out by an appropriately qualified and experienced nurse or doctor

Abdominal palpation	Abdominal masses? Where?
Rectal examination Perineal descent? Faecal soiling?	**Haemorrhoids?** **Internal/external?**
Anal lesions e.g. fissure	**Anal scars**
Anal tone[10] Faecal loading Stool consistency Other findings	**Rectal lesions[11]** **Rectal prolapse** **Prostate**
Further investigations (please tick) Abdominal x-ray[12] FBC Faecal occult blood Thyroid function tests Sigmoidoscopy Barium enema Colonoscopy Other (state)	**Results and date**
What is the problem?[13]	**What factors have contributed to this** **(mobility, hydration, medication, diet, etc.)**
Treatment and date[14] 1. 2. 3. 4. 5. 6. 7.	**Evaluation and date**
Completed by:	

[10] Note particularly if anus is gaping.
[11] Immediate referral if noted! Only the cytology department can tell the difference between a carcinoma and a polyp.
[12] When faecal loading suspected following palpation and rectal examination.
[13] Use English – constipation, diarrhoea, pain, etc.
[14] Be brief – e.g. review medications, increase fluids, alter diet, etc. Not a care plan. Please don't give lactulose. See bowel file.

Chapter 13

Accessing Community Services

Introduction

The official Department of Health response when the issue of nursing homes is raised is to state that they are not part of the NHS and not the responsibility of the Department of Health. This response does not bear scrutiny because the Department of Health have been instrumental in formulating the national minimum standards and the reform of primary care set out in the NHS plan. The people cared for in nursing homes are part of the community and receive primary care services and services from hospitals. In theory older people living in nursing homes have the same right to health services as people living in their own homes. In practice many community services focus on keeping people out of homes and people in homes are viewed as low priority. Nurses in some areas experience great difficulty in obtaining access to services on behalf of older people who require them.

The aims of this chapter are to:

- Explain how changes in the delivery of primary care will affect residents
- Explain how to access services

Creation of Care Trusts

A Care Trust is a new organisation that goes beyond Primary Care Trusts to integrate health and social care in the community. The NHS Plan[1] provided for the establishment of Care Trusts. Care Trusts are designed to enable the integration of commissioning and provision of adult social care and primary health care at a local level. This means that social services departments and Primary Care Groups and Primary Care Trusts need to establish integrated management systems.

At the moment 20 of the 100 local authorities in England are working to become Care Trusts; eventually the Care Trust system will encompass all local authorities. The first wave of 'demonstrator sites' will be able to obtain extra funding, but details of this extra funding have not yet been released.

Care Trusts will affect people requiring health or social care in the following ways:

- There will be one organisation for health and social care
- Care will be more streamlined and integrated

- Joint information about services will be provided
- There will a joint management structure.

Care Trusts will affect the way you access services. Some of the initiatives being trailed at the moment include:

- Allocating a link worker to GP surgeries. The link worker will link social services and health. This means that if a person is having difficulty with moving around because of arthritis, the link worker can link services provided by social services such as home care with health services to provide integrated support for the person.
- Locating social workers, occupational therapists, district nurses and practice staff in the GP's surgery or the health centre. This would mean that you could access services via the GP's surgery rather than via community offices.

Care Trusts will affect staff who work within them and staff who access services for residents in the following ways:

- Quality of services will be improved
- It will be easier to access services because they will located under the same roof
- It will be easier to communicate with staff because there will be one management system
- Staff will work more efficiently because there will be one assessment system
- Communication will be easier because single information systems and joint record keeping will be introduced.

During this period of change, homes within primary care 'demonstrator sites' will begin to provide services in different ways. It is important to work closely with your GP to ensure that you are aware of changes in the way you access services.

Chiropody services

Age-related changes may make older people's nails difficult to cut. Many older people have very tough, thickened toe nails. This is because reduced blood supply to the nails causes changes in the nail bed. Regular cutting of toe nails is important and prevents problems such as ingrowing toe nails. Many older people experience difficulty in cutting their own toe nails because they are unable to bend down or lack the co-ordination to cut nails. Many nurses have never cut toe nails during their nursing careers and a myth has grown up that nurses do not carry out this task. There is no reason why nurses should not cut older people's toe nails.

It is often impossible to cut them with ordinary nail scissors normally used to cut finger nails. Each nursing home should purchase suitable equipment to enable nurses to cut toe nails. A strong pair of toe nail clippers, a pair of toe nail scissors and a selection of files and emery boards are required. It is usually easier to cut tough, thickened toe nails after the individual has had a soak in a warm bath, as this softens the nails. Nails should be cut straight across and any rough edges filed with a nail file or emery board.

Nurses can also cut toe nails in older people who suffer from diabetes. Older people who are suffering from vascular problems should be referred to a chiropodist for treatment. Some older people suffer from corns, bunions, ingrowing toe nails and other problems outside the nurse's sphere of competence. Individuals suffering from such problems should be referred to a chiropodist for treatment.

Obtaining chiropody services

At the moment community-based chiropodists are often based at the local hospital. This will change. Chiropodists work with foot-care assistants to provide services. Chiropodists normally visit housebound older people at home to carry out treatment. Mobile older people are often asked to visit community chiropody clinics, which chiropodists hold in local health centres.

The numbers of older people requiring community chiropody services have increased enormously in recent years. Greater numbers of older people are now living in nursing and residential homes. In many areas, though, chiropody services have not expanded to take account of the greater numbers of people requiring chiropody. Many chiropodists now find that they are able to see older people less frequently than before. An older person who was receiving chiropody services every six weeks may now only receive services every eight weeks.

You can contact your local chiropody department and request chiropody treatment for the older people in the home. The chiropody department will probably send a foot-care assistant for a few hours every eight weeks. It will not be possible for each older person to have nails cut during this session. Staff shortages or illness can mean that a session is missed. If nurses carry out routine footcare and nail cutting for the majority of older people living in the nursing home, the chiropodist or foot-care assistant can concentrate on the individuals who require specialist treatment.

If the nurse does not feel confident about cutting older people's toe nails or would like advice about purchasing suitable nail clippers and cutters, advice and help can be obtained from the local chiropodist. Many chiropodists welcome nurses to their foot-care clinics and will spend a few hours helping the nurse become proficient at cutting what initially appear to be impossible thickened toe nails.

Useful address and telephone number

Local chiropodist

Emergency chiropody

Foot problems seldom occur on the day of the chiropodist's visit. Older people can develop ingrowing toe nails which can be painful and require prompt treatment. Bunions can become painful and infected. An individual can have an accident which leads to bleeding under the nail. Nails can become caught, torn and damaged. In such cases you should contact the chiropodist, who may be able to visit the home that day to offer emergency treatment. Sometimes residents can damage finger nails. It is important to find out if your local chiropodist is willing to work 'above the hip'. Chiropodists normally care for feet but may be willing to treat damaged finger nails in an emergency. Some chiropodists are unable to do this because of insurance reasons. Nurses who carry out routine foot care and have developed a good relationship with the chiropodist normally find chiropodists are willing to visit immediately.

Sometimes the chiropodist may suggest that the older person is brought to a nearby health centre if a clinic is in progress. The nurse who recognises the chiropodist as a fellow professional and builds a good working relationship will find that access to chiropody services is not difficult.

Private chiropody

NHS chiropodists often lack the time to visit frequently enough to ensure that all older people living within the nursing home have their nails cut on a regular basis. Private chiropodists offering nail cutting sessions often approach nurses. In some homes older people themselves pay this charge; in others the home bears the cost. The charges for private chiropody vary but rates from £10 to £20 per resident are not uncommon. It normally takes 10 to 15 minutes to cut an older person's nails and file any rough edges. Sometimes chiropodists offer to work on a sessional basis. The chiropodist charges a set amount per session and will see a set number of people during the session.

If you are purchasing chiropody services for residents it is worth purchasing a mixture of foot care assistant and chiropody sessions. This allows you to use the professional's time more effectively and also contains costs.

Specialist footwear and appliances

Many older people suffer from disabilities, and specialist footwear and appliances can make a real difference to an individual's quality of life. Many older people enter nursing homes after sustaining falls that have resulted in fracture. Surgical treatment of fractured femurs usually involves pinning and plating of the femur. In some cases total hip replacements are carried out. Such surgery often results in the ligaments on the affected leg becoming stretched. The result is that the individual has one leg longer than the other. Older people who fail to make a rapid recovery are often discharged to nursing homes immobile; ensuring that problems are corrected gives the older person the opportunity to regain ability.

You can ask the individual's doctor to complete a referral form and send this to the surgical appliance department, which is usually based at the local hospital. When Care Trusts are established the orthotist may be based at the GP's surgery. The older person will either be visited at the home or given an appointment to see the orthotist. The orthotist measures both legs and either orders specially made shoes that accommodate any shortening or alters the person's own shoes. Providing shoes to correct shortening can make a real difference to an older person's life. It becomes possible for the individual to regain mobility and independence.

Older people who have survived severe strokes often suffer from feet and ankles which tend to turn inwards or outwards (talipes varus or talipes valgus). These foot problems hamper walking and increase the risk of falls. The orthotist is often able to correct such problems by providing shoes with a wedge on one part of the sole. In other cases the orthotist may arrange for a calliper to be provided. The older person's own shoes are sometimes adapted to accommodate a calliper; in other cases shoes and a calliper are supplied.

Some older people suffer from foot deformities such as large bunions and hammer toes. It can be impossible to find shoes to fit and so the older person wears large, wide, ill-fitting carpet slippers. The older woman who takes a size three may wear a pair of size eight men's slippers. These can so easily contribute to accidents and falls.

Some older people suffer from oedema, which prevents them wearing shoes. They tend to wear slippers and in some cases cut the slippers at the front to give them more room. In the morning these slippers are too loose and in the evening when oedema is at its worst they are too tight. These slippers can easily fall off during walking. The orthotist can provide special shoes to accommodate foot deformities and oedema. These shoes fit properly, make walking more comfortable and reduce the risk of accidents.

Some older people suffer from osteoarthritis and when this affects the knee joints they can be painful and can tend to 'give'. This can result in falls. The orthotist can supply knee supports that support arthritic knees and reduce pain on walking.

Older people who have suffered from strokes should be encouraged to exercise hemiplegic or weakened limbs. The nurse should carry out a range of passive movements to affected limbs when an older person is unable to do this. Relatives can also be encouraged to assist in carrying out passive movements. Some older people's limbs tend to contract despite exercise and passive movement, and can easily become deformed. Hands can become tightly clenched and wrists turned inwards. Such deformities can cause older people intense pain.

The individual's doctor may prescribe muscle relaxants in such cases but these are not always effective and can cause unpleasant side effects such as urinary incontinence (by relaxing the detrusor muscle which controls the bladder) or drowsiness (see Chapter 12 for details). The orthotist can examine the individual and provide an appropriate splint for the hand or the hand and wrist. There are a number of different types; some, known as 'lively splints', enable the individual to use the hand while wearing the splint.

Some splints can be worn only at night or when the patient is not exercising. The orthotist will advise nurses about the use of each splint on each patient. Splints can reduce pain, prevent deformity, reduce or eliminate the need for drugs, which can have troublesome side effects, and make a real difference to an older person's quality of life.

Oedema can easily occur in older people who are unable to walk or who are not encouraged and helped to walk. Postural oedema is often treated with diuretics but these can predispose an older person to urinary incontinence; the fear of urinary incontinence can lead older people to become depressed and can reduce mobility. This can lead to a cycle where more drugs are prescribed to treat symptoms.

Older people who suffer from postural oedema should be encouraged and assisted to walk whenever possible. If oedema persists despite mobilisation (where possible) and elevation, the orthotist can measure the individual for surgical stockings. Support stockings are available in four levels of compression from light to extra high. They should be used to prevent recurrence of leg ulcers in individuals who have suffered from varicose ulcers; details are given in Chapter 6. Support stockings are available in a range of colours and the individual can choose the colour she prefers. It is important to ensure that the patient chooses a colour she is happy to wear, otherwise she may not wear them when they arrive. Men are reluctant to wear stockings! Knee length support stockings are available in black and are indistinguishable from men's knee length socks. The nurse who refers to them as support socks may find male patients wear them more readily.

Many orthotists now only supply one pair of support stockings. The measurements are left with the nurse (and kept on record at surgical appliances) so that further supplies can be ordered from the local pharmacist on FP10 prescription.

Wigs

Losing hair is one of the most traumatic experiences an older woman can suffer. Some older women have undergone chemotherapy while others may have suffered from hair loss as a result of undetected thyroid disease. NHS wigs can be supplied and worn until the hair regrows. A wig can make a tremendous difference to morale and the nurse should never assume that just because a woman is in her eighties or nineties she no longer cares how she looks.

Obtaining orthotic services

All the appliances described can be obtained from the surgical appliances department of the local hospital. Normally the individual's doctor writes a referral note that is sent to the department. A letter from a consultant may be required stating the reason for hair loss if a wig is required. GPs are very busy and they can often find it difficult to find the time to write referral letters for appliances. It may be helpful if the home prepares a standard letter. The doctor can then fill in the blank spaces with details of the patient and the type of appliance required, and sign the letter. Hospitals deal with huge volumes of mail and from time to time letters fail to reach their destination. Keeping a photocopy of referrals in the person's notes ensures that if this happens another copy of the referral can be sent to the hospital. This saves time as you do not have to obtain another letter, and it ensures that the patient is seen as quickly as possible.

Many hospitals employ orthotists on a sessional basis and prefer to see people at their outpatient clinics. Individuals attending outpatient clinics will require hospital transport (unless the home has its own transport facilities); using hospital transport can involve long delays waiting for it. This can be exhausting, especially for individuals who have recently undergone major surgery or suffered strokes. It is good practice for the home to send a member of staff to accompany an individual attending an outpatient appointment.

Domiciliary visits can be arranged and if a number of individuals require appliances, domiciliary visits are more cost effective than the hospital budget bearing the costs of both transport and the orthotist's time.

Hairdressing

Most older women enjoyed going to the hairdresser for a weekly or fort-nightly hairdo before admission to the home. Having a shampoo and set or a perm is a real morale booster for most older women. Nursing homes nor-mally have a hairdresser who visits regularly, usually weekly. The hairdresser provides a full range of services. In many homes patients pay the hairdresser for this service; prices are usually lower than in local salons.

Some patients may prefer to visit a local salon and may require the nurse's help to arrange an appointment and get to and from the salon.

Ophthalmic services

Few older people have perfect vision; government statistics indicate that 96% of people over the age of 75 wear glasses. If you have perfect vision you may not appreciate the importance of an older person having regular eye tests and obtaining spectacles that provide the best possible correction.

An older person who has lost their glasses or who has glasses that are no longer appropriate can be at risk of falling. Eating may become difficult. Choosing clothes from the wardrobe may become difficult; dressing can become a struggle. It may no longer be possible to enjoy reading books or daily newspapers. Moving freely around the home can become difficult. The older person who can no longer read the time, read signs, read papers or watch television can easily become disorientated and distressed.

Some older people who enter the home may have been attending one particular optician for many years. If the optician is local, the older person may wish to continue to receive eye care from them. This ensures continuity of care. In some cases the older person does not have a local optician or has not visited an optician in many years. The home should arrange for an optician to provide optical services for older people living in the home.

There are two types of opticians:

(1) Ophthalmic opticians are qualified to examine eyes and detect the presence of disease and also to test sight and prescribe and dispense spectacles to correct visual problems

(2)   Dispensing opticians are qualified to dispense and fit spectacles but not to examine eyes for abnormalities or to test vision and prescribe spectacles.

The home should make arrangements with an ophthalmic optician to provide services to the home. Ophthalmic opticians are independent practitioners. They receive fees from the NHS for providing optical services to individuals who are eligible for NHS ophthalmic services. Individuals who are not eligible for these are charged for ophthalmic services.

There are usually a number of opticians within an area and the nurse can choose which one to arrange services with. Ideally the optician should be located near the home, if possible within walking distance. This makes trips to the opticians more convenient. The optician should have a flexible appointments system and it should be possible to arrange an appointment quickly. If an optician cannot offer an appointment within 48 hours, then choose another optician. It is important to check how quickly an optician can obtain glasses in an emergency. If an older person who is dependent on glasses damages them, it is important to obtain new glasses quickly. Some opticians can obtain new glasses within 24 hours or less, others can take three weeks.

An optician who values the custom of older people resident at the nursing home will normally carry out minor repairs without charge. Some opticians feel that their work is completed when glasses are dispensed. Any decent optician will ensure that glasses are fitted correctly. If you have an optician who is not fitting glasses and ensuring that they sit properly on the nose and are comfortable around the ears you need to make it clear that this level of service is unacceptable. If the optician is not prepared to fit residents' glasses then you may have to find another optician who will provide the level of service that you and I take for granted when we visit an optician.

If an older person is too frail or unwell to leave the home, the optician can make a domiciliary visit. It is preferable to examine eyes at the optician's fully equipped surgery, and domiciliary visits should only be requested if absolutely necessary. Some opticians choose to visit the home and fit spectacles when they are ready, as it is more convenient for an older person to have the fitting at the home. Opticians do not charge for fitting visits.

Eye tests should be carried out each year. The optician will normally have a system that sends out annual reminders to patients advising them that their next eye test is due. An eye test normally takes half an hour. Individuals should be escorted to the opticians and a list of medications and details of medical history should be given, as the optician will wish to take a medical history. The member of staff who escorts the older person may have to help the individual get into the examining chair.

The optician examines the older person's eyes, and may detect signs of eye abnormality or disease. If any abnormality or disease is detected, the optician will write details of his findings on a green form. This form will be given to the older person or the escort. The nurse should photocopy the form and retain the copy in the individual's notes. The original should be given to the individual's GP who will refer to the ophthalmology department of the local hospital. If the optician detects eye disease that requires urgent treatment, such as acute glaucoma, detached retina or retinal haemorrhage, they will normally contact the hospital direct and have the person sent there immediately.

Some opticians offer specialist 'low vision' services which aim to help maximise the vision of people with severe sight defects. Opticians can advise and arrange to supply magnifying glasses, including some with lights, and other aids to vision.

Mobile opticians

Some opticians are now specialising in caring for older people living in nursing and residential homes and are offering a mobile optician's service. The optician has a large, fully-equipped vehicle which is driven to the nursing home. All individuals requiring eye tests are seen and examined in the vehicle, which carries a full range of frames; individuals can choose frames and order spectacles. The vehicle returns when spectacles are ready and all individuals have their spectacles fitted. Opticians offering such services usually offer free eye tests to individuals who are not eligible for NHS eye tests.

Nurses working in rural areas find mobile optician's services very useful. Every visit is a domiciliary visit and such services save time. Mobile opticians now serve many city and suburban areas. They normally make regular visits to the nursing home, usually every three months. Older people who have broken their glasses, who have been admitted to the home between visits or are experiencing problems seeing, should not have to wait weeks or months until the next visit to obtain services. It is important for the nurse to check what arrangements mobile opticians make to provide ad hoc services, before making arrangements with them to provide ophthalmic services to the home.

NHS and private eye tests and spectacles

Older people are eligible for free NHS eye tests. Domiciliary eye tests are available free to those eligible for NHS eye tests.

Individuals on income support are given financial help with the cost of glasses, on a voucher scheme. The voucher can be used towards the cost of frames and lenses. At the time of writing the vouchers are worth between £30 and £154.30 depending on the strength of lenses required. It is usually possible for an older person on income support to obtain an attractive pair of glasses using the vouchers without having to pay any money towards the cost. Individuals may choose to have more expensive frames or expensive high index lenses if they wish, and meet the additional costs. One of my residents supplemented her NHS voucher and bought designer frames and high index lenses stating. 'There's no reason to let yourself go when you get older. It's still possible to be glamorous at 93.'

Individuals who are not on income support do not receive any financial help towards the cost of glasses.

Some older people require glasses for close and distance work. In some cases bifocal glasses are prescribed, but these can be difficult to use; in order to see close up the individual must look out of the bottom half of the glasses and in order to see in the distance the individual must look out of the top half of the glasses. If an individual looks out of the wrong part the vision is poor. Some people (young and old) are unable to cope with bifocal glasses and may require reading and distance glasses. Older people who require two sets of glasses should be advised to choose different frames or different coloured frames to avoid confusion. The optician can engrave an R for reading or D for distance on the inner arm of the glasses, in case the older person or staff mix up the two pairs.

It is possible to have the individual's name engraved inside the arm of glasses. This can help identify glasses when they are put down and forgotten. Many opticians will provide this service free of charge if requested. If you are going to ask the optician to engrave on glasses in microprint make sure that you buy a decent magnifying glass so that you can read what has been engraved.

Further information

The College of Optometrists produces two useful leaflets: *Choosing an Optician* and *Domiciliary Eye Care Services – Guidance for managers of residential care and nursing homes*. The College can provide information and advise on ophthalmic services. These leaflets are not available online so you will need to telephone or write to: The College of Optometrists, 42 Craven Street, London. WC2N 5NG Tel. 020 7839 6000. Fax 020 7839 6800. website:www.college-optometrists.org/

The Department of Health provides information on eligibility for NHS eye tests and details of voucher systems, in patient information leaflet G11. This is available from opticians and GP's surgeries.

Useful address and telephone number

Local optician

Dental services

Most older people wear dentures or partial dentures, while some older people retain their natural teeth. It is important that the home has made arrangements to provide patients with dental care. Some older people are registered with local dentists and should be encouraged to continue to obtain treatment from their dentist. This ensures continuity of care. Some older people may have moved to the area to be near family and friends. The home should make arrangements to ensure that dental services are available for older people who require them.

Dental services can be obtained either from a dental surgeon who is in practice locally or from the NHS community dentist. Many independent dental surgeons are willing to provide dental services to older people but are no longer taking on new NHS patients. In some parts of the UK it can be extremely difficult to find a dentist willing to offer NHS treatment. A list of dentists is also available from the local library and you can telephone and ask if dentists are prepared to offer NHS dental services.

Although some dentists are willing to offer these services they may not be willing to make new dentures for NHS patients. Nurses should clarify this point before considering referring patients to the dentist, as dentures supplied privately cost from £300 to £400. Many older people living in nursing homes, who are on income support, are unable to afford to pay for private dentures.

The government has now pledged that everyone will be able to access an NHS dentist, so if you have problems finding an NHS dentist contact NHS Direct. The dentist(s) offering such services may be some distance away, and this is an important consideration as transport may be required to take individuals to appointments, and escorts may be absent from the home for a considerable time. It can be difficult to organise prompt emergency treatment in such circumstances. Some older people may require domiciliary treatment and dentists may be unwilling to travel considerable distances to offer it.

NHS community dentists are employed directly by NHS Community Trusts to provide dental services to individuals living in the community. In the future NHS community dentists may work for Care Trusts. They provide services in local health centres and offer domiciliary services. Community dentists usually provide specialised dental care to children with special needs and people with learning disability living in the community, as well as other client groups. They normally have a greater expertise in dealing with disabled and cognitively impaired individuals, and can offer a greater range of dental techniques developed to help such individuals.

Community dentists will visit older people in nursing homes and provide all dental care for individuals living in the home. Community dentists normally work with a trained dental nurse and a hygienist. Most dental treatments are carried out within the home. The community dentist carries out routine dental examinations and works with the hygienist and dental nurse to provide older people and nurses with advice and help to ensure good oral hygiene and dental care. Community dentists, unfortunately, are extremely busy and while they provide a superb emergency service, they may have to place older people on a waiting list for dentures. It may be six or eight weeks before the dentist can begin taking impressions and order dentures. Older people are not charged for any treatment or dentures supplied by community dentists; the costs are borne by the Community Trust. Individuals who require new dentures and are unwilling to wait, but can afford to pay, may prefer to pay a local dentist for private treatment.

The local hospital or NHS Community Trust will be able to supply the telephone number of the community dentist for your area.

Useful address and telephone number

Dentist

Hearing aids services

Causes of hearing problems

Hearing loss affects 17% of the adult population and at least 50% of older people living in nursing homes. The commonest cause of hearing loss is wax in the ears. Wax is often visible in the outer ear. Simple treatment such as ear drops or warm olive oil can be put in the ears three times a day for three to five days. This softens the wax and the ears can then be syringed. You can then use an auriscope to check that the ears are completely free of wax. If in doubt you can ask the person's GP to check. Ideally the home should have an auriscope so that you can check ears yourself.

If hearing loss persists, the older person's doctor should be asked to refer to the ENT clinic at the local hospital so that hearing can be checked by carrying out an audiogram. NHS waiting lists for audiograms can be lengthy and some older people have to wait six months for an initial appointment. It is important to ensure that ears are clear of wax prior to an audiogram. If the older person's ears are blocked with wax it is impossible to carry out an audiogram and the nurse is asked to make a further appointment after the wax has been removed.

Hearing aids

Older people who suffer from hearing loss are often supplied with hearing aids. The nurse may assume that hearing aids enable individuals to hear normally. Hearing aids in fact amplify sounds and make them louder.

You should ensure that staff and relatives are aware of the actions they can take to help older people with hearing difficulties to hear. It is important not to shout, as this distorts the voice. People should face the individual and speak slowly and clearly. Plain language should be used and gestures can be used if an individual has difficulty hearing. It is important to cut out background noise; closing doors, turning down the television or closing the window to shut out traffic noise, can help people with hearing impairment to hear.

Older people who do not wear their hearing aids

Some older people do not wear their hearing aids. If they lost their hearing gradually, a hearing aid suddenly exposes them to a great deal of noise, which they may find unbearable. But if they do not use the hearing aid they become cut off from normal life and unable to communicate. The nurse should encourage older people to wear their hearing aids. Suggest that the older person wears the aid twice a day for an hour and gradually encourage it to be used at all times. This allows them to get used to our noisy world again. Some older people find it difficult to put the mould in their ear and to work the controls, but may not wish to ask for help. Nurses should be sensitive to such problems and offer help in a tactful way.

Common problems

Many hearing aids fail to work because the batteries are dead. There are two types of hearing aid batteries available for NHS aids that fit behind the ear. The normal battery will normally last for three or four days if the hearing aid is turned off when the older person goes to sleep. If the aid is left on, the battery will only last for a day or two. Long life batteries normally last about a week if used during waking hours.

Hearing aid batteries are supplied in small blister packs. A dozen ordinary batteries or eight long-life batteries are usually supplied. Unused batteries have a small blue sticker on them that must be removed before use. Occasionally older people and staff open the blister pack and remove the blue stickers; used and unused batteries can then become mixed up. The only way to check batteries when the stickers have been removed is to ask the individual to remove the aid. Place a battery in the aid and turn it up to the highest setting; charged batteries will cause the aid to oscillate and emit a high pitched screeching sound. Charged batteries can then be remarked with sticky tape or labels. Changing hearing aid batteries is a fiddly task and many older people find this difficult; the nurse should offer help if required.

Hearing aids whistle and oscillate at times. Oscillating aids are not functioning properly and the nurse should check them. The commonest cause of oscillation is that the aid is turned up too high; turning it down so that the whistling ceases but the individual is able to hear, is often all that is required. If the aid continues to oscillate even on a low setting such as one or two, you should ask the individual to remove the aid and should check the plastic tube that connects to the ear mould. The tube should be clear and flexible; if it has hardened or yellowed it should be replaced. Spare tubing is supplied with all aids and the nurse cuts a length to size and replaces it. Tubing should normally be changed every two months.

You should also check the mould that fits in the patient's ear. Wax often builds up in the ear drum behind the mould and a small piece of wax can block the mould and cause oscillation. Wax can be removed from the mould with a needle or safely pin. The mould can then be washed in warm water, reconnected to the aid and returned. If wax has blocked the mould, the ears should be checked for wax; any build-up should be removed using ear drops and syringing. If the aid continues to oscillate it is possible that the ear mould no longer fits properly and a new mould is required. You can contact the audiology clinic direct and make an appointment for the individual to be seen.

Individuals who are issued with hearing aids are supplied with a small brown hearing aid book. This book contains details of the type of aid, batteries and tube supplied, and gives the address of the local audiology clinic. When further supplies of batteries are required (usually when half of the supplied batteries have been used) the used batteries are returned to the audiology department with the book and a request for further batteries and tubing; this can be done by post. It is important to return used batteries as these are recharged.

Useful address and telephone number

Hearing aid department

Further information

Counsel and Care produce a free fact sheet (number 21), Helping Residents to Hear. This can be obtained by sending an SAE. They have also produced a study on the needs of older people with hearing loss living in residential and nursing homes. This provides guidance on caring for individuals who have hearing difficulties. It is called Sound Barriers and costs £5 from: Counsel and Care, Twyman House, 16 Bonny Street, London NW1 9PG. Tel. 0171 485 1566 (10 AM –4 PM). Counsel and Care offer information and advice on residential and nursing care. Their website contains lots of useful information and leaflets: http://www.counselandcare.org.uk

Conclusion

Older people may require aids of some kind to prevent deformity developing after illness. Many older people require aids to enable them to walk, see, hear and eat. Older people are often unaware of the range of aids and services available to enable them to participate fully in life. The nurse can work with older people to identify needs, and can then work with other professionals to ensure that these needs are met and older people are able to enjoy a greater degree of independence.

Reference

[1] Department of Health (2000) *The NHS Plan: The Government's response to the Royal Commission on Long Term Care.* Presented to Parliament July 2000. CM4818–II. Available from: The Stationery Office, (Mail, telephone and fax orders only) PO Box 29, Norwich NR3 1GN. General enquiries 0870 600 5522. Also available on website: www.nhs.uk/nhsplan

Chapter 14

Palliative Care

Introduction

Most people would prefer to die at home but in many countries increasing numbers of people die in hospital. In the UK the number of people dying in hospital is falling but the number of people who die in nursing homes is rising[1]. Before the introduction of the Community Care Act in 1993, the average nursing home patient survived for 22 months after admission. Dependency levels have increased and admissions have fallen[2]. Now 60% of older people admitted to nursing homes die within six months of admission and 30% die within six weeks of admission. Increasingly people are admitted to nursing homes 'in the later stages of dying'. Nurses working in nursing homes must now develop a new range of skills in palliative care if they are to meet the needs of the older people admitted requiring palliative care.

This chapter is divided into two sections: offering effective palliative care, and dealing with death and dying.

Offering effective palliative care

This section aims to enable you to:

- Understand the principle of palliative care
- Adopt a palliative care focus when this is appropriate
- Offer humane resident-focused care
- Work with the resident, doctors and other professionals to effectively manage symptoms

What is palliative care?

Palliative care is offered when there is no prospect of cure. The aim of palliative care is to alleviate distressing symptoms and to enable the individual to enjoy the highest possible quality of life.

The palliative care approach

The palliative care approach aims to promote physical and psychosocial well-being. It is a vital part of clinical practice whatever the illness or its stage[3]. The key principles are:

- Caring for the whole person
- Care that encompasses the patient and those who matter to her

- Open and sensitive communication including information about diagnosis and treatment options
- Respecting the patient's autonomy and choice
- Focusing on quality of life and good symptom control.

What kind of care do patients want?

In the US the concept of a dying person's rights has been adopted[4] throughout hospices and nursing homes.

Box 14.1   The dying person's bill of rights.

I have the right to be treated as a living human being until I die
I have the right to maintain a sense of hopefulness, however changing its focus may be
I have the right to be cared for by those who can maintain a sense of hopefulness, however changing this may be
I have the right to express my feelings and emotions about my approaching death in my own way
I have the right to participate in decisions regarding my care
I have the right to expect continuing medical and nursing attention even though cure goals must be changed to comfort goals
I have the right not to die alone
I have the right to be free from pain
I have the right to have my questions answered honestly
I have the right not to be deceived
I have the right to have help from and for my family in accepting my death
I have the right to die in peace and dignity
I have the right to retain my individuality and not to be judged for my decisions, which may be contrary to the beliefs of others
I have the right to discuss and enlarge my religious or spiritual experiences, whatever this may mean to others
I have the right to expect that the sanctity of the human body will be respected after death
I have the right to be cared for by caring, sensitive, knowledgeable people who will attempt to understand my needs and will be able to gain some satisfaction in helping me face my death

Management of distressing symptoms

Research has identified the major symptoms that people (suffering from a range of diseases) found most distressing. Many nurses caring for these people were unaware of symptoms because patients did not wish to complain[5] or felt that little could be done to alleviate symptoms. Symptoms identified in recent research are[6] in order of prevalence:

Weakness	73%
Immobility	71%
Pain	66%
Loss of appetite	61%
Unpleasant taste	55%
Nausea and vomiting	55%
Breathlessness	54%
Lack of bladder control	50%

Other distressing symptoms include constipation, sore mouth, oedema, confusion and pressure sores[7].

Weakness and fatigue

Extreme weakness and fatigue is the most common symptom in terminal illness[8]. People with end stage Parkinson's disease become extremely tired, frozen and weak as the disease progresses and medication become less and less effective. Those with end stage cardiac disease experience reduced blood flow, cardiac hypertrophy and increasing oedema, often affecting the internal organs. Those with end stage renal disease suffer from uraemia, anaemia, oedema, reduced blood flow and drowsiness. The effects of infection to skin and urinary or respiratory tracts can compound electrolyte imbalances caused by end-stage disease processes. It is rarely possible to treat the causes of extreme fatigue and the nurse's role is to enable the person to rest and to arrange visits, outings or activities that the person desires at times when energy levels are highest.

Immobility

Older people who feel utterly exhausted quickly lose the ability to move around. Immobility puts a person at risk of developing urinary incontinence, constipation, deep vein thrombosis, pressure sores and a host of other complications. Encouraging the individual to retain some mobility for as long as possible contributes to the person's physical and emotional well-being. Some nursing solutions include:

- Supplying wheeled Zimmer frames which require less effort than conventional frames
- Gutter frames
- Supplying a self-propelled wheelchair
- Supplying an electric wheelchair
- Teaching the person to transfer from chair to toilet and chair to bed
- Helping the person to transfer
- Supplying aids such as raised toilet seats, EZE rise chairs, monkey poles, grab rails and one cot side – which the person can use for turning or pulling herself up in bed
- Ensuring that our practice enables rather than disables the dying person.

Pain

Pain is all embracing and pain control is one of the most important aspects of palliative care. This will be dealt with later in the chapter.

Loss of appetite, unpleasant taste, nausea and vomiting

These symptoms are all related. A number of factors can cause anorexia. These factors can be divided into two categories: those affecting the person directly and other influencing factors.

Factors affecting the person directly include:

- Advanced renal disease – this leads to uraemia
- Advanced cardiac disease – this can lead to oedema around the internal organs
- Advanced cancer – this can lead to hypercalcaemia and changes to amino acid levels and causes changes in taste
- Delayed digestion
- Electrolyte imbalance
- Psychological stress and emotional state.

Other influencing factors are:

- Pain
- Fatigue
- Sore mouth
- Swallowing difficulties
- Requiring help to eat
- Taste changes

Taste changes

Many people who are dying suffer from 'blind mouth' – a loss of taste or altered taste caused by biochemical changes such as hypercalcaemia, uraemia and changed amino acid levels. Nursing measures that can enable people to enjoy their food include:

- Adding extra sugar to drinks and foods
- Adding extra spices – but avoid adding extra salt if oedema is a problem
- If meat tastes 'off' then offer fish, cheese, vegetable proteins, beans, pulses, soya, tahini, and Quorn.
- If tea and coffee taste 'like metal' avoid them and offer fizzy drinks (many people suffering from altered taste and nausea enjoy Coca Cola and find it reduces nausea)
- Fruit juices refresh the mouth and stimulate production of saliva (avoid acidic juices such as orange and grapefruit if the person has an ulcerated mouth as acid juices sting)
- Herbal teas can be offered instead of tea and coffee
- Offer a glass of sherry before meals, or gin with Angostura Bitters; both stimulate the flow of saliva and gastric juices
- Offer a beer or glass of stout with the meal – these are rich in calories, high in B vitamins and a useful way of encouraging fluid intake.

Causes of nausea and vomiting

It is important to identify the cause of nausea and vomiting, as it is only possible to give effective treatment if the cause has been identified. The most common causes of nausea and vomiting are discussed here.

Drugs/uraemia and hypercalcaemia

A simple blood test will identify uraemia and hypercalcaemia. Nurses can usually identify drug induced nausea and vomiting fairly easily. If possible ask for any medication that is inducing nausea and vomiting to be reviewed. This type of nausea responds well to phenothiazines and a small dose of chlorpromazine or one of the other phenothiazines often controls nausea effectively. Phenothiazines can be given in suppository form if vomiting prevents oral administration.

Squashed stomach syndrome

Problems with the abdominal viscera, external pressure (perhaps from gastric tumours, liver metastases), chronic cardiac failure with oedema of the internal organs, and sub-acute bowel obstruction (perhaps because of bowel cancer) all cause patients to complain that they feel as if their stomach is being squashed. These problems respond well to metoclopramide because it increases the rate of gastric emptying, enabling the person to eat more with less discomfort and little risk of nausea and vomiting. It can be given orally; the usual dose is 10 mg six-hourly but it can be increased to 20 mg every six hours. It can also be given by subcutaneous injection if the person is too ill to swallow. Domperidone suppositories (10 mg) can be given four to six-hourly.

Nausea and vomiting on movement

The person complains of nausea or vomits when she sits up or moves her head. This nausea is caused by problems affecting the vestibular centre and responds well to antihistamines. Drugs normally used include Cyclizine – the recommended dose is 50 mg three times daily, but half the recommended dose, i.e. 25 mg eight-hourly, is often sufficient to control nausea in frail older people who are dying, and reduces side effects of dry mouth and blurred vision. Promethazine is also used – this is more sedating than cyclizine; again, the recommended dose is 25 mg eight-hourly but half the recommended dose is often effective. In some cases 12.5 mg twelve-hourly is sufficient to control nausea in the very frail. Antihistamines potentiate the effect of alcohol.

Nausea and vomiting brought on by the sight or smell of food

This is usually the result of anxiety and responds well to a small dose of haloperidol, which is available in tablet and liquid form. Initially, 500 mcg twelve hourly is given; this may be increased to eight hourly if nausea and vomiting is not controlled. The books suggest larger doses but frail older people are very sensitive to haloperidol. Haloperidol can build up in frail older people and it may be possible to reduce the dose when nausea and vomiting are under control. This prevents drowsiness and unwanted side effects but controls nausea.

Complementary therapies to treat nausea and vomiting

Aromatherapy

Aromatherapy is: 'a form of treatment using essential oils extracted from plants for therapeutic effect'. The first recorded use of aromatherapy was 4500 BC by Kiwant Ti, a Chinese emperor[9]. Aromatherapy has been used by people all over the world for thousands of years; it has been used by

Australian Aboriginals, people of the Indus valley, Jews, Greeks and Romans, and was widely used in England and France in the middle ages[10]. Interest in the twentieth century followed the publication of a book by a French chemist R.M. Gattefosse in 1931 and research by Dr Jean Valet that commenced in the 1960s[11].

Oils from flowers and plants are distilled to produce essential oils. These oils can be administered in a number of ways:

- *Massage* – the essential oil is diluted in a carrier oil such as almond oil and massaged into the skin. *Essential oils must never be applied undiluted on to the skin.*
- *Inhalation* – the oil is used in a burner, a ring attached to a light bulb, a container attached to a radiator, or on a tissue, linen, pillow case, secondary dressing, or bandage.
- *In a bath* – a few drops of essential oil (usually 3–6 drops) are added to bath water.

Although limited research has demonstrated that aromatherapy is effective, researchers have not yet discovered what causes the effect, how it works or why it works. The olfactory nerve fibres are directly connected to the limbic system of the brain and although we know very little about the limbic system we do know that it controls emotions. Emotions such as anxiety and insomnia affect quality of life. Aromatherapy oils that may help the patient with nausea and vomiting include neroli (Citrus aurantim)[12] and bergamot, which helps relieve nervousness, anxiety and depression.

Aromatherapy, like other therapies, can be potentially dangerous in unskilled hands. It is important that nurses are trained before practising aromatherapy. Any treatment should be documented with the aims and objectives of treatment in nursing records. In some nursing homes a consent form has been introduced so that the patient gives written consent to treatment.

Finally, remember that smells bring back memories – some of them good and some of them unpleasant. Ask the patient if they like the scent of the oil before using it.

Acupuncture

Acupuncture has been proven to be effective in controlling nausea resistant to drug therapy[13]. Chemists sell bands that are worn on the wrists and have small studs which stimulate acupuncture pressure points and can effectively control nausea and vomiting brought on by movement.

Insomnia

The reasons for insomnia include pain, nausea, anxiety, noise, temperature and light.

Adopting a problem solving approach will enable you to find solutions for the individual's insomnia. Ensuring that pain and nausea are controlled is essential. Hypnotics can cause daytime drowsiness and contribute to general fatigue. Measures to decrease anxiety, and complementary therapy, can aid sleep. Lavender oil has been proven to help elderly people sleep[14,15].

Camomile has anti-inflammatory properties and calms and aids sleep. Bergamot is useful for nervousness, anxiety and depression. Graham Canard used a commercial blend of basil, lavender, juniper and sweet marjoram to help patients sleep. He put one drop on each of the top corners of the sheets – this avoided contact with the eyes. If the person was still awake 1–2 hours later a hand massage was given. If the person was still awake at midnight and was distressed by this, night sedation was given. This reduced night sedation from 90% to 36%[16].

Sore mouth

Ensuring that mouth care is maintained is an important indicator of the quality of nursing care. We use our mouths to taste, feel and kiss. Older people who are dying can easily develop sore, infected, dry mouths, foul breath, coated tongues and cracked dry lips.

Candida infection can develop in frail older people. Steroid and antibiotic therapy increases the risk of candida. This can be treated either by oral nystatin (1 ml four times a day) or by offering live natural yoghurt.
Sore gums can be caused by ill-fitting dentures. A temporary soft liner can be inserted into dentures to improve fit and enable the person to wear dentures. Bonjela and other analgesic pastes can relieve discomfort.
Mouth ulcers can be caused by broken dentures or natural teeth; conservative dental treatment can rectify these problems. Tablets retained in the mouth can also cause mouth ulceration; ensuring that tablets are washed down with water or giving medication in liquid form can prevent this. Some mouthwashes, e.g. benzydamine, contain analgesic agents and can be used to relieve pain.
Dry mouths can be caused by drugs such as phenothiazines, antispasmodics, antihistamines, anticholinergics, and antidepressants, and by poor fluid intake. Frequent mouthcare stimulates the flow of saliva – clean the patient's mouth before meals as well as after. Use fruit juices, ice chips and give small amounts of fluids frequently. Glycerine is no longer recommended in mouth care because it causes the mucosa to dry out. Use synthetic saliva to maintain moisture in the mouth.

Mouth cleaning
Research indicates that the most effective way of removing plaque and dealing with furred tongues is to use a toothbrush and toothpaste. Soft, small-headed toothbrushes designed to clean babies' and toddler's teeth are easy to use and less traumatic than large, hard, adult toothbrushes[17]. If this cannot be tolerated, swabbing gauze wrapped around the finger and dipped in clean water is effective.

Antibacterial mouthwashes normally contain antiseptics such as chlorhexideine. These disturb the natural balance of the mouth and alter pH; they can predispose patients to candida infection.

Helping people who are unable to clean their dentures is essential if mouthcare problems are to be avoided. Research on the dental hygiene of older people in hospital found evidence of inadequate cleaning of dentures.

Swabs taken from dentures showed heavy contamination; 53% grew yeasts, 27% *Staphylococcus aureus* and 21% coliforms[18]. Researchers recommend that dentures are brushed twice daily and soaked in denture cleaning fluid overnight to remove bacteria and yeasts[19].

Respiratory problems

Causes of respiratory problems include accumulation of secretions in final hours of life (death rattle), infection, pulmonary oedema, chronic obstructive airways disease and malignant tumour. The aims of care are to administer medication to alleviate symptoms and to provide nursing care to increase comfort.

Cough is treated with expectorants if productive. These act by loosening sputum and decreasing sputum viscosity. Ensuring that fluid intake is as high as possible and offering inhalations to loosen sputum help improve patient comfort. Using backrests and pillows to support the person in an upright position aids breathing. In the end stage when the person is too weak to clear secretions, local anaesthetics and anticholinergics can be used; antibiotics are rarely appropriate and do not relieve suffering. Anticholinergics reduce the volume of secretions. Hyoscine hydrobromide can be given subcutaneously or via a patch. It can be combined with diamorphine in a syringe driver. Some older people become very agitated and confused if given hyoscine. If this occurs then glycopyrronium 0.2 mg can be given four hourly; this is less likely to cause confusion.

Dry cough is treated with cough suppressants, and morphine is often used as an analgesic because it suppresses cough and reduces dyspnoea. Bupivacaine (a local anaesthetic) 2.5 ml given in a nebuliser suppresses distressing coughs when the patient is too weak to clear secretions. Using suction is very rarely appropriate and can cause great distress to the older person, family and nursing staff. Salbutamol nebulisers can ease breathing and diazepam can be used to reduce anxiety.

Pulmonary oedema and oedema of the internal organs and abdominal viscera are treated with diuretics. In the final days of life when the person is taking little fluid these are usually discontinued as they are no longer necessary.

Sometimes nurses feel that there is little they can do to make sure distressing symptoms are treated. Hopefully this section has given you some information that will enable you to enhance care. Alleviating distressing symptoms such as immobility, pain, loss of appetite, taste changes, vomiting and breathlessness enables older people who are dying to experience the best possible quality of life.

Pain management

Recently a colleague asked older people in the nursing home where she works if they suffered from pain. Three-quarters of the individuals replied that they were frequently in pain but only 20% of these individuals told nursing staff about their pain. Most individuals who did not report pain felt that little could be done to help and there was no point in bothering the nurses.

Pain can affect *every* aspect of an individual's life. Individuals suffering from unrelieved pain may not wish to eat, move around or talk to others, and can become extremely depressed. Controlling pain can enhance an older person's quality of life and enable them to enjoy life once again. Nurses cannot always rely on older people to report pain and they should observe individuals for signs of pain. Nurses should always ask if they suspect patients are in pain. The nurse is in a unique position to monitor the effectiveness of prescribed analgesia and should inform the individual's doctor if analgesia is ineffective.

Around 10% of adults suffer from pain lasting longer than three months[20,21]. Chronic pain affects a greater percentage of women than men. Chronic pain limits mobility and many older people with chronic pain have difficulty walking, getting out of chairs unaided, dressing and bathing[22]. Older people with chronic pain are more likely to require care in homes. Pain can be overwhelming and can dominate every aspect of a person's being. Pain can lead to isolation, depression and feelings of despair[23]. Good pain management can break the cycle of depression, disability and despair. The nurse's role in breaking this cycle is crucial. It involves assessment of pain and working with the multidisciplinary team to determine appropriate pharmacological and non-pharmacological treatments.

Pain assessment

The aim of assessment is to identify the cause of pain, type of pain and its clinical characteristics, and then to develop management strategies. There are three main types of pain:

- *Somatic* – this is localised to an area on the body surface such as a wound or pressure sore. It is mediated via the somatic nerves.
- *Visceral* – this is a diffuse poorly localised pain such as colic or angina.
- *Neuropathic or neurogenic pain* – this is caused by a number of conditions such as disc compression, diabetic nerve damage or bone infiltration by tumours.

It is important to identify the clinical characteristics of the pain. Generally there are four different types of pain:

- *Inflammatory* – described as aching, throbbing, and painful to touch. Acute rheumatoid arthritis and infections such as cellulitis are typical examples.
- *Neuralgic* – described as burning, shooting, pins and needles, stinging. Sciatica and neuralgia are typical examples.
- *Nociceptive* – described as a dull sickening ache. Angina and organ tumour are typical examples
- *Colic* – described as gripping, coming and going in waves. Renal colic, constipation and bowel obstruction are typical examples.

It is important to document your assessment and any treatment prescribed. In many homes a pain assessment tool is used. Box 14.1 provides an example.

Principles of pain management

The most important principle of pain management is to treat the underlying cause whenever possible. The case history below illustrates how staff

Box 14.1   Sample pain assessment tool.

Site	Where is the pain?
Radiation	Does it go anywhere?
Duration	How did it start? How long have you had it?
Intensity	Is it mild, moderate, severe?
Type	What type of pain is it? Is it there all the time?
Modification	What makes it better or worse?
Relationships	Is it affected by exercise, movement, diet, defecation, urination?
Past history	Have you had it before?
Response to treatment	Have you had any tests for it? What did these show? Have you had any treatment? What was it? How did it work?
Observation	Facial expression, respiration, agitation, restlessness, pallor, sweating
Examination of site	Rash, signs of inflammation, tissue damage, swelling, muscle wasting
Rating scale	If zero was no pain and ten the worst pain you have ever experienced, what number is your pain now?

balanced long-term goals of removing the cause of pain and short-term goals of treating the pain.

Case history

Mrs Dorothy Latham had been admitted to hospital with extensive ulceration to her legs. Her ulcers had been treated with bed rest and paraffin tulle dressings. On admission to the nursing home, assessment reveals that she has extensive oedema to both legs. They ache and throb constantly, making it difficult for her to sleep. Mrs Latham is tearful and upset.

Doppler ultrasound investigations reveal that it is safe to use compression therapy. Compression therapy reduces leg oedema and the heavy, throbbing, dragging pain that accompanies oedema. The leg ulcers are treated with appropriate dressings that are changed twice weekly. The dressings chosen reduce the frequency of dressing changes and trauma on change.

Pain is treated with an appropriate analgesia and Mrs Latham is helped to regain mobility. Walking further reduces swelling and improves circulation reducing pain and helping the healing process.

It is important to treat the pain and then to assess how effective the treatment is. There are two main treatment options – pharmacological treatment and non-pharmacological treatment. Both pharmacological and non-pharmacological treatments can be used together.

Pharmacological treatments

Medication prescribed will depend on the intensity of pain and the type of pain. It is important to give the right type of analgesia to deal with a particular type of pain. Table 14.1 outlines commonly used analgesia.

Non-pharmacological treatments

It is important to treat the person with pain and not simply supply analgesia. Mind and body are linked and there is evidence that people who are

Table 14.1 Commonly used analgesics.

Drug	Use	Comment
Aspirin	Mild to moderate pain and inflammation	Doses of 75–360 mg daily have been shown to reduce risk of death from strokes and heart attacks by 25%[24]. Regular use of aspirin halves the risks of colon cancer[25] and delays the onset of Alzheimer's disease[26]. May cause gastric irritation and acid base changes in therapeutic doses
Paracetamol	Mild to moderate pain and inflammation	Heavy drinkers vulnerable to liver damage when taking therapeutic doses[27]
Non-steroidal anti-inflammatory drugs (NSAIDs)	Pain with an inflammatory component, e.g. active arthritis	Ineffective in treating visceral pain. Side effects of gastric irritation and bleeding are thought to be responsible for up to 2500 deaths a year[28]
Antidepressants/anticonvulsants	Pain with a neurogenic component, e.g. trigeminal neuralgia or sciatica	Antidepressants such as amitriptilline are often used as an adjunct to analgesia as they appear to affect the perception of pain
Opiods	Severe pain such as ischaemic pain and cancer pain	Cause nausea, constipation, respiratory depression; tolerance occurs

depressed experience higher levels of pain than those who are not[29,30]. High levels of pain and fear of injury lead to a cycle of immobility and physical decline[31]. Non-pharmacological treatments include efforts to treat the pain and the underlying causes and also efforts to reverse the physical and psychological decline that the person has experienced. Table 14.2 outlines non-pharmacological treatment.

Specialist pain control services
If an individual's pain cannot be controlled, specialist help should be sought. Many hospitals run pain control clinics. Individuals can visit the clinic if they are able, or a member of the community or hospital pain control team can visit the home. Pain control teams use a range of surgical and medical treatments in addition to drugs, and can normally ensure that individuals remain free of pain.

Specialist palliative care nurses normally work alongside medical staff and provide help, advice and support to individuals suffering from pain and nursing staff caring for them. In some areas palliative care nurses who work

Table 14.2 Non-pharmacological treatment.

Treatment	Benefits	Comments
Physiotherapy	Treatment and rehabilitation in muscular-skeletal conditions	Improves strength, stability and morale
Occupational therapy	Ensuring provision of aids and adaptations that improves the person's ability to function independently	Improves ability and reduces dependency
Transcutaneous nerve stimulation (TENS)	Interrupt the pathways conveying the sensation of pain by using a small electric current through the skin	No known side effects. Puts patient in control of pain
Acupuncture	Small needles placed in specific sites realign energy fields or 'chi' within the body and eliminate pain	Some patients complain that they feel dizzy or faint, but often effective with severe pain
Aromatherapy	Essential oils burned or diluted with carrier oils and massaged into the skin, thought to affect the limbic centre and reduce/eliminate sensation of pain	Effective in treating pain and depression in many patients
Activities and interests	This can be anything from taking up a hobby to making new friends	Can help as part of the process of the person taking control of his or her own life

at the pain clinic work in both hospital and community settings. In other areas there are two teams, one for the hospital and another for the community. The local hospital and trust will be able to provide details of pain clinics and specialist palliative care nurses.

Useful addresses and telephone numbers

Pain clinic

Dealing with death and dying

At the beginning of the twentieth century most people died at home. Infant mortality rates were higher then; people died from infectious diseases, complications of childbirth; diseases such as diabetes that are now treatable, and war, claimed the lives of young men. Death or the threat of death was ever present. Rituals existed to enable people to come to terms with death and to grieve. Society recognised that the bereaved person required a period of adjustment before getting on with life.

In the early twenty-first century all this has changed. Most people die away from their family and friends. People now die in hospitals, hospices and nursing homes. Medical advances, improved living conditions and the absence of major wars have all combined to make early death less likely. Death has become remote and is hidden in our society. Rituals developed to help people cope have disappeared. Now people are expected to have a day or two off to bury their parent and then return to work as though nothing had happened. Families are no longer as united as they once were and so support from within the family is reduced. The extended family is now rare; many marriages now end in divorce and the number of children born outside marriage increases every year.

Death and the process of dying now occur mostly in the very old. Most adults have never seen a dead body until their parents die. Then the parent is often in their late eighties or nineties and the bereaved person is often elderly. The process of dying has become increasingly professionalised. As nurses we are the professionals who have the most contact with the dying and their families. We are expected to provide intimate physical care and to care psychologically for the patient, the patient's family and our junior colleagues. The general expectation is that we cope with all these roles while remaining untouched by it all. Yet we live in this same society where death is such a taboo. Remember when you first saw a dead person? How could you ever forget? Your first introduction to death was probably as a junior student nurse. Nursing the dead and dying takes an emotional toll on all nurses.

This section aims to:

- Enable you to understand the process of dying
- Enable you to understand how relatives grieve
- Help you to support staff
- Enable you to cope with the emotional impact of caring for people who are dying
- Enable you to understand the formalities of dealing with a death
- Explain when cases must be referred to a coroner

First we look at the ways in which we as nurses can try to meet the needs of patients, families and our colleagues while maintaining our humanity and being gentle on ourselves.

Dying trajectories

Each dying person is following a dying trajectory[32]. This trajectory can be graphed: for some people it plunges quickly and inexorably downwards; for others it changes slowly moving slightly down then up, and then hits a plateau before finally plunging towards death. The person lingers. Nurses find that caring for the person who lingers is more stressful.

Critical junctures

In dying trajectories there are a series of clinical junctures:

(1) The patient is defined as dying
(2) Staff and family make preparations for death. The patient (if aware) makes preparations for death
(3) The patient reaches the point where 'nothing more can be done'
(4) The process of dying takes hours, days, weeks or months
(5) The last hours of life
(6) The death watch
(7) Death.

During this process staff must provide physical and psychological support.

Stages of dying

Elizabeth Kubler Ross was one of the first people to identify stages which dying people go through. The stages she identified were[33]:

● Denial and isolation
● Anger
● Depression
● Bargaining
● Acceptance

Different researchers all identify different stages[34]. All agree that individual reactions to dying vary. Not everyone reaches acceptance – some die in denial, angry, depressed or hopeful. An understanding of the stages of dying enables nurses to understand what each individual is going through. We can then help dying people to work through these stages. Hopefully our increased understanding will enable us to help people work through emotions such as anger without feeling that the anger is our fault.

Spiritual needs

Spirituality is an important aspect of many people's lives. Other people find it less important but may welcome the opportunity to talk about their fears and hopes with a minister of religion. It is important to recognise the spiritual dimension of care and enable the older person to meet those needs.

Supporting families

Research carried out in 1985 showed that a quarter of relatives involved in caring for dying people were themselves over 70 years of age[35]. Older people admitted to nursing homes have normally been supported and cared for by family and friends until a crisis occurs. Usually the older person is admitted to hospital for a short period of treatment and then admitted for nursing home care. Once the older person is admitted we 'take over' care and do everything in our power to meet the individual's physical and psychological needs. Often we meet relatives who 'camp out' in the home – arrive at dawn and depart at dusk – and we wish they would go home and leave us to it. Often we make special efforts to meet patient needs yet relatives appear critical and carping. We feel that relatives' expectations become higher every year. Let's look at it from the relatives' point of view.

Stages of grieving

Relatives often go through stages of grieving – before the person dies. Research has identified these stages as[36]:

- Shock
- Anger
- Disorganisation
- Volatile emotions
- Loss
- Loneliness
- Relief
- Re-establishment

Family guilt

Many families feel guilty about being unable to cope – often the older person blames the family for admission to the nursing home. As nurses we encourage families to hand over care to us and we effectively shut them out. Without thinking, we ask a daughter who has cared for her mother for years to leave the room while we deliver intimate care. Then we wonder why that daughter becomes either disinterested, tailing off visits, or hostile and critical of nursing care.

Involving families in care

Nurses can find ways to include families in decisions about treatment and care. Nurses can enable families to continue to give physical care (if they wish) and help families to remain involved. This can help families to feel more comfortable about the decision to admit the older person and to come to terms with the individual's impending death[37].

Supporting staff

Although most of us were taught 'to keep our distance' and warned 'not to get too involved' we do get involved in nursing homes.

'That's the difference in long term care. You get to know them as well as your children. You can tell something is wrong just by the look on their face or the way they are walking. We perform the most intimate acts over time.'

(Nursing Home manager)

Staff do get close to people. A research study examining the quality of care in nursing homes found that when staff were close to residents and treated them 'like family', the quality of care was better[38]. Caring for people who are dying, meeting their physical and emotional needs, and supporting them and their families is demanding. Nurses are not bottomless wells; they too need support and help in caring for dying people. In order to function effectively we need to:

- Take measures to minimise the stress and strain
- Recognise it when it occurs
- Offer help and support.

Ensuring adequate levels of staff are available to meet patient needs is vital. This can only be accomplished if we develop measures to demonstrate our workload to our managers. Ensure that staff training is given priority. Well-educated staff will have the skills to ensure symptoms are controlled and complications prevented[39]. Nurses who provide care of the highest quality feel less stressed. They can console themselves with the knowledge that the person died peacefully and without pain and that the death was 'good'.

It is important to give staff 'permission' to express their feelings about caring for dying people. Be open about your feelings. Be gentle with yourself and your staff. Share your feelings and encourage your staff to share theirs. This can be done formally through team meetings, informally at handover and on a one-to-one basis. Often junior staff do not understand why the person has died or do not understand about some aspects of treatment. If you are open about the stress that caring for dying people places on staff they are more likely to come to you and give you the opportunity to discuss things. Admit that you do not know all the answers. Recognise that some times there are no answers. Learn as much as possible about the physical and psychological aspects of dying.

Useful address

Specialist palliative care nurse

Treatment decisions

Listening to the resident

In your home you have people at differing stages of the dying trajectory. What are you going to do if a crisis occurs? If Mr Jones, with end stage dementia, develops a chest infection – will this be treated or not? What would Mr Jones have wanted? What do his relatives expect? Does the nurse in charge ring the GP? Is the GP 'expected' to prescribe antibiotics? Is the

GP expected to send Mr Jones to hospital for IV antibiotics? In the US, information on such issues is commonly recorded on nursing documentation[40]. If information about treatment decisions is recorded this will reduce staff uncertainty and reduce stress and strain.

Many older people living in nursing homes come to regard the home as 'home' and fellow residents and nursing staff as friends. Many individuals wish to die in familiar surroundings and among friends. Nurses should make every effort to ensure that the wishes of older people who wish to end their days in the nursing home are respected.

Case history

Charles Scott lived in a nursing home. One morning the nurse who was bathing him noticed that his feet were rapidly turning navy blue. Both Charles' legs were navy blue up to the knees by the time the ambulance arrived a few minutes later to take him to the local hospital. Surgeons at the hospital diagnosed a saddle embolus which was completely blocking the arteries supplying Charles' legs. The surgeons felt that Charles would not survive any attempt to remove the large embolus. Intravenous morphine administered via a syringe driver controlled pain. Charles told his primary nurse and his family that although he realised he was dying, he had no wish to die in a busy hospital ward surrounded by strangers. He asked to return home to die. The nurse specialist responsible for pain control accompanied Charles back to the nursing home and showed nursing staff how to operate the syringe driver and deal with any problems. Staff were given a number so that the nurse specialist could be contacted if problems arose. The pain control specialist visited the night staff and checked that Charles remained free of pain. Charles died three days later, in the place he had come to regard as home, surrounded by family and friends. His death was peaceful, dignified and in accordance with his wishes.

Case history

Rosie Beckford was no nurse's idea of a typical old lady. She lived life to the full in a nursing home despite appalling deformities caused by osteo and rheumatoid arthritis. Rosie normally had her hair dyed bright orange but occasionally had it dyed pink, blue or mauve to match her latest outfit. Rosie always wore far too much make-up and was a noisy and exuberant person. One winter she became quieter and quieter and took to her bed. She appeared to be in great pain although she never complained. Analgesia did not appear to be effective and Rosie winced and flinched when turned. The pain control specialists visited; potent analgesia was prescribed; relatives, fellow patients and staff prepared themselves for Rosie's death. Rosie, though, free at last from the excruciating pain that had drained her reserves, rose from her bed like a phoenix from the ashes and enjoyed a further two years of life before dying.

Supporting the family of a dying resident

No one is ever really prepared for the death of their father, mother or close relative. Death and bereavement are things that happen to other people. The family of a person who is dying can experience a whole range of emotions:

Denial – 'Dad will be all right, he's rallied before'
Mitigation – 'well, he is 84'
Anger – 'why mum, she's really enjoying life?'

Blame – 'if my sister hadn't taken mum out in the cold . . .'
Guilt – 'I should never have gone away on holiday'.

You need to be aware of these emotions and should understand the devastating effect that the death of a loved one can have. You should offer to spend time with the family if they wish to talk about their feelings. The family should feel free to visit at any time and to stay for as long as they wish. Some families take turns to sit with an individual so that the individual always has a family member present during the final days of an illness. Providing tea, coffee, snacks and meals is a way of showing concern. Families may wish to contact one of the organisations listed at the end of this chapter, which offer support and advice after the older person has died.

Spiritual needs

Spirituality is an important part of many people's lives. The home should make arrangements to enable older people to have their spiritual needs fulfilled. Many homes arrange for ministers of religion to visit the home on a regular basis, usually weekly, to see individuals.

One survey carried out by a nurse working in a nursing home discovered that although older people appreciated ministers visiting the home, they would prefer to visit the church, synagogue or mosque if at all possible. Older people enjoy going to church, mixing with other members of the congregation and taking part in church activities. It is often possible to arrange for them to attend church services. Many churches have some form of transport; some even have mini-buses with ramps or tail-gate lifts. In other cases church members have cars and will arrange to pick up an individual or a group of individuals and take them to church.

It is essential to check that either the home, church or individual has insurance that covers such journeys. Older people who attend services not only benefit from going out and worshipping with others but they are often able to participate in other church activities. Invitations to activities such as coffee mornings, church bazaars, plays and other activities can enrich an older person's life. Church members often become friends and in the case of older people who have no family they can visit and act as an advocate for the individual. Church members often continue to visit the home when the older person becomes too unwell to continue to visit the church.

Case history

Miss Lucy Tucker was a lifelong church member. She had been a music teacher, played the organ and taught the junior choir for 53 years. She became frail, weak and bed bound in her final days and told her primary nurse that her greatest regret as she approached death was that she would never again hear the junior choir sing Christmas carols. On 23 December, the day before Miss Tucker died, the junior choir slipped into her room to sing for her, as many of their parents and grandparents had. Her primary nurse said that the look on Miss Tucker's face as the choir began to sing was the highlight of her nursing career.

Older people who live in nursing homes come from a variety of backgrounds and may be of the Jewish, Muslim, Hindu or other faith. It is important that the home can help people of all faiths to continue to practise their faith within the home and to attend their usual place of worship when possible. Ministers and members of the Jewish, Moslem, Hindi, Zoroastrian and other faiths are willing to offer assistance in enabling an older person to continue to take their place in the social and religious aspects of faith. The Jewish Passover celebrations are as important to members of the Jewish faith as Christmas is to Christians. Eid, the festival which celebrates the end of Ramadan, is equally important to Muslims. Diwali, the Hindu festival of light, is of prime importance to Hindus. Many families will wish to celebrate these occasions with the older person, and the nurse should offer to help, perhaps by helping the individual to get ready to go out with the family for a special meal or religious service, or preparing the older person so that family and friends can visit to celebrate this special day within the home.

Useful address and telephone number

Local ministers of religion

The role of the GP in certifying death

Older people living in nursing homes are normally cared for by their own GP. In practice many older people will be cared for by either a single-handed GP or one from a group practice. When a death occurs the doctor normally visits and pronounces death. If the GP is able to issue a death certificate, permission is given to remove the body to a local chapel of rest. The GP may issue the death certificate immediately or, if busy, may return later to do this. In recent years homes have sometimes found GPs reluctant to come out to pronounce death. There is no legal requirement for a doctor to pronounce death. A nurse or indeed anyone could pronounce death. When death is pronounced the person may be sent to the chapel of rest. In some cases local undertakers are happy with this arrangement; in other cases they will not remove a body until a doctor has pronounced death. A person's body may not be buried or cremated unless a death certificate has been issued.

A doctor may only issue a death certificate in certain circumstances. The doctor must have seen the individual within the last two weeks, must be satisfied about the cause of death, and the individual must not have had surgery within the last 12 months. If a locum doctor is on duty, perhaps because the doctor is having an evening off, and the GP should be able to issue a death certificate on return to duty, then permission is given to remove the body to a chapel of rest. If the GP is off duty and a partner from the GP practice is on call, permission is normally given to remove the body. The death certificate will be issued by the normal GP on return to duty.

If a GP is going away for more than a few days, both the GP and the doctor who will be caring for the patients during the GP's absences should visit the home, see the residents and have a handover session. This not only ensures continuity of care but also prevents the locum being forced to refer deaths to the coroner. It avoids the risk of unnecessary post mortem examinations that can cause great distress to the older person's family.

Referring deaths to the coroner

Doctors must consult the coroner in a number of circumstances:

- If the doctor has not seen the individual in the last two weeks
- If the individual has had an operation in the last 12 months
- If the doctor does not know the cause of death
- If the death is sudden, possibly the result of an accident
- If there are any suspicious circumstances.

The coroner or the coroner's officer (normally a serving police officer who has been seconded to the coroner's office for a period of time) usually discusses the circumstances of death with the GP on the telephone. The coroner normally decides if a post mortem will be required.

Post mortem examinations

The decision to carry out a post mortem examination to determine the cause of death rests with the coroner, not the individual's doctor. The coroner will take into account the circumstances of death, the doctor's opinion and the wishes of the family wherever possible. In a case where the GP has not seen the individual for more than two weeks but the individual has a long-standing illness (such as terminal cancer or a heart condition) which the GP feels has caused death, the coroner may decide that a post mortem is not required. In a case where the individual has had surgery in the last 12 months but the GP is satisfied that the operation did not directly lead to death, the coroner may decide that a post mortem is not required. In a case where an older person has suddenly died and the GP is not able to ascertain the cause of death, a post mortem is required. Coroners will take into account any religious views of the deceased and his or her family. In a case where death has followed an accident or there are suspicious circumstance a post mortem is required.

Removal of the body

If a person dies following an accident or in suspicious circumstances, the body is not normally touched until the coroner has given permission. The coroner and/or the coroner's officer may wish to visit the home to see the body, perhaps take photographs or talk to nursing staff. The coroner normally only visits if the death may have occurred as a result of an accident or in suspicious circumstances.

When a post mortem examination is required the body is washed and dressed in a nightgown or pyjamas. Catheters, colostomy bags, dressings, etc. are left untouched and the orifices are not normally packed. The nurse should consult the local coroner and check procedure in the local area. This procedure may change when one corcner leaves and another takes up post.

The body is removed by undertakers nominated by the coroner, at the coroner's expense, to the coroner's office to await post mortem. Post mortem is normally carried out within two or three working days of death. The home and family are normally notified of the result by telephone. In most cases a death certificate is issued by the coroner, the body is transferred to the firm of undertakers dealing with the arrangements, and the family can arrange burial or cremation.

Coroner's informal enquiries and inquests

In some cases the coroner may wish to ask the nursing staff a few questions relating to the circumstances of an individual's death. Many nurses become very worried and upset by the thought of being questioned informally by a coroner. The coroner is merely trying to find out about the circumstances relating to the death and is not blaming the nurse in any way. Nurses, though, often prefer to have a member of their professional organisation or a friend present in such circumstances and this is perfectly reasonable.

Case history

Mr George Blackstone had lived in a nursing home for some years. After lunch each day he walked back to his room accompanied by a nurse. One day Mr Blackstone fell backwards, struck his head on a radiator and was dead when the nurse bent down. The coroner visited the home and photographs were taken before Mr Blackstone could be moved. The coroner spoke to the nurse, Paul Henry (in the presence of Mr Henry's professional representative) asking if Mr Blackstone had complained of being unwell before falling or if the nurse had noticed any difference in Mr Blackstone's condition that day. A post mortem revealed that Mr Blackstone had suffered a massive heart attack and had been dead before he struck his head on the radiator.

Inquests are normally to establish the circumstances, actions or inactions which led to an older person's death. Inquests take place in the coroner's court. Nurses asked to attend an inquest should consult their professional body for further advice and support.

Last offices

The home should have a policy for last offices, which respects the individual's faith. People of the Muslim faith are not normally touched by non-Muslims after death and last offices are carried out by a person from the local mosque. For other individuals the eyes should be closed, dentures placed in mouth and a pillow placed under the jaw for support. The body is normally left for an hour before last offices are performed. The supporting pillow is removed from the jaw. Dressings are normally removed and wounds covered with gauze and an opaque occlusive dressing material to prevent leakage. Any catheters, drains or tubes are removed and dressings applied if required to contain leakage. The rectum may require packing with cotton wool if leakage is occurring. The body is normally washed by two members of the nursing staff, then dressed in clean night clothing, the hair is combed, and the bed remade with clean linen. Nursing staff may wish to read a prayer or poem or merely say goodbye at this stage. Members of the family may wish to see the body at this stage and say their last goodbye. The nurse must judge whether it is appropriate to remain with the family or to leave them alone. Undertakers then remove the body to a chapel of rest until burial or cremation is arranged.

Cremations

Usually people wish to be buried or cremated locally, but in some cases an individual indicates a wish to be cremated some distance from the home. When an individual is to be cremated two doctors must examine the body of the deceased and complete a cremation form before cremation can take place. The GP usually carries out an examination, completes the first part of the form and arranges for a colleague to visit the local chapel of rest to carry out an examination and complete the second part of the form. If arrangements have been made to carry out a cremation some distance away from the home, the cremation form must be completed by both doctors before the body can be transported some distance. Arrangements can usually be made either for both doctors to complete their examination and fill in the cremation form before the body is transported, or for the body to remain in a local chapel of rest until these formalities have been completed.

Funerals

Many older people have come to terms with their own mortality and have made arrangements for their own funeral. A widow may wish to be buried in the family plot with her husband or to have her ashes scattered in the garden of remembrance as her husband's were. Another individual may wish to be buried in the family plot. Many older people have nominated undertakers, and made arrangements for and paid for their funerals. Older people who have families normally involve or inform the family of their plans. The nurse should enquire about the individual's wishes sensitively and with great tact. Any funeral arrangements should be recorded in the individual's records so that all staff are aware of them.

Some older people have no relatives and wish to make arrangements for their own funeral. They often ask the nurse for advice about organising and paying for a funeral from their savings. The nurse should ask the older person if they wish to be buried or cremated and can then ask a number of funeral directors to provide quotations for a prepaid funeral. There is an enormous variation in the cost of a funeral from different funeral directors within the same area. If an older person wishes to be buried in a family plot the undertaker's quotation will include the costs of re-opening the grave, placing an additional inscription on the head stone and replacing the headstone. In some cases a family plot has no further space for burial and the older person may wish to have their ashes scattered over the family plot.

If an older person wishes to be buried in a cemetery they must purchase a plot. Cemeteries are either owned by churches or local authorities or are privately owned. Charges for plots vary and cemeteries will provide brochures giving details of these.

Prepaid funerals

Many older people wish to pay for their funerals from their savings. A number of schemes exist which enable an older person or their family to make such arrangements.

The Age Concern Funeral Plan can be contacted at Spencer House, 62a The Parade, Sutton Coldfield, West Midlans B72 1GT. Freephone: 0800 731 0651.

Help the Aged offer their own range of prepaid funeral plans. For details call Freephone 0800 169 1112. Help the Aged also produce a free information sheet explaining what pre-paid funerals are and offering advice on what to look for when thinking of buying one. Contact details are given of other organisations/companies offering this type of plan, including the Co-operative Funeral Bond, Funeral Planning Services, Golden Charter (who are recommended by the Society of Allied and Independent Funeral Directors) and Golden Leaves Ltd. The information sheet gives other useful addresses, such as the National Association for Pre-paid Funeral Plans. It can be read and downloaded from the website: www.helptheaged.org.uk and bulk copies can be ordered using the order form from the website, or contact: Help the Aged, 207–221 Pentonville Road, London N1 9UZ. Tel. 020 7278 1114.

Financial help with funeral costs

Some older people and their families do not have sufficient money to pay for a funeral. In some circumstances the family of an older person may be able to get help from the Department of Social Security's social fund to help with the costs. The person applying for this grant must fulfil certain criteria. The person taking responsibility for the funeral (not the older person who has died) must be in receipt of income support, family credit, disability working allowance, housing benefit or council tax benefit, or be the partner of someone receiving these benefits. Assets of the deceased are taken into account, together with any savings of the person making the arrangements. If the older person has no savings and no family, the home will be unable to claim the costs of a funeral from the DSS social fund. When a person who has no family dies, the home should seek legal advice regarding possessions.

Funeral arrangements for individuals who have no assets and no family

Local authorities have a legal duty under the Public Health (Control of Diseases) Act 1984 (section 46) to arrange the burial or cremation of any person who has died in their area with no assets and no family. A simple burial or cremation is arranged and a minister of religion is present. The local authority normally has an agreement with a local undertaker who organises the funeral. These funerals usually take place early in the morning but the nominated undertaker will normally change the time if nursing staff wish to attend to pay their last respects.

When an individual dies in such circumstances the nurse should contact the local authority who will give details of the nominated undertaker and ask the home to liaise with the undertaker. Often such events occur during holidays or at weekends and it can be difficult to contact the local authority. It is sensible to inform the local authority in advance of any individuals in the home without savings, family or friends, and to obtain and keep details of the nominated undertaker.

It may not always be possible to inform the local authority in advance about individuals without savings as many older people do not wish to discuss their financial affairs with nursing staff. In such circumstances, if it is not possible to inform the local authority, the nurse can contact the nominated undertaker direct. The body can be taken to the chapel of rest and the local authority contacted when their offices are open.

When an individual without savings or family dies in hospital the health authority has a duty (HSG(92)8) to arrange and meet the cost of the funeral.

Useful address and telephone number

Local undertaker nominated by local authority

Legal formalities

When a death certificate has been issued, the death must be registered. This is normally within five days of death. A member of the family usually registers the death. If the individual has no family or close friends, the nurse may have to register the death. The death should be registered in the area where the person has died and not the area where the family live or where the older person lived prior to admission to the nursing home. The death certificate and the individual's medical card are given to the registrar of births, deaths and marriages. The registrar will ask for certain information that will be included in the register of births and deaths: the full name, place and date of birth, occupation, maiden name and husband's occupation (in the case of a married woman).

The Department of Social Security produce a useful leaflet, *What to do after a death* (leaflet no D49). This contains detailed information and advice and you may wish to give a copy to families and friends who are arranging funerals and dealing with the affairs of someone who has died. The leaflet can be obtained free from local benefit offices. Bulk copies can be obtained from: BA Storage and Distribution Centre, Manchester Road, Heywood, Lancashire OL10 2PZ. Remember to quote the reference number and state the number of copies required.

The home must keep a register of deaths. Registration and inspection officers routinely ask how many deaths have occurred since the date of the last annual inspection. Although details of deaths are normally kept in the admission and discharge register, many homes also keep a separate book or computer record that states the individual's name and date of death. Each home must provide registration and inspection officers with details of individuals who have died. Many health authorities produce a standard form and it is the duty of the nurse in charge of the shift to complete this form and post it to the local registration officers. Most health authorities and primary care trusts have introduced new forms to be completed when a self-funding resident dies. The information about the self-funding resident's death goes to the accounts department of the health authority or primary care trust who are paying for the registered nursing element of care.

Discussing a resident's illness and death with other residents

Older people form deep friendships with other residents in the home. When an individual becomes ill other residents often ask how the person is. The nurse should inform the person who is ill (or the family if the individual is unable to speak) that other residents are enquiring about them, and should obtain permission to inform other residents about the individual's condition without breaching confidentiality. Some residents may wish to visit, and if the individual welcomes these visits the nurse should help residents to the room and leave them to speak privately or simply sit with the individual.

When an individual dies it is important that other residents do not see the body leave the home, as this can be distressing. Residents should be informed that the individual has died. Some may wish to attend the funeral. The nurse should work with the family and friends of those who wish to attend the funeral and should make arrangements for residents to pay their last respects.

Conclusion

The nurse's role in supporting older people and their families and ensuring that an older person's last days are without pain, is of vital importance. Sensitive care attuned to the needs of the individual enables older people to experience a dignified death and to have their needs met. The nurse's role in helping older people and their families prepare for and come to terms with death is a demanding one. It is important that death, one of the last great taboos, is acknowledged and that residents who wish to discuss the deceased person's life are not discouraged from doing so. Residents may wish to pay their last respects and the nurse should work with relatives to enable them to do so. Nurses are only human and need to support each other and talk openly about their feelings after the death of an older person they have cared for.

Useful address and telephone number

Local coroner

Further information

Aromatherapy

Aromatherapy Organisations Council, Po Box 19824, London SE25 6WF. Tel. 020 8251 7912.

International Federation of Aromatherapists, 182 Chiswick High Road, Chiswick, London W4 1PP.

International Society of Professional Aromatherapists, ISPA House, 82 Ashly Road, Hinkley, Leicestershire LE10 ISN. Tel. 01455 637987. Fax 01455 890956.

Palliative care services

Macmillan Cancer Relief, 15/19 Britten Street, London SW3 3TZ. Tel. 020 7351 7811.

Marie Curie Cancer Care, 89 Albert Embankment, London SW1 7TP. Tel. 020 7599 7777.

Support

Cruse offers counselling, support and advice after bereavement. Cruse Bereavement Care, Cruse House, 126 Sheen Road, Richmond, Surrey TW9 1UR. Tel. 020 8939 9530.

National Association for Staff Support, 9 Caradon Close, Woking, Surrey GU21 3DU. Tel. 01483 771599.

National Association of Bereavement Services, 2 Plough Yard, London EC2A. Tel. 020 7247 1080.

Age Concern (England), Astral House, 1268 London Road, London SW16 4ER. Tel. 020 8765 7200. http://www.ace.org.uk. email:infodep@ace.org.uk

Age Concern Scotland, 113 Rose Street, Edinburgh EH2 3DT. Tel. 0131 220 3345.

Age Concern (Cymru), 4th Floor, 1 Cathedral Road, Cardiff CF1 9SD. Tel. 029 2037 1566.

Age Concern Northern Ireland, 3 Lower Crescent, Belfast BT7 1NR. Tel. 0298 9024 5729.

References

[1] Higginson, I.J., Astin, P. & Dolan, S. (1998) Where do cancer patients die? Ten year trends in the place of death of cancer patients. *Palliative Medicine*, **12**(5), 353–363.

[2] Crawford, V. *et al.* (1999) Comparison of residential and nursing home care before and after the 1993 community care policy. *British Medical Journal*, **318**(7180), 366.

[3] National Council for Hospice and Specialist Palliative Care Services (1995) *Specialist Palliative Care, A statement of definitions*. Occasional Paper no 8. NCHSPCS, London.

[4] Barbus, A. (1975) The dying person's bill of rights. *American Journal of Nursing*, **1**, 99–100.

[5] Hockley, J. (1983) An investigation to identify symptoms of distress in the

terminally ill patient and his/her family. Unpublished research report. Cited in: *Nursing Issues and Research in Terminal Care* (1988) Wilson Barnett, J. & Rainman, J. John Wiley & Sons, Chichester.

6 Davis, B.D., Cowley, S.A. & Ryland, R.K. (1996) The effects of terminal illness on patients and their carers. *Journal of Advanced Nursing*, **23**, 512–520.

7 Wilkes, E. (1984) Dying now. *The Lancet*, **1**, 950–952.

8 Working Party on Clinical Guidelines in Palliative Care (1997) *Changing Gear – Guidelines for Managing the Last Days of Life in Adults*. National Council for Hospice and Specialist Palliative Care, London.

9 Arcier, M. (1990) *Aromatherapy*. Hamlyn, London.

10 Williams, D. (1989) *Lecture notes on essential oils*. Eve Taylor, London.

11 Valet, J. (1990) *The Practice of Aromatherapy*. C.W. Daniels, Saffron Walden, UK.

12 Stevenson, C.J. (1994) The psychological effects of aromatherapy following cardiac surgery. *Complementary Therapies in Medicine*, **2**, 27–31.

13 Knapman, J. (1993) Controlling emesis after chemotherapy. *Nursing Standard*, **7**, 38–39.

14 Gillemain, J., Rouseau, A. & Delaveau, P. (1989) Neurodepressant effects of Lavandula augustifolia. *Annales Pharmaceutiques Francais*, **47**, 337–343.

15 Hardy, M. (1991) Sweet scented dreams. *International Journal of Aromatherapy*, **3**(1), 11–13.

16 Canard, Graham (1996) The effect of aromatherapy in promoting relaxation and stress reduction in a general hospital. *Complementary Therapies in Nursing and Midwifery*, **2**, 38–40.

17 Crosby, C. (1989) Method in mouthcare. *Nursing Times*, **85**(35), 38–41.

18 McSweeney, M.P., Shaw, A. & Yip, B. (1995) Oral health in elderly patients. *British Journal of Nursing*, **4**(20), 1204–1209.

19 Abelsen, D.C. (1985) Denture plaque and denture cleansers; review of the literature. *Gerodontics*, **1**(5), 202–206.

20 Crooke, J. *et al.* (1984) The prevalence of pain complaints in a general population. *Pain*, **18**(3), 299–314.

21 Bowsher, D. *et al.* (1991) The prevalence of chronic pain in the British population; a telephone survey. *The Pain Clinic*, **4**(4), 223–231.

22 Cooper, J.K. & Kohlman, T. (2001) Factors associated with health status of older Americans. *Age Ageing*, **6**, 495–501.

23 Smith, A. & Friedmann, M. (1999) Perceived family dynamics of person's with chronic pain. *Journal of Advanced Nursing*, **30**(3), 543–551.

24 Antiplatlet trails collaboration (1994) Collaborative overview of randomized trails of antiplatlet therapy. *British Medical Journal*, **308**(6921), 81–106.

25 Giovannuci, E. *et al.* (1995) Aspirin and the risk of colorectal cancer in women. *New England Journal of Medicine*, **333**(10), 609–614.

26 Rang, H. *et al.* (1999) Pharmacology, 4th edn. Churchill-Livingstone, London.

27 Stockley, J. (1999) Drug interactions, 5th edn. Blackwell Science, Oxford.

28 Hawkey, C. (2000) Management of gastroduodenal ulcers caused by non steroidal anti-inflammatory drugs. In: Balliere's Best Practice and Research, *Clinical Gastroenterology*, **14**(1), 173–192.

29 Creamer, P. & Hochberg, M.C. (1998) The relationship between psychosocial variables and pain reporting in osteo-arthritis of the knee. *Arthritis Care and Research*, **1**(1), 60–65.

30 Casten, R.J. *et al.* (1995) The relationship among anxiety, depression and pain in a geriatric institutionalised sample. *Pain*, **61**(2), 271–276.

31 Covington, E.C. (1991) Depression and chronic fatigue in the patient with chronic pain. *Primary Care*, **18**(2), 341–358.

32 Straus, A. (1971) *Anguish; the Case History of a Dying Trajectory*. CA Sociology Press, San Francisco.

33 Kubler, Ross (1969) *On Death and Dying*. Tavistock Publications, London.

34 Parkes, C. Murray (1986) *Bereavement: Studies of Grief in Adult Life*. Penguin, Harmondsworth.

35 Scott, T. (1985) National Association of Health Authorities. *Conference on Care for the Dying*. DHSS, The Stationery Office, London.

36 Kavanagh, R. (1972) *Facing Death*. Penguin, Baltimore.

37 Bloomfield, K. (1986) Ask the family. *Nursing Times*, 12 March, 28–30.

38 Wilson, S.A. & Daley, B.J. (1998) Attachment/Detachment: Forces influencing care of the dying in long term care. *Journal of Palliative Medicine*, **1**(1), 21–33.

39 Arner, S., Killander, E. & Westerberg, H. (1999) Poor leadership behind poor pain relief. Medical audit of cancer related pain treatment. *Lakartidningen*, **96**(1–2), 33–36. (Information taken from English abstract)

40 Levin, R., Wenger, N.S., Ouslander, J.G., Zellman, G., Schnelle, J.F., Buchanan, J.L., Hirsch, S.H. & Reuben, D.B. (1998) Life sustaining treatment decisions for nursing home residents who discusses, who decided and what is decided. *Journal of the American Geriatric Society*, **47**(1), 82–87.

Chapter 15

Diabetes

Many older people living in nursing homes have diabetes. The National Service Framework on diabetes sets out new evidence-based standards on diabetic care. These standards include setting up diabetic registers and providing evidence-based care. The National Service Framework will impact on the way people with diabetes are cared for. You can download a copy from the Department of Health website[1]. The incidence of diabetes is growing and diabetes is one of the major health issues of the twenty-first century[2]. Diabetes is the fourth leading cause of death in the UK[3]. The incidence of diabetes rises with age[4] but older people with diabetes have fewer symptoms of diabetes than younger people[5]. Half of all older people with diabetes remain undiagnosed. Those who are diagnosed have often been diabetic many years before diagnosis[6].

This chapter is divided into five sections: causes and consequences of diabetes, medical treatment of diabetes, managing diabetes, skin problems, and visual problems. The first section aims to enable you to understand that diabetes is not simply a disorder of carbohydrate metabolism but a chronic disease that affects every aspect of a person's body.

Causes and consequences of diabetes

This section will:

- Review the anatomy and physiology of diabetes
- Discuss type I – insulin dependent diabetes
- Discuss type II – non-insulin dependent diabetes
- Explain how diabetes affects vision
- Explain how diabetes affects renal function
- Explain how diabetes affects arterial circulation
- Explain the neurological affects of diabetes

What is diabetes?

Diabetes mellitus means sweet diabetes. Many years ago, before it was possible to test urine for sugar, physicians diagnosed by tasting the urine. The high sugar content of diabetic urine gave it a sweet taste.

'The term diabetes mellitus describes a metabolic disorder of multiple aetiology characterised by chronic hyperglycaemia with disturbances of carbohydrate, fat and protein metabolism resulting from defects in insulin secretion, insulin action or both.'[7]

'Diabetes mellitus is a metabolic disorder in which the body has a deficiency of, and or a resistance to insulin.'[8]

The World Health Organisation classification of diabetes[9] is shown in Box 15.1.

Box 15.1   WHO classification of diabetes.

Diabetes mellitus
- Type I – insulin dependent diabetes (IDDM)
- Type II – non-insulin dependent diabetes (NIDDM)
  - Non obese
  - Obese
- Other types of diabetes associated with specific conditions and syndromes
- Gestational diabetes

Impaired glucose regulation
- Non-obese
- Obese
- Associated with certain conditions and syndromes

Statistical risk classes
- Previous abnormality of glucose tolerance, e.g. past history of gestational or steroid induced diabetes
- Potential abnormality of glucose tolerance, i.e. people at risk of diabetes such as those with islet cell antibodies or with an identical twin who has type I diabetes.

How insulin acts

Insulin is a hormone. It is produced in the pancreas by the beta cells of the islets of Langerhans. The pancreas is part of the endocrine system. Endocrine glands release hormones directly into the bloodstream. Insulin is released directly into the bloodstream and acts quickly. Insulin is the body's mechanism for regulating blood glucose levels. When we eat carbohydrate the body breaks this down into glucose. Blood glucose levels rise. The pancreas responds to this by producing insulin and releasing it directly into the bloodstream. Insulin allows the body to convert surplus glucose into glycogen and fat. Glycogen is stored in the liver and muscles. When blood glucose levels fall to a certain level the glycogen in the liver is broken down and converted back into glucose. This process is called *glycogenolysis*. When glycogen stores have been exhausted the body begins to break down fat to produce glucose. When fat stores have been exhausted the body begins to break down muscle. This process is known as *gluconogenisis*. This homeostatic process enables healthy people to maintain stable blood glucose levels of 3–8 mmol/l.

Type I diabetes

Fewer than 20% of diabetics have type I diabetes. There are between 138 000 and 345 000 people with type I diabetes in the UK. Type I, insulin dependent diabetes mellitus, is a disease that leads to the destruction of the beta cells of the pancreas. In type I diabetes no insulin is produced by the beta cells of the pancreas[10]. There are two types of type I diabetes: rapidly progressive and slowly progressive[11]. In rapidly progressive type I diabetes, the rate of beta cell destruction is rapid. This rapidly progressive form of type I diabetes is common in children but can also occur in adults. The slowly progressive form of diabetes usually occurs in adults and is sometimes referred to as latent autoimmune diabetes adult (LADA). People with slowly progressive type I diabetes may have sufficient beta cells to prevent keto-acidosis for many years[12]. However their diabetic control can rapidly deteriorate when the body is stressed by infection, trauma or surgery[13]. People with slowly progressive type I diabetes will eventually become insulin dependent. Often professionals consider that type I diabetes only occurs in young people. This is a mistaken view; type I diabetes can occur in all age groups.

We do not yet fully understand the causes of type I diabetes. There appear to be several factors. Type I diabetes is primarily an autoimmune disease. People with autoimmune diseases such as Graves' disease, Hashimoto's thyroiditis and Addison's disease have an increased risk of developing diabetes. Some people are more genetically susceptible than others to developing antibodies that lead to the destruction of the beta cells. Viral infections such as congenital rubella, mumps Coxsackie's B3 or B4 can trigger diabetes in people who are genetically susceptible. Environmental factors are also thought to play a part in the development of type I diabetes, but the relationship between environmental factors and the development of diabetes is not yet fully understood. Some people who have diabetes have idiopathic diabetes – that means that we do not yet understand why the diabetes has developed and there is no evidence of autoimmune disease.

Type II diabetes

Over 80% of diabetics have type II diabetes[14]. There are between 1 million and 1.2 million adults in the UK who have type II diabetes, half remaining undiagnosed. Different races have different incidences of diabetes. In the adult population, 4% of white people, 20% of black people, 25% of Asians and 5% of Chinese have diabetes[15]. The incidence of diabetes increases with age and 20% of elderly Caucasians are diabetic[16]. Type II diabetes is more common in overweight people. The incidence of diabetes in the US is twice that in the UK. It has been described as 'A collision between thrifty genes and an affluent society'[17].

In type II diabetes the beta cells of the pancreas produce insulin normally when the disease begins. This insulin is released into the bloodstream but the body is unable to use the insulin effectively. Normally circulating insulin is taken up by glucose receptors. There are glucose receptors in muscle, fat and the liver. The body's reduced ability to use insulin effectively is known as *insulin resistance*[18]. Insulin resistance leads to high blood glucose levels. The beta cells respond to high blood glucose levels by producing more insulin in an effort to reduce blood glucose levels. The pancreas goes into overdrive. This excessive glucose production fails to maintain normal blood glucose levels and the pancreas works harder and harder. Eventually the beta cells are exhausted by the overproduction of insulin and begin to fail. The diabetes worsens.

Insulin resistance syndrome

Insulin resistance is worse in overweight people. It is linked to a number of other abnormalities. These include hyperinsulaemia, central obesity, defective lipid metabolism and blood coagulation and disturbances in blood pressure homeostasis. These abnormalities are known as insulin resistant syndrome (IRS)[19]. IRS increases the risk of macrovascular damage and arterial disease.

Consequences of diabetes

Diabetes leads to elevated blood glucose levels – hyperglycemias. Hyperglycaemia leads to:

- *Lack of energy* – This is because glycolysis, the process that enables sugar to be broken down into adenosine triphosphate (ATP), is affected. ATP enables cells and tissues to obtain energy.
- *Lack of reserves* – This is because glycogen, normally stored in the liver, is broken down. High blood glucose prevents the body drawing on emergency reserves of glycogen.
- *Increased risk of tissue damage* – This is because hypoglycaemia leads to high levels of circulating amino acids and urea.

Undiagnosed or poorly treated diabetes leads to premature death. At least 20 000 people in the UK die prematurely each year because of diabetes. Undiagnosed or poorly controlled diabetes has the following effects:

- Increases the risk of cerebrovascular disease and stroke by twelve times
- Increases the risk of coronary heart disease by twelve times
- Increases the risk of peripheral neuropathy by sixteen times[20]
- A quarter of all people with type II diabetes suffer nephropathy though they usually die of cardiac problems before they reach end stage renal failure[21]
- Increases the risk of blindness – almost everyone who has been diabetic for 20 years has retinopathy.

Diabetes and vision

Diabetes affects vision and increases the risk of blindness[22]. It affects vision in a number of ways. Hyperglycaemia reduces vision, and good diabetic control enables people to see more clearly. Often diabetic people know that their blood sugar is high because vision is poor. People with diabetes are five times more likely than non-diabetics to develop cataracts. The incidence of glaucoma is also higher in diabetics. The commonest cause of visual problems is diabetic retinopathy. The number of people who lose their sight because of diabetes is not known. An estimated 2% of diabetics are registered blind[23] but only a third of people eligible to be registered blind actually register[24] so the figure could be 6%. Retinopathy occurs when the small blood vessels supplying the retina become diseased and close off. Other vessels dilate and attempt to provide the retina with sufficient blood. These dilated vessels leak. This causes diabetic maculopathy, a small swelling of the macula. The macula is the small area of the retina where best vision is concentrated. Vision gradually fails as macular oedema spreads[25]. Visual problems are discussed later in this chapter.

Diabetes and renal function

Diabetic nephropathy is a common complication of diabetes. In diabetic nephropathy the small vessels in the kidneys become abnormal and protein leaks into the urine. In the early stages only small amounts of protein leak into the urine. As the disease progresses more protein is lost in the urine and eventually the person will develop end stage renal failure.

Diabetes and arterial disease

People with diabetes are more likely to develop hypertension and arterial disease and to suffer from cardiac problems and stroke. People with type II diabetes are most likely to die prematurely because of arterial disease. We'll discuss ways of minimising risk factors later.

Diabetic risk factors

The risk of developing diabetes varies according to ethnic group, weight and genetic factors. Diabetic risk factors are:

- Obesity – body mass index more than $30\,\text{kg/m}^2$
- Parent, sibling or child with type II diabetes
- Hyperlipidaemia
- Hypertension
- Coronary artery disease
- Cerebrovascular disease
- Peripheral neuropathy
- Peripheral vascular disease
- History of gestational diabetes
- History of having a baby weighing more than 4 kg
- History of skin infections.

Clinical features

The clinical features of diabetes are well known:

- Thirst
- Weight loss
- Tiredness and irritability
- Rapid deterioration of vision
- Urinary problems: polyuria, nocturia, urinary incontinence
- Fungal infection: candida, interigo, balanitis
- Cellulitis, poor wound healing and boils.

Ageing affects the presentation of diabetes and older people have fewer symptoms than younger people[26]. Diabetes is insidious and many of the changes associated with diabetes are less marked in older people. The thirst mechanism is less efficient in old age so the older diabetic may be less aware of a raging thirst. Older people tend to be thinner than middle-aged people so weight loss may be considered 'normal'. The older person, family and professionals may put tiredness down to old age when the real reason is a blood glucose of 22 mmol. Rapid deterioration in vision may not be picked up as it may be considered to be part of the ageing process. Urinary problems are still not taken seriously and investigated and an older person developing continence problems is still more likely to receive pads than a continence assessment. If the older person develops a fungal infection we are more likely to blame the last course of antibiotics than suspect diabetes. When an older person develops cellulitis, medical and nursing staff rarely think of a urine test. At least half of all cases of diabetes in older adults are undiagnosed. Many older adults diagnosed diabetic have had undiagnosed diabetes for years[27]. Delayed diagnosis is dangerous and increases the risk of complications.

Disease progression

Type II diabetes is often thought of as mild but it is not. Many people with type II diabetes progress to insulin therapy. The rate at which diabetes deteriorates is related to ethnicity. Twenty years after diagnosis of type II diabetes most Caucasians require insulin therapy. The disease progresses more rapidly in other ethnic groups. Ten years after diagnosis most Asians require insulin therapy[28].

Conclusion

Diabetes is one of the major health issues of the twenty-first century. The number of people with diabetes is growing, and good diabetic control reduces the severity and risk of complications and improves quality of life.

Key points

- The number of people with diabetes is rising
- The incidence of diabetes rises with age
- Around 20% of diabetics have type I diabetes
- Around 80% of diabetics have type II diabetes
- An estimated 50% of older people with diabetes are undiagnosed
- Diabetes increases the risk of blindness, renal failure, stroke and circulatory problems
- Undiagnosed or poorly managed diabetes reduces the length of life and impairs quality of life.

Medical treatment of diabetes

The aims of medical treatment are to maintain normoglaecemia (a blood sugar within normal limits), to relieve symptoms, maintain or improve quality of life and to prevent complications associated with diabetes.

This section aims to:

- Explore dietary management of diabetes
- Examine different hypoglycaemic agents
- Discuss the advantages and disadvantages of oral hypoglycaemic agents
- Discuss when insulin therapy is required
- Explore the advantages and disadvantages of insulin
- Discuss when to switch from oral hypoglycaemics to insulin
- Update you on research and development of new treatments for diabetes

Holistic care

The older person with diabetes probably has a host of problems. The aim of care is to ensure that the person experiences the highest possible quality of life, not the perfect blood sugar level. Sometimes you have to make fine judgements about how to meet that aim – those judgments should be made on the basis of your knowledge of the whole person and not just their diabetes.

Dietary treatment

In type II diabetes dietary treatment is begun before any other treatment is considered. The aim of dietary treatment is to control symptoms, to control hyperglycaemia and to keep weight within normal limits. It is important not to start drug treatment too early, while dietary changes are reducing blood sugar levels. If oral hypoglycaemics are started too early there is a risk of hypoglycaemia. Oral hypoglycaemics should not normally be given until the person has been on a diabetic diet for three months. However, if the person is unwell and has a fasting blood glucose of 12 mmol or above, tablets may be started a month after the diet[29]. Few patients with type II diabetes respond to dietary modification alone and drug treatment is often necessary.

Oral hypoglycaemics

There are four groups of drugs used to treat type II diabetes:

- Sulphonylureas
- Biguanides
- Alpha-glucosidase inhibitors
- Glitazones

The decision about which drug or which combination of drugs to use must be based on the individual's health status. Each group of drugs is examined in detail here.

Sulphonylureas

Sulphonylureas work by stimulating the beta cells in the pancreas to produce more insulin, by reducing glucose production from the liver and by increasing insulin uptake. Sulphonylureas have differing half-lives and that is important when treating frail older people. Chlorpropramide has a half-life of 24 to 72 hours in healthy young adults. Glibenclamide has a half-life of 20 to 24 hours. Sulphonylureas are excreted by the kidneys, so half-life is prolonged in older people who have poorer renal function because of age-related changes. Renal failure, a common complication of diabetes, further extends half-life. Chlorpropramide is rarely used now. Glibenclamide is not now recommended for older people. Older people are best treated with shorter acting drugs such as tolbutamide or gliclazide as these are excreted by the liver.

Side effects

The main side effect of sulphonylureas is hypoglycaemia. Severe hypoglycaemia can cause death. Another major side effect is weight gain. One of the reasons for weight gain is overtreatment – the person overeats to prevent hypoglycaemia. Many doctors prefer to avoid prescribing sulphonylureas to obese diabetics as they lead to further weight gain. Overweight increases insulin resistance and makes diabetes more difficult to control[30]. Other side effects are rare but include skin rashes, nausea, vomiting, headache and blood disorders.

Dosage and administration

Sulphonylureas should be given 30 minutes before a meal – this lowers blood glucose levels most effectively. If you give sulphonylureas with a meal, blood glucose levels do not respond so well to the drug. Dosage should be increased gradually *only* if lower doses are ineffective. There is a narrow therapeutic range for sulphonylureas and some doctors consider larger doses ineffective. A pancreas can only take so much stimulating. Table 15.1 gives details of common sulphonylureas.

Table 15.1   Common sulphonylureas.

Drug	Dose	Half-life
Chlorpropramide (diabiese)	100–500 mg daily	24–72 hours
Glibenclamide	2.5–15 mg daily	20–24 hours
Tolazamide	100–1000 mg daily	16–24 hours
Gliclazide	40–320 mg daily	10–15 hours
Glipizide	2.5–40 mg daily	12–14 hours
Tolbutamide	500–2000 mg daily	6–10 hours

Biguanides

Metformin is the only biguanide available in the UK. Its mode of action is not clear. It is thought to have multiple effects including inhibiting glycogenesis and reducing hepatic glucose output[31]. Metformin reduces weight and elevated blood lipid levels. It is suitable for overweight diabetics.

Side effects

The most serious risk is of lactic acidosis. The risk of lactic acidosis is greater when renal, hepatic or cardiac failure is present. Some doctors consider it is best avoided in older people. Others point out that the risk of lactic acidosis is small. There has never been a single reported case of lactic acidosis in an older person with normal renal, cardiac and hepatic function[32]. Judgements on whether or not to use metformin should not be based solely on age[33].

Gastrointestinal effects are common. Metformin affects the salivary glands and people taking Metformin sometimes complain of a metallic taste in their mouths. Metformin may reduce the absorption of vitamin B_{12}.

Administration and dosage
Metformin should be given half an hour after meals; this reduces gastro-intestinal side effects. The starting dose is 500 mg daily or 500 mg b.d. The maximum dose is 3 g daily but few doctors prescribe more than 2 g. Metformin may be given with sulphonylureas or an alpha-glucosidase inhibitor.

Alpha-glucosidase inhibitors

Acarbose is the only alpha-glucosidase inhibitor available in the UK. It acts on the small intestine and reduces carbohydrate absorption. This reduces blood glucose levels. Acarbose, like metformin, does not cause weight gain. It is now recommended as first line therapy for type II diabetes. It is especially suitable for obese diabetics. Acarbose does not cause hypoglycaemia.

Side effects
Acarbose is contraindicated in renal and hepatic impairment. It is also contraindicated when the person has a history of inflammatory bowel disease. The main side effects are flatulence, abdominal distension and pain.

Dosage and administration
The initial dose of acarbose is 50 mg daily. This is chewed with the first mouthful of food. The dose is reviewed after two weeks and can be increased to 50 mg b.d. if required, provided there are no severe gastrointestinal symptoms. The maximum dose is 200 mg t.d.s. Acarbose may be combined with a sulphonylurea. When this combination is used hypoglycaemia can occur. You must treat this with glucose as acarbose prevents metabolism and absorption of sugar. Sugar is useless in treatment of hypoglycaemia when acarbose is given.

Limitations of existing hypoglycaemics
Existing oral hypoglycaemics work by stimulating the beta cells in the pancreas and preventing the liver from producing glucose. They do not treat insulin resistance[34]. Existing oral hypoglycaemics may make diabetes worse by increasing insulin resistance[35]. Existing oral hypoglycaemics work by stimulating the beta cells to work harder. Many people with diabetes require up to three different drugs to maintain blood glucose control[36]. When multiple oral hypoglycaemics are required hypoglycaemia becomes common[37].

Glitazones

In the late 1990s a new type of oral hypoglycaemics was developed. These drugs are known as glitazones or thiazolinediones or proliferator activated receptor gamma agonists (PPARγ). Glitazones were developed especially to treat insulin resistance. They act by enhancing the action of insulin in adipose tissue, skeletal muscle and the liver[38]. Research suggests that Glitazones preserve pancreatic function and protect the beta cells from further damage[39]. The first glitazone, troglitazone, was introduced in October 1997 but withdrawn a month later because it caused severe liver damage. New glitazones, rosiglitazone and pioglitazone, have been approved for use in the UK.

Glitazones are suitable for older people. They reduce blood sugar and blood lipid levels and reduce the amount of albumen excreted in the urine[40].

NICE Guidance

The National Institute for Clinical Excellence (NICE) recommends that people who are not able to take metformin and sulphonylurea combination therapy, and people whose blood sugar remains high despite combination therapy, should be given rosiglitazone in combination with a sulphonylurea or metformin as an alternative to injected insulin.

NICE recommend that obese people are offered metformin and rosiglitazone because it helps weight loss.

Side effects

It will take time before the full range of side effects are known. There are rare reports of liver problems so doctors should monitor liver function before beginning treatment and then every two months for the first 12 months of treatment. Known side effects include headache, anaemia, fatigue, dizziness, rash, hair loss, weight gain, dyspnoea, altered blood lipids and blood disorders.

Dosage and administration

The recommended starting dose for rosiglitazone is 4 mg daily when given in combination with metformin or a sulphonylurea. This may be increased to 8 mg daily (given in single or divided doses) after eight weeks if control was not established on the lower dose.

Insulin therapy

Sooner or later most people with type II diabetes will require insulin therapy. Insulin therapy may be required as a temporary measure because the person is ill. Illness increases demands on the body and causes blood sugar control to deteriorate. Insulin therapy is often required in such circumstances and can usually be discontinued when the crisis has passed.

Type II diabetes is a progressive disease and eventually all beta cells may cease functioning and insulin is required. In other cases the need for insulin is less clear-cut. The older person may be poorly controlled on oral hypoglycaemics and doctors may consider insulin. The decision to move an older person with poor diabetic control from oral therapy to insulin should not be taken lightly. Table 15.2 outlines factors that should be considered. If insulin

Table 15.2 Factors to consider before switching to insulin therapy.

Investigate	Consider
Does the patient have symptoms?	If there are no symptoms insulin will not make the person feel better
Does she have complications?	Will insulin remove these complications?
Does she have poor healing?	Insulin therapy will improve control and improve wound healing
Does she have an infection?	Infections will destabilise diabetes – insulin will improve control and may only be required temporarily
Is she confused, tired and unwell?	Good control will improve these symptoms
How old is she?	Are there compelling reasons for starting a 90-year-old on insulin?
Are tablets taken at correct time in correct dose?	Check compliance before insulin
What is she really eating?	Do not treat the relatives (bearers of chocolates)
How does she feel about insulin?	Quality is about choice and control

is required, diabetic specialists will work out the most suitable regime for the individual.

Future therapies

In the last century, until insulin was discovered people died because of diabetes; now they die prematurely because of the complications of diabetes. Current research is set to revolutionise the way we treat diabetes. The most important research at the moment is on insulin patches, transplants, artificial pancreases and immunisation.

Insulin patches

Insulin is given by injection because it is destroyed by the digestive process. The development of insulin patches could make insulin injections a thing of the past. Conventional skin patches are now used routinely to deliver some drugs. Their use is limited because they rely on diffusion to get drugs through the skin. Researchers are now trialling patches with an integrated electrical circuit. The electrical circuit delivers a small amount of current to the skin and enables drugs to cross through the skin into the body. Drugs such as insulin have large molecules and this charge is not effective in getting the drug through the skin. Researchers have now developed a way of incorporating small blades a tenth of a millimetre long into the patches. These blades are so tiny that they cause no pain. Patches with microscopic blades and an electrical circuit can effectively deliver the volume of insulin required to control diabetes.

Pancreatic transplants

In the last ten years pancreatic transplants have moved from the experimental to the established. Graft survival rates have increased and are now 75% at a year and 65% at five years. Patients who have pancreatic transplants must take immunosuppressants for the rest of their lives. Normally pancreatic transplant is restricted to patients who also require renal transplant. A dual transplant increases the rate of kidney survival and does not carry an additional risk to the patient. In exceptional cases when it is impossible to control diabetes with conventional treatment, pancreatic transplant alone may be considered. Criteria for transplant are very strict[41].

Islet cell transplants

Islet cell transplantation is an experimental procedure. It involves injecting islet cells into the portal vein. These are seeded in the liver. Immunosuppressive therapy is currently required to prevent rejection. Researchers are working on a membrane to enclose the islet cells. This membrane is to protect the islet cells from autoimmune attack. If researchers are successful, immunosuppression will no longer be required.

Dr Shapiro of the University of Alberta in Edmonton, has developed a way of taking islet cells from a donor and injecting them into the diabetes sufferer's liver. The treatment takes half a day and can be done under local anaesthetic. After two injections, the cells kick-start the body's insulin production and no more treatment is needed. Those patients who have already had the revolutionary treatment have to take a mixture of anti-rejection drugs for the rest of their lives to stop their bodies destroying the transplanted cells. Diabetes UK (formerly the British Diabetic Association) are funding research that will enable ten Islet cell transplants to be carried out each year. The treatment will initially be targeted at people with severe diabetes who often lapse into coma: 'We have to balance the risks of the treatment procedure and anti-rejection drugs against the risks these patients face every day. These patients have a 25 times greater risk of kidney failure, heart attacks, strokes and blindness, and have an average of 15 years sliced off their life span.'

Stem cell research

Islet cells, found in the pancreas, could theoretically be developed from stem cells. Stem cells taken from the person with diabetes could be treated so that they develop into islet cells. If these were developed and injected there would be no need for the person to take immunosuppressants because the person would be receiving their own cells. It may take 5 to 10 years to complete this work but ultimately it could prove to be the cure for diabetes and people would no longer be forced to take insulin or tablets to stay alive.

Artificial pancreas

Researchers in the US are working on an implantable artificial pancreas. This uses sensors to monitor blood glucose levels and is linked to an implanted, refillable insulin pump. The system also has a hypoglycaemia alarm. Trials began in 2002.

Vaccination

Animal studies have proven that it is possible to vaccinate diabetes-prone rodents against diabetes. Researchers are now working on vaccines to prevent diabetes in humans.

Continuous glucose monitoring

The Glucowatch monitors blood sugar levels throughout the day by using an electric current. It sits on a disposable gel disc containing the enzyme used to monitor blood glucose with test strips. The watch draws glucose from the skin into the gel disc by using a small electric current that flows between the two terminals in the watch body. It takes three hours for the watch to warm up and hydrate the pad. Once the watch has warmed up glucose levels are measured every 20 minutes for 12 hours. If blood sugar levels rise or fall too much the watch beeps. The Glucowatch was developed in the US and is now available in the UK for around £200.

Conclusion

At the moment people with diabetes suffer ill health and die prematurely because of their diabetes. Medical treatment of diabetes is far from perfect but future advances may improve the health of people with diabetes. It is important to remember though that an ounce of prevention is worth more than a ton of 'cure'. People who eat a healthy diet, keep their weight down and exercise regularly are less likely to develop diabetes than those who do not. People developing diabetes who take responsibility for their health are less likely to develop complications. The people who are admitted to nursing homes generally are people who are less able to reduce the complications of diabetes.

Key points

- Dietary management and weight control are the first treatment for diabetes
- Oral hypoglycaemics should be given after diet begins to reduce blood sugar
- Traditional oral hypoglycaemics act by increasing insulin production and inhibiting glycogenesis
- Glitazones enhance the action of insulin and lower raised blood lipids
- Most diabetics will require insulin at some stage
- New treatments have the potential to prevent diabetes and to treat existing diabetics.

Managing diabetes

Diabetes care in the UK is poor. Most primary care services do not meet recommended levels of specialist nurse cover. Practice nurses who have only a rudimentary knowledge of diabetes management run a third of diabetic clinics[42]. People living in homes receive fewer services than those of the same age living in their own homes. That is set to change with the introduction of the National Service Framework and for the first time people with diabetes will receive coherent diabetic care that aims to avoid complication and improve health.

Often older people receive poorer diabetic care because professionals mistakenly believe that good diabetic management does not matter at this stage of life. This section aims to enable you to offer high quality diabetic care.

This section will explore:

- What is good diabetic control?
- The benefits of good diabetic control
- Diabetic diet
- Diabetes and infection
- Hyperosmolar non-ketotic coma (HONK)
- Hypoglycaemia and how to treat it
- Managing relatives

What is good diabetic control?

In younger people we aim to maintain physiological glucose levels. This tight control means maintaining glucose levels of 3–8 mmol. Tight control minimises complications and improves quality of life, but there are dangers to tight diabetic control. Attempts to maintain normal blood sugar levels carry the risk of hypoglycaemia. The risk of hypoglycaemia increases with age. Older people get less warning of hypoglycaemia and are more severely affected by it. Severe hypoglycaemia can be fatal in old age[43]. The principle aims of tight diabetic control are to relieve symptoms and avoid long-term complications. Symptoms are often less marked in older people so there is often less need to control symptoms. Many people with diabetes admitted to nursing homes have already developed complications of diabetes. Those who have not probably will not live long enough to develop these complications, which take years to develop. It is considered inappropriate to aim for the same blood sugar levels that you would aim for in a young adult. Most specialists believe that blood sugar levels of 5–11 mmol are acceptable in older people with diabetes. It is important though not to ignore diabetes in older people.

The benefits of good diabetic control
Diabetes has a real effect on older people's lives. Older people with poorly controlled diabetes are more likely to feel depressed. Consistently high blood sugar levels reduce mental functioning. The hyperglycaemic older person can become forgetful, lack concentration and become confused[44]. Stabilising blood sugar and improving diabetic control improves memory, concentration and ability[45]. Good diabetic control improves quality of life and minimises the risk of hypoglycaemia and HONK.

Achieving good diabetic control
Good diabetic control is achieved by dietary management, exercise whenever possible and ensuring prescribed medication is taken. Three-quarters of

people concerned are aged 65 or over. Most older people with diabetes do not take medication as prescribed when living at home. Researchers in Dundee studied almost 3000 people with diabetes and found that only a third of people prescribed a single medication for diabetes took it as prescribed. Only 13% of people prescribed both metformin and a sulphonylurea took medication as prescribed. When doctors find an older person's blood sugar is poorly controlled they tend to think the diabetes is worsening and may prescribe more medication. The real problem may be that the patient is not taking the tablets! You may find that you need to monitor carefully newly-admitted people on hypoglycaemics. The older person who has not been taking tablets at home suddenly receives regular doses in your home and may suffer severe hypoglycaemia.

The aims of diabetic management

The aims of good diabetic management in older people are:

- To maintain a reasonable body weight
- To avoid hypoglycaemia
- To avoid hyperglycaemia
- To avoid infection
- To improve quality of life.

The mainstay of good diabetic management is providing an appropriate diet.

Diabetic diet

The diabetic diet has changed dramatically in the last 25 years. Once diabetics were encouraged to restrict carbohydrate and make up calorie deficits by eating fats and proteins. We now know that a high intake of fats leads to arterial disease and contributes to obesity. Once diabetics were encouraged to have a 'no sugar' diet and eating a cake was a cardinal sin. All that has changed. The following paragraphs discuss the recommendations that Diabetes UK (contact details at the end of the chapter) now recommend.

Dietary assessment

Diabetes UK recommend that every person with diabetes is assessed by a dietician. The dietician can advise about energy requirements. It is important to get energy requirements right. You may think that the obese diabetic requires a reducing diet but if she has a pressure sore or a leg ulcer calorie requirements may be high. It is also important that the obese diabetic person does not lose weight too quickly. Weight loss should be slow and steady. The ideal weight loss is around 0.5 kg a week. It is important that weight loss is no more than 2 kg a week. Weight loss of more than 2 kg a week indicates that muscle is being metabolised[46].

The dietician will calculate the body mass index (BMI) by dividing the weight in kilograms by the height in metres squared. Details of BMI are given in Chapter 11. You can obtain tables and charts from the dietician to enable you to do this. The aim of diet is to enable the person to maintain or regain an acceptable BMI. The ideal BMI is between 20 and 25 kg/m^2. The typical diabetic cared for in homes is overweight and has type II diabetes. The diet devised for this person will be a reducing diabetic diet.

Obtaining dietary advice

People living in nursing homes have the same right to community services as people living in their own homes. You need to obtain a referral from the person's GP as dieticians can only accept referrals from doctors. Your GP can supply you with referral forms and you can complete these and ask him to sign them when a referral is required. This speeds up the referral process.

Regular food intake

People with diabetes need to eat three widely-spaced meals a day. This is particularly important for people taking sulphonylureas as a missed meal can lead to a hypoglycaemic attack. If the evening meal in your home is served early the person on sulphonylureas may require a bedtime snack. People on insulin therapy generally require snacks between meals[47].

Sugar

People with diabetes should have a diet low in sugar. The person may have up to one ounce (25 g) of sugar daily. Sweet foods such as chocolates and sweets are restricted, not eliminated from the diet. Sugary drinks such as Coca Cola and Lucozade should normally be avoided. Diet drinks such as Diet Coke can be used as substitutes. Saccharine or Canderel can be used instead of sugar in tea and coffee.

Carbohydrate

People with diabetes are now encouraged to eat carbohydrate – half of the ideal diabetic diet should be carbohydrate. The recommendation for non-diabetics is 45%. Carbohydrate intake should be complex carbohydrates. There are two types of carbohydrate:

- *Monosaccharides* or refined carbohydrates or simple sugars – such as honey, sweet drinks and sweets
- *Polysaccharides* or complex carbohydrates – foods such as bread, potatoes, pasta, rice and fruit.

Refined carbohydrates are rapidly digested and boost blood sugar levels quickly but their effect is short lived. Complex carbohydrates are digested slowly and blood sugar levels rise in a slow sustained way. This staves off hunger and leads to improved blood sugar levels.

Fibre

A high fibre diet improves blood sugar levels and prevents constipation. There are two types of fibre:

(1) Soluble fibre reduces blood glucose and cholesterol levels. Foods such as peas, sweet corn, beans, lentils and oats contain soluble fibre.
(2) Insoluble fibre reduces hunger and helps weight loss. Foods such as Weetabix, All Bran, wholemeal bread and flour, wholemeal pasta and brown rice are good sources of insoluble fibre.

Suggested foods to increase dietary fibre are:

- Porridge, Weetabix, All Bran, Fruit and Fibre
- Prunes, compote of fruits
- Fresh fruit (cut, peeled, stewed, juiced)
- Jacket potatoes, potato skins
- Wholemeal pasta (in sauce)
- Carrot cake and banana bread (sweetened with Canderel)
- Rice and peas
- Wholemeal chapattis and rotis
- Soups with barley, lentils, peas, corn (purée if swallowing is difficult)
- Vegetables (purée if necessary).

Fat

There is evidence that reducing fat intake reduces the risk of complications in younger people, but there is no evidence that it helps reduce complications in older people. However, reducing fat intake reduces calorie intake and can help the obese diabetic to lose weight. There are three types of fats in food:

(1) *Saturated fats* – found in red meat, fat on red meat, dripping, lard, butter and cheese.
(2) *Polyunsaturated fats* – found in vegetable oils such as sunflower oil, corn oil and soya oil and margarines and spreads made from these oils. Oily fish such as herrings and pilchards are high in polyunsaturates. Oily fish also contain omega 3 fatty acids and these are known to protect against heart disease.
(3) *Monounsaturated fats* – found in olive oil and rapeseed oil and margarines and spreads based on these. Olivio is made from olive oil.

Fat reduction can be done subtly so that no one notices. It is important not to reduce the fat from dairy products in frail older people because dairy products contain the fat soluble vitamins A and D. Many frail older people living in our homes rarely go outdoors. Half an hour's winter sunlight on the hands and face enables the body to make vitamin D and this helps maintain strong bones. In 1991 researchers found that 40% of people living in long-stay hospitals, residential and nursing homes suffered from vitamin D and calcium deficiency due to inadequate exposure to sunshine. People with dark skins require greater exposure to sunlight to manufacture vitamin D. Inadequate intake of calcium and vitamin D deficiency increases the risk of osteoporosis and fracture. Researchers have found that treating older people with vitamin D increases bone strength and reduces the risk of fractures. Suggested ways to decrease fat in the diet are:

- Reduce the amount of red meat eaten
- Choose chicken (without the skin)
- Choose fish
- Grill, boil, steam or microwave foods
- Use more pulses and vegetables and less meat in stews and casseroles
- Serve lean meat and trim off fat (e.g. serve back bacon, not streaky)
- Serve fewer pies and sausages
- Serve more fruit and fewer cakes and pies.

Protein

Diabetes UK recommend that people with diabetes avoid eating more protein than that in the normal diet. People with nephropathy may be advised to restrict protein; the dietician can advise you of this.

Salt

Hypertension is common in diabetics. Hypertension increases the risk of stroke. Men with a systolic blood pressure of above 180 mmhg have six times the risk of stroke than normotensive men. Men with a systolic blood pressure of 160–180 mmhg have four times the risk of stroke of normotensive men. Hypertension is of greater significance in black people whose risk factor is even higher at the same levels. Reducing salt intake helps lower the blood pressure and reduce the risk of stroke. Suggested ways to decrease salt intake are:

- Use less processed and packaged food
- Avoid salty foods like crisps, peanuts and smoked bacon
- Use less salt in cooking, use herbs and spices instead
- Use less salt at the table.

Diabetic foods

Many older people with diabetes, and their families, think that if food has the word 'diabetic' on it, that means it can be eaten freely. This is not true. Diabetic foods are unsuitable for overweight diabetics. They are sweetened with sorbitol or fructose and are high in calories. Sorbitol and fructose can cause severe diarrhoea. Diabetic foods are expensive and unnecessary additions to a diabetic diet. Low sugar and low calorie jams and marmalades are cheaper and more suitable for overweight diabetics. If the person with diabetes wants a little chocolate then ordinary chocolate (preferably after a meal rich in complex carbohydrates) is fine.

Alcohol

Alcohol increases the risk of hypoglycaemia in people treated with sulphonylureas because it inhibits gluconeogenesis. Sweet wines and sherry should be avoided. If a drink is taken with a mixer, the mixer should be low calorie. A moderate amount of alcohol can be taken (but not on an empty stomach) as part of a diabetic diet. Liqueurs such as Bailey's, Drambuie and Grand Mariner should be avoided because of their high sugar content.

Avoiding infection

The immune system becomes less effective with age[48]. The inflammatory response is less efficient. Older adults have greater difficulty in destroying invading micro organisms and limiting their spread. Many older people with diabetes have immune system abnormalities and are more at risk of infections than non-diabetic older people. These infections can lead to disability or even death. The Department of Health now recommend that all older people are vaccinated against flu and pneumococcal infections. Vaccination is effective in reducing life-threatening disease in vulnerable older people[49].

Hypoglycaemia

When blood sugar falls to around 3.6 mmol in healthy adults, glucagons, cortisol and adrenaline are released. These hormones cause release of glycogen stores, and gluconeogenesis and blood sugar is restored to normal levels. In diabetes these normal homeostatic responses do not function and blood glucose continues to fall. When blood sugar falls to 3 mmol the person is unable to think clearly or carry out everyday tasks. At 2 mmol the person becomes confused and drowsy. When blood sugar is around 1 mmol the person falls into a coma. In coma the person may fit or develop a hemiplegia. Hypoglycaemia is very dangerous in older people and it is important to maintain blood sugar above 4 mmol to avoid the dangers of hypoglycaemia.

Signs and symptoms of hypoglycaemia

The signs and symptoms of hypoglycaemia vary from person to person. Some people are good at detecting the warning symptoms, but some older people are not. You need to observe carefully to detect hypoglycaemic symptoms. Table 15.3 outlines hypoglycaemic symptoms. The person with hypoglycaemia can present in different ways. Some people have personality changes. Sometimes the person is rude and aggressive, sometimes a person is giggly or tearful. Some people behave as though they are drunk. Sometimes the person continues automatic behaviour. Noting and recording how the person presents when having a hypoglycaemic attack helps to recognise hypos early.

Table 15.3   Hypoglycaemic symptoms[50].

Autonomic	Neuroglycopenic	General
Tremor	Dizziness	Hunger
Feeling hot	Confusion	Weakness
Sweating	Tiredness	Blurred vision
Anxiety	Difficulty speaking	Drowsiness
Nausea	Inability to concentrate	Shivering
Palpitations	Headache	
	Visual disturbance	

Treating hypoglycaemia

Treating hypoglycaemia is a three-step programme:

- Raise blood sugar as quickly as possible by giving quick acting carbohydrate. Examples of quick acting carbohydrate are: two or three glucose tablets, tea with two spoonfuls of sugar, 50 ml of Lucozade or 100 ml of Coca Cola or 25 g (a mini-bar) of chocolate. If the patient is semi-conscious give hypostop gel. If the patient is unconscious give 1 ml of glucagons. It takes 15 minutes for glucagons to work. If the patient is still unconscious 15 minutes after glucagons, an intravenous injection of 25–50 ml of 50% dextrose is required. Make sure that there is someone available to give this.

- Prevent blood glucose falling quickly by giving 10 to 20 g of slowly absorbed carbohydrate. Examples of slow acting carbohydrate are: a sandwich, two plain biscuits or an apple. Give normal meal at normal mealtime.
- Find out why the hypo occurred. Did the person miss a meal? Did the person take more exercise than usual? Has medication been increased? Does the person have an infection? Does medication need reviewing?

Hyperglycaemic coma

There are two types of hyperglycaemic coma: diabetic ketoacidotic coma (DKA) and hyperosmolar non-ketotic coma (HONK). Illness can upset diabetic control and cause blood glucose levels to rise. However, because the person feels unwell and does not feel like eating, insulin or tablets are omitted. Blood sugar levels rise and coma may follow.

Diabetic ketoacidotic coma

DKA is much more common in people with type I diabetes. It is rare in people with type II diabetes. In DKA urine testing shows that the person is ketotic. If the person is dehydrated, vomiting for more than four hours and unable to take oral fluids, hospital admission may be required. Clinical features of DKA are:

- Blood glucose may be only slightly elevated, is always under 40 mmol
- Moderate to large amounts of ketones in urine
- Develops over a few days
- May have vomiting
- Sodium plasma levels low.

Hyperosmolar non-ketotic coma (HONK)

HONK usually affects older people and around 60% of people who develop HONK are undiagnosed diabetics[51]. Over 40% of older people who develop HONK will not survive. Thiazide diuretics, infection and high glucose drinks can lead to HONK developing. People with HONK develop it slowly over a period of weeks. The person is often severely dehydrated, uraemic and drowsy. Diagnosis is easy – check blood sugar. Clinical features of HONK are:

- Hyperglycaemia – blood glucose over 50 mmol
- High sodium levels
- No evidence of ketones in urine
- Slow onset over weeks
- Middle aged or elderly
- No vomiting
- No hyperventilation
- Dehydrated.

HONK is treated with fluid replacement; half strength normal saline is used due to high sodium levels. Insulin is used to reduce blood glucose. People with HONK are treated in hospital.

Managing relatives

Relatives can sabotage attempts to improve glaecemic control in older people. Relatives can smuggle in Cherry Bakewells, Quality Street and high energy drinks designed for Olympic athletes and give them to the resident when you are not looking. Communicating with relatives and explaining what the aims of treatment are and how you aim to achieve them, does get many relatives to work with you. Sadly you will always have a hard core who delight in bringing in foods that can (in excess) be harmful. Strategies to deal with such relatives include:

- Explaining the consequences of poor control.
- Providing information leaflets from the Diabetes UK. The relative may take these more seriously than they do you.
- Asking the dietician to review and asking the relative to attend the review
- Asking other members of the family to intervene.

Conclusion

It is possible to manage diabetes well in nursing homes. Good diabetic management increases quality of life by avoiding distressing hypoglycaemic attacks and enabling the person to function to capacity.

Key points

- Tight diabetic control is inappropriate in older people
- Diabetic management aims to maintain blood sugar between 5 and 11 mmol
- Good diabetic control enables the individual to function to capacity
- Dietary assessment enables you to ensure an appropriate diet is provided
- Infection risks are high in diabetes and vaccinations should be offered
- Hypoglycaemia should be promptly treated and the reasons for occurrence investigated
- If coma occurs in an older patient check blood sugar
- Educated and informed relatives can help you with dietary management

Skin problems

People with diabetes are more vulnerable to skin damage. When skin damage does occur, diabetes impairs healing and increases the risk of complications.

This section will explore:

- How diabetes increases the risk of skin damage
- Diabetic foot
- How to prevent skin damage
- How diabetes impairs wound healing
- Treatment of skin ulcers
- Future therapies

How diabetes increases the risk of skin damage

Around 50% of people over 60 who have type II diabetes develop nerve damage[52]. Peripheral neuropathy causes a loss of sensation. Limbs with reduced sensation are vulnerable to damage because the person does not feel pain. Pain warns us that damage is occurring and enables us to prevent further damage. Loss of sensation can lead to severe soft tissue damage.

People with diabetes are likely to develop arterial problems. Arterial problems in the lower limbs affect blood flow. Tissue damage is more likely to occur when blood flow is poor because poorly oxygenated tissues are more easily damaged[53].

Diabetes is more common in poor people and poor diabetics are more likely to develop complications of diabetes such as peripheral neuropathy and peripheral vascular disease than more affluent diabetics[54]. Older people have the lowest incomes in our society.

As diabetes care has improved, the risk of amputation for gangrene or ulceration has fallen from 15 times[55] that of non-diabetics to 12 times that of non-diabetics[56]. People of Afro-Caribbean descent have a higher incidence of vascular problems and amputation than Caucasians. Afro-Caribbean people are twice as likely to require amputation as Caucasians[57]. The mortality risk following amputation is dependent on the level of amputation; the higher the amputation, the greater the mortality becomes. However, Afro-Caribbean people, because of their greater risk factors, are more likely to die following amputation than people of other races[58].

Diabetic foot

Diabetic foot disease is different from ischaemic foot disease. A diabetic may have warm, pink feet but those feet may still be at risk of skin damage. Some diabetics have peripheral vascular disease in addition to diabetic foot disease. This increases the risk of damage. Table 15.4 outlines the clinical

Table 15.4 Clinical features of diabetic and peripheral vascular disease (based on Jerreat L. (1999) *Diabetes for Nurses*. Whurr, London).

Neuropathic (Diabetic)	Neuro-ischaemic
Absent or greatly reduced sensation	Normal or slightly reduced sensation
Warm	Cool
Pink or normal colour	White or greyish in dark-skinned people
No cyanosis	Cyanosed (check nail beds in dark-skinned people)
No pain during the day. May hurt at night	Pain at rest
Pulses palpable	Pulses absent
Callus under head of first metatarsal	No callus
May develop ulcer on sole of foot	May develop ulcer on margins of foot
May develop Charcot's joint	May develop gangrene

features of diabetic foot disease and peripheral vascular disease. Some of the people you care for will have clinical features of both diseases.

Risk factors

All diabetics are not equally at risk of developing diabetic foot problems. The risk factors are:

- Aged 65 plus
- Obese
- High lipid levels
- Macrovascular disease elsewhere in the body
- Neuropathy
- Peripheral vascular disease
- Foot deformity
- Infection
- Poor foot hygiene
- Poor foot care
- Smoking
- Oedema
- Poor diabetic control.

The people with the highest factors are exactly the type of people cared for in nursing homes. It is important to do everything possible to prevent people with such high risk factors developing skin damage.

How to prevent skin damage

In order to prevent skin damage you need to adopt a problem solving approach. There are factors that you cannot change. You cannot make the person younger; you cannot reverse diabetic neuropathy or peripheral vascular disease. You can however improve hygiene, improve diabetic control, ensure that the person with foot deformity has appropriate foot-wear and minimise or eliminate oedema. Ways to prevent foot damage are:

- Wash feet daily and dry carefully. Apply cream if skin is dry
- Do not soak feet
- Inspect feet for signs of damage
- Toenails should be cut straight across
- Ensure person does not walk barefoot
- Never use corn plasters (these contain salicylic acid and can damage feet)
- Shoes should have broad toes and low heels
- Avoid excessive hot or cold
- Avoid hot water bottles
- Keep feet away from fires and radiators.

Foot assessment

Diabetes UK recommends that everyone with diabetes has their feet examined once a year by a doctor with expertise in diabetes[59]. Patients at high risk of developing foot problems should be given appropriate treatment. Research suggests that tight, ill-fitting shoes cause 83% of foot ulcers. Poorly fitting shoes increase plantar pressures and can lead to ulceration[60].

Providing specially fitted shoes reduces the risk of foot ulcers recurring from 83% to 26%[61].

Chiropody

People at high risk of developing foot problems should be referred to a specialist chiropodist who has expertise in diabetes. Specialist chiropodists are often part of the team at the diabetic clinic. The diabetic chiropodist's role will vary from hospital to hospital but will involve:

- Education of patient and people caring for the patient
- Initial assessment
- Investigation and treatment of people at high risk of developing foot problems
- Treatment of people who have developed foot problems
- Assessment of footwear
- Altering existing footwear to minimise risk of damage
- Fitting new or specially made footwear to prevent damage
- Follow-up treatment of high-risk patients.

How diabetes impairs wound healing

The people who live in our homes do not just have diabetes. They are old, and ageing affects the ability of the body to heal. Details of how ageing affects wound healing are provided in Chapter 6. Diabetes can compromise circulation and hyperglycaemia can delay healing[62]. The presence of a wound, especially an infected wound, can lead to poor diabetic control and further inhibit healing. Individuals suffering from diabetes who develop a leg ulcer require close monitoring of their blood glucose and may require additional medication to control diabetes because of the wound. It is essential to ensure that the diabetes is well controlled as high glucose levels will not only inhibit healing but also predispose to infection, which will further destabilise diabetic control. People with diabetes heal more slowly than non-diabetics. Animal studies indicate that diabetes doubles healing time. When tissue damage occurs, the body releases cortisol to aid healing. Cortisol release is less effective in diabetics. When tissue is damaged, collagen is produced and this acts as the scaffolding for wound repair. Collagen produced by people with diabetes is weaker than that in non-diabetics. Experiments in rats show that if the adrenal glands are removed and hydrocortisone given, then collagen metabolism and wound strength improves[63].

Treatment of skin ulcers

Assessment is the key to treating skin ulcers. You need to know what kind of ulcer you are dealing with. You need to know why it has developed before you have any hope of treating it. You can only begin to treat effectively when you know what the problems are. When you have identified the problems (and there is never a single problem), you can begin to treat them. Details of general assessment are provided in Chapter 6. The main features of treatment specific to diabetes are:

- Assessment of ulcer – Doppler ultrasound is indicated
- Expert chiropody if foot is involved
- Assessment of person including HB, electrolytes
- Correction of abnormalities, e.g. treat anaemia
- Antibiotic or larval therapy if infection present
- Tight blood sugar control – insulin may be required for the first time
- Good dietary intake
- Good fluid intake
- If a foot ulcer, stop the damage – non-weight bearing if footwear was to blame and no suitable footwear
- Do not compress limbs
- Regular reassessment
- Treat pain – pain impairs healing
- Reassure – stress impairs healing
- Ensure good quality sleep – lack of sleep impairs healing
- Use appropriate dressings
- Avoid tape on skin – can cause further damage.

Future therapies

Diabetes reduces the number of macrophages produced and this reduction slows healing. Animal experiments demonstrate that insulin, like growth factor, improves healing in diabetics. Researchers are now trialling insulin-like growth factors on people with diabetes.

In the US researchers are using low dose electrical stimulation and have found that this increases wound healing in diabetics by 60%[64]. In Israel researchers are using hyperbaric oxygen to improve wound healing in diabetics. Hyperbaric oxygen increases the levels of oxygen reaching the affected tissues. Increased oxygen levels have an antiseptic effect, reduce oedema and increase collagen production. This improves wound healing and can save limbs from amputation[65]. Austrian researchers are using low intensity laser treatment to stimulate cell growth and tissue repair. They are using low intensity laser light three times a week to improve healing rates. Healing time is related to the size and cause of the ulcer[66].

Conclusion

Although older people with diabetes are more at risk of infection, tissue damage, amputation and death, there are many ways to prevent tissue damage. As our knowledge of how diabetes affects healing increases, the incidence of complications is falling.

Key points

- Diabetes increases the risk of skin damage
- People with peripheral neuropathy are at greatest risk
- Peripheral vascular disease increases risk of damage
- Diabetes impairs wound healing and increases the risk of infection

- Assessment and treatment of people at risk reduces skin damage
- Prompt treatment of damaged skin reduces the risk of complications.

Visual problems

Diabetes is the leading cause of blindness in the UK. Diabetes affects the ability to see colours and contrasts. People with diabetes are more likely to develop cataracts and glaucoma. The most sight-threatening complication of diabetes is diabetic retinopathy. As our knowledge of the causes of retinopathy increases and treatment methods improve, the incidence of blindness can be reduced.

This session will explore:
- How diabetes affects vision
- How retinopathy affects vision
- How retinopathy can be prevented
- Screening for retinopathy
- Treatment of diabetic retinopathy

How diabetes affects vision

Diabetes affects the ability to see colours and contrasts. People with diabetes (including people who have been newly diagnosed) have difficulty distinguishing certain colours. The colours most difficult to distinguish are blues and yellows[67]. Difficulty in distinguishing colours and contrasts is associated with poor diabetic control and high glucose levels[68]. Retinopathy is the most sight-threatening eye condition associated with diabetes.

How retinopathy affects vision

Retinopathy occurs when the small blood vessels supplying the retina become diseased and close off. Other vessels dilate and attempt to provide the retina with sufficient blood. These dilated vessels leak.

Non-proliferative retinopathy
When the small blood vessels to the retina block, other vessels dilate in order to compensate. These vessels leak serous fluid and this forms into hard exudate. The dilated capillaries are weakened and the walls of the vessels leak, causing small haemorrhages in the retina. The person has no symptoms. Non-proliferative retinopathy does not endanger sight and does not require laser treatment.

Proliferative retinopathy
As the blood supply to the retina fails, the retina becomes ischaemic. New blood vessels develop in an attempt to provide a blood supply to the retina. These new blood vessels are fragile and bleed easily. They may bleed into

the vitreous body of the eye. They can lead to the formation of scar tissue. This scar tissue can cause the retina to detach as the scar tissue contracts. Proliferative retinopathy leads to painless loss of vision. If proliferative retinopathy is untreated it will lead to blindness within five years[69].

Diabetic maculopathy
Maculopathy is a form of diabetic retinopathy. The macula is the small area of the retina where best vision is concentrated. Hard exudate and oedema damage the macula. Vision gradually fails as macular oedema spreads[70].

Preventing retinopathy
The key to preventing retinopathy is to detect diabetes early; 40% of people with newly diagnosed type II diabetes have retinopathy. Early detection of diabetes would prevent complications[71]. The factors that lead to the development of retinopathy are:

- Longstanding diabetes
- Uncontrolled hypertension
- Chronic renal failure
- Poor diabetic control.

Preventing blindness

Twenty years after diabetes is diagnosed almost all insulin dependent diabetics have retinopathy. Almost two-thirds of people with type II diabetes have retinopathy[72]. Around 5% to 10% of people with retinopathy are in danger of losing their sight[73]. Control of hypertension reduces the risk of diabetic retinopathy. It also reduces the risk of stroke and renal damage. Ways to control hypertension are:

- Reduce salt in diet
- Reduce cholesterol
- No smoking
- Avoid obesity
- Increase physical activity
- Use ACE inhibitors to reduce blood pressure if above measures unsuccessful.

Chronic renal failure may well be established by the time the older person enters a nursing home. Good diabetic control will reduce the risk of retinopathy. Our aim must be to detect and treat retinopathy early before it progresses and sight is lost.

Detection and screening

One of the key features of the National Service Framework for diabetes is regular checkups for people with diabetes. The National Service Framework recommends annual eye screening to detect diabetic retinopathy. A screening programme should feature:

- Annual screening recall
- Measure visual acuity

- Dilate pupils to detect maculopathy
- Use retinal photography to examine retina
- Document results and inform consultant
- Emergency ophthalmology referral if sight-threatening retinopathy detected
- Refer to ophthalmologist if significant progression of retinopathy.

Treatment of retinopathy

Treatment of retinopathy is laser photocoagulation. Laser light is applied to a large part of the peripheral retina and destroys the new vessels. Most patients require several sessions to treat retinopathy. On an average course of treatment around 2000–5000 burns are required. Laser coagulation is uncomfortable and can be frightening. There is a blinding flash and a dreadful smell. An anaesthetic is often given to reduce pain. Laser therapy very seldom improves vision but in 90% of cases it prevents blindness[74].

Many people who have laser coagulation for retinopathy develop poor night vision. This can contribute to the risk of falls. Patients may also find bright sunlight intolerable and may need to wear sunglasses on sunny days. Some people suffer a loss of part of the visual field. Some people report that the overall quality of vision is reduced and that things look dull. One diabetic patient described it as 'looking through a dirty windscreen'.

Treating maculopathy

Less extensive laser treatment is required to treat maculopathy. Usually treatment takes 5 to 10 minutes. The laser seals off the leaking capillaries that are causing exudate and oedema in the macula. Around 50 to 200 burns are required. Laser treatment enables most patients to retain existing vision. The patient requires close follow up as further treatment may be required.

Conclusion

Improved diabetic control and screening procedures are reducing the incidence of blindness caused by diabetes. Early detection of diabetes and improved diabetes management are required to enable people with diabetes to retain their sight.

Key points

- Diabetes affects the ability to distinguish colours and contrasts
- Diabetes increases the risk of cataract
- Diabetic retinopathy is common
- Untreated diabetic retinopathy is sight-threatening
- Laser therapy preserves existing vision but can affect quality of vision
- Maculopathy can cause blindness
- Laser therapy preserves existing vision.

Further reading

Diabetes and your Eyes (1995) British Diabetic Association (now Diabetes UK), London.

Diabetes and Visual Impairment (1995) Information for people with diabetic retinopathy. British Diabetic Association (now Diabetes UK), London.

Prevention of Visual Impairment. Incorporating a report on a recommended minimum data set for collection in diabetic patients. A National Clinical Guideline recommended for use in Scotland by the Scottish Intercollegiate Guidelines Network (SIGN). Pilot edition, March 1996. Available from SIGN Secretariat, 9 Queen Street, Edinburgh EH2 1JQ.

Report of the Visual Handicap Group of the BDA/Department of Health St Vincent Joint Taskforce for Diabetes. *Diabetic Medicine* (1996) 13 (Suppl. 4), S13–S26.

Further information

Diabetes UK (formerly British Diabetic Association), 10 Parkway, London NW1 7AA. Tel. 020 7424 1000. Fax 020 7424 1001. website: www.diabetes.org.uk This organisation produces a number of useful publications including: *Diabetes and You. A guide for the older person. Diabetes Care Today: a guide for residential and nursing home managers and staff.* These are available free.

The Royal College of Nursing, 20 Cavendish Square, London W1M OAB Tel. 020 7409 3333. website: www.rcn.org.uk Produces a number of useful publications including: *Quality Assurance in Diabetes Nursing.* Royal College of Nursing Diabetes Nursing Forum. *Diabetes Clinical Guidelines for Practice Nurses,* 3rd edn (1994) Royal College of Nursing. (RCN publications are not yet available on its website.)

References

[1] Department of Health (2001) *National Service Framework for Diabetes Standards.* Department of Health, London. www.doh.gov.uk

[2] Stout, R.W. (1997) Old age and diabetes mellitus: 741–74–11. In: Pickup, J. & Williams, G. (eds) *Textbook of diabetes,* 2nd edn. Blackwell Science, Oxford.

[3] Alberti, K.G. (1997) The costs of non insulin dependent diabetes mellitus. *Diabetic Medicine,* **14**(1), 7–9.

[4] Meneilly, G.S. & Tessier, D. (1995) Diabetes in the elderly. *Diabetic Medicine,* **12**, 949–960.

[5] Sinclair, A.J. (1994) Diabetes care in the aged: time for a reappraisal. *Practical diabetes,* **11**(2), 60–62.

[6] Harris, M.I., Klein, R., Wellborne & Knuiman, M.W. (1992) Onset of non insulin dependent diabetes occurs at least 4–7 years before clinical diagnosis. *Diabetes Care,* **15**, 815–819.

[7] World Health Organisation (1999) *Definition, diagnosis and classification of Diabetes Mellitus and its complications.* Report of a WHO consultation. World Health Organisation, Department of Noncommunicable Diseases Surveillance, Geneva.

[8] Jerreat, Lynne (1999) *Diabetes for Nurses.* Whurr, London.

[9] World Health Organisation (1999) *Definition, diagnosis and classification of Diabetes Mellitus and its complications.* Report of a WHO consultation. World Health Organisation, Department of Noncommunicable Diseases Surveillance, Geneva.

10 Vadheim, C.M. & Rotter, J.I. (1992) Genetics of diabetes mellitus: 31–98. In: Alberti, K.G.M.M., De Fronzo, R.A., Keen, H. & Zimmer, P. (eds) *International Textbook of Diabetes Mellitus*. John Wiley & Sons, Chichester.

11 Zimmet, P.Z., Tuomi, T. & McKay, R. *et al.* (1994) Latent autoimmune diabetes in adults (LADA): the role of antibodies to glutamic acid decarboxylase in diagnosis and prediction of insulin dependency. *Diabetic Medicine*, **11**, 299–303.

12 Willis, J.A., Scott, R.S., Brown, L.J., Forbes, L.V., Schmidli, R.S. & Zimmet, P.Z. *et al.* (1996) Islet cell antibodies and antibodies against glutamic acid decarboxylase in newly diagnosed adult onset diabetes mellitus. *Diabetes Res. Clin. Pract.*, **33**, 89–97.

13 Zimmet, P.Z. (1995) The pathogenesis and prevention of diabetes in adults. *Diabetes Care*, **18**, 1050–1064.

14 Marks, L. (1996) *Counting the Cost. The real impact of non insulin dependent diabetes*. Kings Fund Policy Institute and British Diabetic Association, London.

15 British Diabetic Association (1996) *Diabetes in the United Kingdom*. A report by the British Diabetic Association, London.

16 Meneilly, G.S. & Tessier, D. (1995) Diabetes in the elderly. *Diabetic Medicine*, **12**, 949–960.

17 Group, C. & Tuomi, T. (1997) Non insulin dependent diabetes – a collision between thrifty genes and an affluent society. *Annals of Medicine*, **29**(1), 37–53.

18 Donnelly, R. & Garber, A. (1999) Proceedings of worldwide insulin resistance editorial board meeting. *Diabetes, Obesity and Metabolism*, **1**(suppl. 1), SV–S16.

19 Took, J. (1999) The association between insulin resistance and endiotheliopathy. *Diabetes, Obesity and Metabolism*, **1**(suppl. 1), S17–S22.

20 Currie, C.J. *et al.* (1996) Patterns of inpatient and outpatient acuity for diabetes; a district survey. *Diabetic Medicine*, **14**, 273–280.

21 Kings Fund (1996) *Counting the Cost. The real impact of non insulin dependent diabetes*. A report by the Kings Fund Policy Institute commissioned by the British Diabetic Association. Kings Fund, London.

22 Rohan, T.E., Frost, C.D. & Wald, N.J. (1989) Prevention of blindness by screening for retinopathy, a quantitative measurement. *British Medical Journal*, **299**, 1198.

23 Fox, C. & Pickering, A. (1995) *Diabetes in the Real World*. Class Publishing, London.

24 Bruce, J., McKennell, A. & Walker, E. (1991) *Blind and partial sighted adults in Britain: The RNIB Survey 1991*. The Stationery Office, London.

25 McKinnon, M. (1999) Type 2 Diabetes. *Nursing Standard*, **14**(10), 39–45.

26 Sinclair, A.J. (1994) Diabetes care in the aged: time for a reappraisal? *Practical Diabetes*, **11**(2), 60–62.

27 Harris, M.I., Klein, R., Wellbourne, T.A. & Knuiman, M.W. (1992) Onset of NIDDM occurs at least 4–7 years before clinical diagnosis. *Diabetes Care*, **15**, 815–819.

28 Burden, A.C. (1996) Quality of care, past present and future. Indo Asian Diabetics practical ways of improving care. *Practical Diabetes International Supplement*, **13**(3), 52–53.

29 Groop, L.C. (1997) Drug treatment of non insulin dependent diabetes mellitus. In: Pickup, J. & Williams, G. (eds) *Textbook of Diabetes*, 2nd edn. Blackwell Science, Oxford.

30 Grant, J. & Marsden, P. (1991) Module three oral hypoglaecaemic therapy. In: *Diabetes Care in General Practice*. Eli Lilly, Basingstoke.

31 Groop, L.C. (1997) Drug treatment of non insulin dependent diabetes mellitus. In: Pickup, J. & Williams, G. (eds) *Textbook of Diabetes*, 2nd edn. Blackwell Science, Oxford.

[32] Meneilly, G.S. & Tessier, D. (1995) Diabetes in the elderly. *Diabetic Medicine*, **12**, 949–960.

[33] Sinclair, A. (1995) Initial management of non insulin dependent diabetes mellitus in the elderly. In: Finucane, P. & Sinclair, A.J. (eds) *Diabetes in Old Age*. Wiley, Chichester.

[34] Reasner, C.A. (1999) Promising new approaches. In: Donnelly, R. & Garber, A. Proceedings of a Worldwide Insulin Resistance Editorial Board Meeting. *Diabetes, Obesity and Metabolism* (suppl. 1).

[35] Lehman, J.M. et al. (1995) An antidiabetic thiazolinedione is a high affinity ligand for peroxisome proliferator activated receptor gamma (PPARy). *Journal of Biological Chemistry*, **270**(22), 12953–12956.

[36] UK Prospective diabetes study (1998) (UKPDS 33) Intensive blood glucose control with Sulphonylureas or insulin compares with conventional treatment the risk of complications in patients with type 2 diabetes. *Lancet*, **352**, 837–853.

[37] UK Prospective diabetes study (1998) (UKPDS 34). Effect of intensive blood glucose control with Metformin on complications in overweight patients with type 2 diabetes. *Lancet*, **352**, 854–865.

[38] Patel, J. et al. (1998) Rosiglitazone (BR49653) monotherapy has a significant blood glucose lowering effect in type 2 diabetic patients. *Diabetes* (suppl. 1) A17 abstract 0067.

[39] Lister, C.A. et al. (1999) Rosiglitazone increases pancreatic islet area and number and insulin content but not insulin gene expression. *Diabetologia*, **42**(suppl. 1) abstract 869.

[40] Charbonnel, B. et al. (1999) Rosiglitazone is superior to glyburide in reducing fasting plasma glucose after 1 year of treatment in type 2 diabetic patients. The 59th scientific sessions of the American Diabetes Association. *Diabetes*, **48**(suppl. 1) abstract 0494.

[41] Robertson, R.P., Davis, C., Larsen, J., Stratta, R. & Sutherland, D.E.R. (2000) Pancreas and islet transplantation for patients with diabetes mellitus. Technical review. *Diabetes Care*, **23**, 112–116.

[42] Audit Commission (2000) *Testing Times*. Audit Commission Publications, Oxford. For summary see website: www.audit-commission.gov.uk

[43] Meneilly, G.S. & Tessier, D. (1995) Diabetes in the elderly. *Diabetic Medicine*, **12**, 949–960.

[44] Palinkas, L.A., Barrett-Connor, E. & Wingard, D.L. (1991) Type 2 diabetes and depressive symptoms in older adults: a population study. *Diabetic Medicine*, **8**, 532–539.

[45] Meneilly, G.S. & Cheung, E. (1993) The effect of improved glaecemic control of cognitive functions in the elderly patient with diabetes. *Journal of Gerontology*, **48**, M117–M121.

[46] Ha, T. & Lean, M.E.J. (1997) Diet and lifestyle modification in the management of non insulin dependent diabetes mellitus. In: Pickup, J. & Williams, G. (eds) *Textbook of diabetes*, 2nd edn. Blackwell Science, Oxford.

[47] Gale, E.A.M. (1996) Insulin Lispro: the first insulin analogue to reach the market. *Practical Diabetes International*, **13**(4), 122–124.

[48] De Week, A.L. (1992) Immune response and ageing. Constitutive and environmental aspects. In: Munro, H. & Schlierf, G. (eds) *Nutrition and the Elderly*. Raven Press, New York.

[49] American Diabetes Association (2000) Immunisation and the prevention of influenza and pneumococcal disease in people with diabetes. *Diabetes Care*, **23**(suppl. 1), 1–7. Clinical Practice recommendations 2000.

[50] Gatling, W., Hill, R. & Kirby, M. (1997) Hypoglycaemia prevention and treatment. In: *Shared Care for Diabetics*. Isis Publishing, Oxford.

51 Lewis, M.J., Ferguson, S.C., Campbell, I.W. & Nowroz (1996) A very unusual case of hyperosmolar coma. *Practical Diabetes International*, **13**(6), 195–197.

52 Kings Fund (1996) *Counting the Cost. The real impact of non insulin dependent diabetes*. A report by the Kings Fund Policy Institute commissioned by the British Diabetic Association. Kings Fund, London.

53 Yudkin, J.S., Blauth, C., Drury, P.L., Fuller, J., Henley, T., Lankester, M. & Lean, M. *et al.* (1996) Prevention and management of cardiovascular disease in patients with diabetes mellitus: an evidence base. *Diabetic Medicine*, **13**, S101–S121.

54 Yudkin, J.S., Blauth, C., Drury, P.L., Fuller, J., Henley, T., Lankester, M. & Lean, M. *et al.* (1996) Prevention and management of cardiovascular disease in patients with diabetes mellitus: an evidence base. *Diabetic Medicine*, **13**, S101–S121.

55 Neil, H.A.W., Gatling, W., Mather, H.M., Thompson, A.V., Thorogood, M., Fowler, G.H., Hill, R.D. & Mann, J.L. (1987) The Oxford Community Diabetes Study: evidence for an increase in the prevalence of known diabetes in Great Britain. *Diabetic Medicine*, **4**, 539–543.

56 Morris, A.D., McAlpine, R., Steinke, D., Boyle, D.I., Ebrahim, A.R., Vasudev, N., Stewart, C.P., Jung, R.T., Leese, G.P., MacDonald, T.M. & Newton, R.W. (1998) Diabetes and lower limb amputations in the community. A retrospective cohort study. DARTS/MEMO Collaboration Diabetes Audit and Research in Tayside Scotland/Medicines Monitoring Unit. *Diabetes Care*, **25**(5), 738–743.

57 Lavery, L.A., Ashry, H.R., van Houtum, W., Pugh, J.A., Harkless, L.B. & Basu, S. (1996) Variation in the incidence and proportion of diabetes related amputations in minorities. *Diabetes Care*, **19**(1), 48–52.

58 Lavery, L.A., van Houtum, Armstrong, D.G., Harkless, L.B., Ashry, H.R. & Walker, S.C. (1997) Mortality following lower limb amputation in minorities with diabetes mellitus. *Diabetes Res. Clin. Pract.*, **37**(1), 41–47.

59 British Diabetic Association (1997) *Diabetes Care: What you should expect*. British Diabetic Association, London.

60 Mueller, M.J., Strube, M.J. & Allen, B.T. (1997) Therapeutic footwear can reduce plantar pressure with diabetes and transmetatarsal amputation. *Diabetes Care*, **20**(4), 637–641.

61 Edmonds, M., Boulton Buckingham, N. & Every, J. *et al.* (1997) Report of the diabetic foot and amputation group. *Diabetic Medicine*, **13**, S27–S42.

62 Rosenburg, C.S. (1990) Wound healing in the patient with diabetes mellitus. *Nursing Clinics of North America*, **25**, 247–261.

63 Bitar, M.S. (1998) Glucocorticoid dynamics and impaired wound healing in diabetes mellitus. *American Journal of Pathology*, **152**(2), 547–554.

64 Baker, L.L., Chambers, R., DeMuth, S.K. & Villar, F. (1997) Effects of electrical stimulation on wound healing in patients with diabetes. *Diabetes Care*, **20**(3), 405–412.

65 Weisz, G., Ramon, Y. & Melamed, Y. (1993) Treatment of the diabetic foot by hyperbaric oxygen. *Heureuah*, **124**(11), 678–681.

66 Schindl, M., Kerschan, K., Schindly, A., Schon, H., Heinzyl, H. & Schindl, L. (1999) Induction of complete wound healing in recalcitrant ulcers by low intensity laser irradiation depends on ulcer size and cause. *Photodermatology, Photoimmunology and Photomedicine*, **15**(1), 18–21.

67 Ismail, G.M. & Whitaker, D. (1998) Early detection of changes in visual function in diabetes mellitus. *Ophthalmic Physiol. Opt.*, **18**(1), 3–12.

68 Ewing, F.M., Deary, I.J., Strachan, M.W. & Frier, B.M. (1998) Seeing beyond retinopathy and psychophysical abnormalities. *Endocrine Review*, **19**(4), 462–476.

[69] Marks, L. (1996) *Counting the Cost. The real impact of non insulin dependent diabetes*. Kings Fund Policy Institute and British Diabetic Association, London.

[70] McKinnon, M. (1999) Type 2 Diabetes. *Nursing Standard*, **14**(10), 39–45.

[71] Effective Health Care Bulletin (1999) Complications of diabetes. Screening for retinopathy, management of foot ulcers. *Effective Care Bulletin*, **5**, 4.

[72] Sjølie, A.K., Stephenson, J., Aldington, S., Kohner, E., Janka, H., Stevens, L. & Fuller, J. (2001) Retinopathy and vision loss in insulin-dependent diabetes in Europe. The EURODIAB IDDM Complications Study. *Ophthalmology*, **104**(2), 252–260.

[73] Effective Health Care Bulletin (1999) Complications of diabetes. Screening for retinopathy, management of foot ulcers. *Effective Care Bulletin*, **5**, 4.

[74] Kohner, E., Allwinkle, J., Andrews, R., Baker, R., Brown, F., Cheng, H. & Gray, M. *et al.* (1996) Report of the visual handicap group. *Diabetic Medicine*, **13**(suppl. 4), S13–S26.

Chapter 16

Respite Care

Introduction

When I wrote the first edition of this book, *Nursing in Nursing Homes*, in 1995 I hoped that social services departments would realise the importance of respite care. The eligibility net has drawn ever tighter and people who would once have been admitted to nursing and residential homes are cared for at home. This policy saves social services departments money but increases the pressure on relatives. An estimated seven million people care for older people at home. The majority of older people receiving care are in their eighties and nineties and are cared for by daughters, sons and other members of the family. Most carers are themselves in their sixties and seventies and may have health problems. Most carers provide care week after week and month after month without help or respite. Many carers have not had a night's unbroken sleep for years. Carers often find themselves unable to do things which we take for granted, such as go shopping, without a great deal of planning and organisation. Carers who provide care without help eventually find that their own physical and psychological health suffers. Many older people are admitted permanently to nursing homes because the carer has become ill or can no longer continue to provide care.

The aim of respite care is to ensure that carers have a break from caring. This break may be on a regular planned basis. The older person may have two weeks respite care followed by six weeks at home. In some cases respite care is organised because the carer can no longer cope, perhaps because of illness or exhaustion. The aim of respite care is to enable an older person to return home.

At the moment much attention, energy and funding are being directed to rehabilitation (see Chapter 17 for details). Rehabilitation is very important but it is equally important that we do not forget that respite care often enables carers to care for longer, and delays or prevents permanent admission to homes.

This chapter aims to enable you to:

- Understand the older person's fears and anxieties
- Understand the carer's view
- Provide care that allays fears and anxieties and promotes confidence
- Avoid problems associated with respite care

The older person's view of respite care

Older people can feel extremely anxious about the prospect of being admitted to a nursing home for respite care. The older person would usually prefer to remain at home. The prospect of entering a home rarely appeals. The home may be clean, bright and nicely decorated but the older person often feels they are being 'put away'. In an emergency situation when the carer is no longer able to cope, admission can take place within a few hours. The older person who was happy at home is suddenly told that they have to be looked after in a home until the situation is resolved. Many older people fear that they will never again leave the nursing home and that they have been dumped. You must be sensitive to the older person and must be aware of the fears and anxieties that often accompany such admissions. You must, however, be careful not to reassure an older person that they will definitely return home if this may not be possible. The nurse should be open and honest with the older person; giving assurances about circumstances that are outside the nurse's control can be unethical and will adversely affect the nurse/patient relationship.

Planned respite care is less traumatic for the older person. The individual has an opportunity to meet the staff and residents, see the room and find out about the home before admission. The older person may still fear that respite care may become permanent; these fears are normally allayed after the first successful period of respite care. Older people often benefit enormously from a period of respite care. Assessment by the nurse often uncovers ongoing problems or unmet needs that can begin to be met during the period of respite care. This care can be continued on discharge.

Case history

Betty McKay was admitted to a nursing home for respite care while her daughter attended her son's wedding in Australia. On admission Betty was wearing incontinence pads. She visited the toilet every 15 minutes but leaked in between. Her daughter explained that Betty had not had a proper night's sleep for some months because she had to keep going to the toilet. Betty's doctor had said it was due to her age and the fact that she had had six children. A continence assessment revealed that Betty was faecally impacted and a urine specimen sent for culture and sensitivity indicated that she also had a urinary tract infection. Disimpaction, dietary advice and a diet rich in fibre ensured that Betty opened her bowels regularly and did not suffer from constipation.

Antibiotic therapy, advice about fluids, an adequate fluid intake and advice on wiping herself from front to back to avoid reinfection resolved the urinary tract infection. Betty found that she only needed to go to the toilet every couple of hours and only had to get up once in the night to pass urine. Her general health improved and she was no longer forced to rely on pads for protection. Betty enjoyed meeting people of her own age and taking part in the activities of the home. She returned home having benefited from her period of respite care.

The carer's view of respite care

Carers often only consider asking for respite care when they have reached the end of their tether. The carer is often exhausted and angry that he or she has been left to care alone for so long without help. At the same time the carer often feels guilty that she is no longer able to cope and she is convinced that no one will be able to provide care of the same standard as that given at home. Carers are sometimes criticised by other family members for seeking respite care.

The carer enters the nursing home with mixed emotions and can appear prickly and extremely critical. The empathic nurse will be aware of the carer's feelings and will do everything possible to allay fears, anxieties and guilt. Some carers fear that nurses will secretly condemn them for being weak and unable to cope. Nurses who recognise the carer's achievement in caring for the older person, perhaps saying, 'You've done a marvellous job but you must be looking forward to a break', can help the carer to come to terms with fears and anxieties.

Carers benefit from a break and from having time to do what they want without having to worry about caring for the older person. Carers who have access to respite care are able to continue providing care for longer. Often respite care enables the carer to continue providing care at home without ever seeking long-term admission. Nurses are also aware of services that would help a carer when the older person returns home. They can help carers gain access to services or can persuade carers to accept services which have been offered but declined.

The nurse's view of respite care

Respite care is a new, challenging and rewarding development in nursing homes. In the past, many older people entered nursing homes and remained there until death. Even older people who had recovered well after illness were unable to return home because the services they required in the community did not exist or because the person's home had to be sold to pay for care. Respite care enables nurses to assess and offer care to older people and their carers. Older people often show physical and psychological improvement when they receive skilled nursing care. Carers also benefit, changing from the terse individual who appears strained almost to breaking point, to a more contented and relaxed individual.

Nurses looking after individuals on regular respite schemes find that it takes the older person some time to settle into the home and build a relationship with staff and patients. If a few individuals are using the same respite bed on a rota basis, a number of things can help each individual settle into the home more easily on admission and readmission. Carers can be asked to provide personal possessions which remain in the home. A colour photocopy (or a print if the negative is available) in a picture frame, like the one the older person has at home, a bedspread, a table lamp and other treasured items as similar as possible to the ones at home, can be supplied to the nursing home. These items can be placed in the room prior to admission so that it looks as if they have been brought from home and the room has been undisturbed since the individual's last stay. Surrounding the older person with belongings from the home environment makes the room homely and welcoming.

When the individual is returning home these items can be placed in a cardboard box with the person's name on it and stored until re-admission The room can then be repersonalised for the next re-admission. The use of primary nursing ensures that the older person is able to build up a relationship with the primary nursing team more readily than with a large group of nurses. Admissions should, whenever possible, be planned so that the primary nurse (or a member of the primary nursing team) is present. This ensures continuity of care and both older adults and their carers find this reassuring.

Respite care can make a real difference to the physical and psychological health of older people and their carers. Providing that care is incredibly rewarding and is a real morale booster for nurses.

Social services' view of respite care

Social Services Departments (SSDs) are currently responsible under the Community Care Act (CCA) for identifying need and purchasing services to meet the identified need. They have been allocated funds from central government to enable them to purchase care.

Respite care is crucial if SSDs are to meet their responsibilities under the CCA. SSDs or the new Care Trusts must develop a strategy that offers a range of care to take account of the needs and wishes of older people and their carers. Respite care allows SSDs to use resources prudently. Funds which would provide one long-term care place can be used to provide four respite care places if two weeks respite is offered every eight weeks. Respite care enables carers to continue to provide care for as long as possible and can postpone or eliminate the need for long-term care. Older people are able to remain where they want to be – at home – and carers who are able to have regular breaks are less likely to suffer ill health themselves.

SSDs that offer regular respite care will be informed by care managers of an individual's condition and how the family are coping. Extra services can be offered to support carers who are experiencing difficulties. Respite care can be increased, a stay of a few months organised, or permanent care planned if this is required. SSDs can plan budgets more effectively, and can plan a programme of care that will reduce the need for crisis interventions which are traumatic for older people and their carers and disrupt care managers' normal work patterns.

Problems associated with respite care

Respite care should be planned and every effort should be made to ensure continuity of care on each admission. NHS respite services ensured that the older person always returned to a designated respite bed on the same ward. Social services respite care used a similar system. Social services departments (SSDs) are currently responsible for respite care. This will change as Care Trusts develop. Some SSDs have made every effort to ensure that older people receiving respite care in nursing homes receive such continuity of care. They have contracted with one or more homes to provide respite beds.

The SSD purchaser negotiates and agrees a price with the nursing home, which provides a respite bed for the use of the SSD. The home is paid an annual fee for the bed, which is reserved exclusively for the use of the SSD for respite care. Care managers meet their team leader and determine which of their clients require rotating respite care and the frequency of respite required.

The individuals and the carers are invited to visit the home, meet residents and staff and decide if they wish to take the place offered. A rota of three or four individuals and dates of admission and discharge is drawn up. A copy of this rota is given to the home, to the individuals who are booked for respite care, and to carers. Regular planned respite care in the same home ensures continuity of care and enables nurses, older people and carers to build up a relationship.

Unfortunately, some SSDs have not yet contracted with homes for regular respite care and organise it on an ad hoc basis. This is time consuming as care managers can spend hours searching for a bed that is booked for a set period, usually a fortnight. There is no opportunity for nurses to build up a relationship with the individual in such circumstances. In some cases the bed is booked for another individual for a fortnight but the same individuals rarely return to the home due to poor management. This conveyor belt system of respite care is fraught with difficulty, and older people can feel unhappy and unsettled by frequent changes of home. This system does not enable carers to plan a break and does little to allay their anxieties at leaving their loved one. Nurses find such respite care less rewarding than planned, rotating respite care.

Sometimes rotating respite care fails to work to plan. A carer may telephone at 11 AM to say they feel unable to continue to provide care. The next planned respite admission is due at 2 PM. The carers of the individual who is due for admission have booked their first holiday abroad in five years and there are no empty beds in the home. Intervention and the offer of respite care before carers reach breaking point can help avoid such problems.

Sometimes an individual can become ill and is too unwell to be discharged or transferred. In such circumstances the care manager, team leader or duty social worker should be contacted immediately.

Innovative models of care

Some social service departments have developed innovative schemes to enable carers to plan respite. In Bradford the local social services department assess the needs of older people and their carers and give out respite care vouchers. The vouchers enable the carer and the older person to purchase care in local nursing homes. The individual arranges admission with the home and pays with a voucher. If the home has a vacancy, one or more nights of care can be booked. Most carers are provided with 14 vouchers a year. If the older person and the carer are happy with the home, they return; if they wish to try another home they simply book in using the voucher scheme. The home submits the vouchers to social services for payment. Most homes find that older people return and are able to build up relationships with staff.

This scheme, like ad hoc purchasing arrangements, is dependent on homes having spare capacity when it is required. Many nursing homes are having a difficult time. As homes close there are fewer spare beds available for respite. In areas where there are bed shortages, social services may have to contract with homes to ensure that there are beds available for emergencies, otherwise the older person may have to be admitted to hospital.

Contracting with social services

Some social services departments advertise the fact that they wish to contract with nursing homes for respite care. Usually a set number of beds is advertised for individuals who require elderly mentally infirm (EMI) and elderly infirm care. Homes apply for a copy of a form, complete it, and the home is visited prior to contracting.

SSDs who are arranging care on an ad hoc basis may welcome an approach from a home willing to contract to provide respite services, especially if there is a shortage of beds in the area. It is important to establish who will be responsible for providing transport to and from the home. It is also important to determine who will be responsible for deciding which individuals will be admitted to the home and for ensuring that the SSD provides written notice of such admissions. This can easily be done using fax or email if this is an emergency admission.

If an SSD merely contracts with a home and circulates all care managers with details of the respite provision at the home, problems may arise. Each care manager may work out a rota and the number of respite places booked may far exceed the number contracted. The home may receive calls from several care managers who have all promised carers respite care over the same period. Care managers may compete with each other for places or book 26 patients into the home over a year so that each of their carers has a break. A break of two weeks a year is of little use to carers and may lead to increased demand for long-term care.

The contract should include contingency plans if an individual is unable to be discharged due to illness or if the carer is unable to continue providing care. Contracts are normally placed for one year but some social services departments are now contracting for longer periods because of uncertainty about the number of nursing home beds that will be available in the future.

In the future it seems likely that Care Trusts will be responsible for contracting.

Funding for respite care

Older people who are eligible for income support normally have respite care funded by social services. Older people with savings or property above income support levels were in the past expected to fund their own respite care. This changed when the NHS Plan and the government response to the Royal Commission on Long Term Care was released. Chapter 2 provides details of funding arrangements. Now the value of an older person's house is disregarded for the first 12 weeks of admission. Local authorities are interpreting this in different ways. Some will fund care (at social services rates) for up to 12 weeks; other local authorities insist that their care man-agers carry out complete assessments on the older person as though she were entering long-term care. This means that assessments can take many weeks to carry out. If the situation is desperate, families sometimes bypass the system and pay for care. Sometimes families cannot afford to do this and the older person is admitted to hospital because the system is so cumber-some that it cannot react to an urgent situation. The creation of Care Trusts will hopefully end such problems and prevent people being admitted unnecessarily to hospital beds when they require care and not treatment.

Supporting carers

Some carers find that their lives are empty when the older person enters the nursing home for respite care. Such carers normally visit within a few days of admission and stay for hours. They often offer to help nursing staff not only with caring for their own loved one but also with other residents. They offer to lay tables, serve meals, give out tea and help in any way possible. Some carers, especially those who have been living alone with the older person, have gradually lost touch with their friends. Leisure interests have been dropped and the carer's life has centred around the loved one. Carers can suddenly feel that their life has lost all purpose when the older person is admitted for respite care.

Planned respite care gives carers an opportunity to rebuild their lives and to expand their horizons once again. Carers may feel that they should come to the home and offer help; this situation should be handled with great care and tact. You do not want the carer to feel that she is unwelcome but must not make her feel that she *must* visit daily and help out. In some cases the carer wants you to give her 'permission' not to visit daily. The carer needs to come to terms with her wish to rebuild her own life without feeling that she has failed to care for the older person.

Most areas of the country have local carer support groups. Details are available from care managers, the local community health council or the local library. Carer support groups meet regularly and in addition to pro-viding support also have social functions. They usually offer a 'sitter scheme' and a volunteer gets to know the older person and the carer. The volunteer arranges to come and stay at the house while the carer attends carer support meetings or goes out. Carer support groups usually have volunteer drivers who can give carers lifts to local meetings. Many carers find that attending carer support groups helps to combat the terrible sense of isolation which can affect them. It also helps them to work through feelings of guilt and anxiety and provides a support network.

Useful address and telephone number

Local carers' support network

Liaising with other professionals and organising services

The nurse may discover that an older person admitted for respite care has been experiencing problems that require ongoing care. The older person may be unable to get into the bath at home, even with the carer's help. The procedures for organising assistance with bathing vary from area to area. In some areas the district nursing team are responsible for organising baths; in other areas district nursing services only take responsibility for 'medical baths' and social services departments take responsibility for 'social baths'. 'Medical baths' are baths that are required for medical reasons, for example because an individual has a continence problem, and are provided as part of NHS care. Individuals receiving 'social baths' are charged a fee if they have savings above income support levels.

The individual may require special footwear to accommodate oedema or bunions. The individual may be deaf and require an audiology appointment. Physiotherapy may help to improve mobility or reduce pain. Speech therapy may be required to help an individual to communicate. The older person may benefit from a walking aid. Details of how to obtain these services are given in Chapter 13.

It is important when accessing these services that the nurse writes a letter that is enclosed with the doctor's letter, giving details of the older person's whereabouts. This can state, for example, 'Mrs Daniels will be at her own home from 1 February until 14 March; from 14 to 28 of March she will be resident at the nursing home'. Both addresses and contact numbers should be given. This prevents individuals missing appointments because the letter has been sent to the home address and the individual is in the nursing home while the carer has gone away. Arranging ongoing services is extremely difficult if respite care is arranged on an ad hoc basis and the individual is admitted to a number of different homes.

The older person may have enjoyed mixing with others and may confess that she sometimes feels lonely at home and will miss the company. She may benefit from attending a luncheon club, a social services day centre or a day hospital once a week. The choice available will be dependent on the individual's ability, the facilities available at each place and availability of places. Some SSD-run day centres will not accept any older people who have continence problems or difficulty in walking, or require help going to the toilet, while others accept individuals requiring such help. Some NHS day hospitals have strict admission criteria and will only accept individuals requiring active treatment for limited periods. Nurses should check what facilities are available locally and on the criteria for acceptance.

Arranging discharge

In a planned, rotating, respite scheme, discharge dates are agreed prior to admission. If the older person becomes ill and is too unwell to return home, this should be discussed with the individual, the carer (if available), the doctor and the care manager. If respite was arranged for a limited period on an emergency basis, perhaps because the carer was ill, and the carer is still unwell, this should be discussed. It may be possible in these circumstances to extend the stay or to delay a planned admission.

The nurse should ensure that if the individual is taking prescribed medication, enough to last at least a week is given to the individual or the carer on discharge. If a district nurse has been treating the person at home, the district nurse should be informed of discharge. A letter should be sent if a wound has improved or changed significantly, or if different dressings are being used. If they are, a few dressings should be supplied for the district nurse to use. The nurse should ensure that the individual's doctor is aware of the person's whereabouts; providing details of the dates of planned respite can reduce paperwork.

Conclusion

Every Social Services Department should offer respite care as part of a range of facilities that fulfil the needs and respect the wishes of older people who wish to live at home, and of carers who wish to continue providing care at home. Respite care should normally be planned and offered on a regular basis. This enables older people to live at home while benefiting from ongoing assessment and care from nurses. Older people and carers are often anxious when respite care is first offered. Nurses should make every effort to allay anxieties and ensure continuity of care. Working with older people, carers and other professionals to ensure that older people can continue to live at home, is rewarding for the nurse.

Chapter 17

Rehabilitation

Introduction

When I wrote the first edition of this book, *Nursing in Nursing Homes*, I stressed the value of rehabilitation and said that failure to provide rehabilitation services was leading to unnecessary permanent admissions in nursing homes. Government has now recognised the value of rehabilitation and is investing £600 million into enabling older people to recover and return home[1].

This chapter aims to:

- Examine the evidence on rehabilitation
- Explain how purchasers should contract for rehabilitation
- Explain how to organise rehabilitation services within your home

---

Why is rehabilitation necessary?

In the early twentieth century few people survived long enough to pick up the newly introduced old age pension. Most people who lived beyond pension age died within a few years. Now people can look forward to 25 to 30 years of life after retirement. Figure 17.1 illustrates the rising numbers of people surviving into extreme old age in the UK.

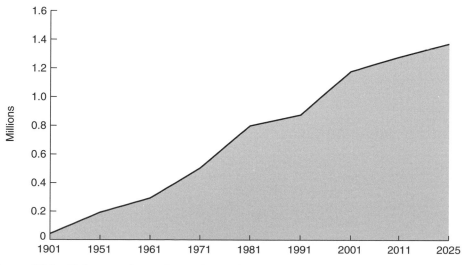

Figure 17.1 Rising numbers of people aged 85+.

Improved nutrition and sanitation and medicines such as antibiotics increased lifespan. Sometimes some of the additional years of life that individuals gained were marred by disability and loss of function. In the late twentieth century policymakers were alarmed by 'the rising tide of elderly' and worried that their demands would swamp the NHS. Government policy concentrated on moving older people through the system at speed. This policy of discharging people 'quicker and sicker' was an exercise in futility. Older people who had the potential to recover were denied the opportunity to do so and were forced into permanent nursing home care[2]. Readmission rates soared; in one study 33% of older people discharged from hospital were readmitted within a month[3]. One study found that 43% of older people discharged home were readmitted within two months[4].

Community care was set up to offer low levels of assistance to large numbers of older people, not to provide high levels of care to people who had not fully recovered from illness or injury. Social services departments changed their focus and began to concentrate on providing care to highly dependent older people in their own homes to avoid nursing home placements. In many cases this meant that people with lower levels of need and people with carers found that they were unable to access help that they needed.

Social services departments, lacking expertise in health care, sought to provide care without considering an individual's potential to recover lost abilities. We returned to the situation of the 1930s when the 'chronic sick' were written off. The challenge of adding life to years and enabling older people to function to capacity was ignored for decades because policy makers could not see the big picture. In 2000 government announced that it would invest in giving older people the same opportunities to rehabilitate after accident and injury that younger people have always taken for granted.

What is intermediate care?

Intermediate care aims to reduce avoidable hospital admissions, to enable older adults to function to capacity and to prevent avoidable institutionalisation. The NHS Plan considers that intermediate care will provide a bridge between home and hospital. Intermediate care units will function by 'helping people recover and resume independent living more quickly'[5]. Intermediate care can function in a number of ways, as outlined in Table 17.1.

Defining rehabilitation

Government appear to be using the terms rehabilitation and intermediate care as though they were the same thing, but they are different. When government speak of intermediate care they refer to both step down and rehabilitation services. Step down and rehabilitation services are both rehabilitation services; the main differences lie in the severity of disablement and the complexity of care required to re-enable. Generally people suitable for fast stream rehabilitation have simple rehabilitative needs. The lucid person who fractures a femur requires straightforward care to enable them

Table 17.1   Types of intermediate care.

Type	Use	Examples
Subacute	Prevention of hospital admission	<ul><li>Care of an older person with a chest infection in a nursing home setting avoiding the need for hospitalisation</li><li>Providing emergency care and support when primary carer unwell or unable to cope</li></ul>Duration approximately 2 weeks
Step down (fast stream rehabilitation)	Freeing up hospital beds	<ul><li>Early discharge following repair of fractured femur</li><li>Providing skill care and support to enable person to return home</li></ul>Duration approximately 2 weeks
Rehabilitation (slow stream rehabilitation)	Preventing acute hospital beds being blocked because people require ongoing rehabilitation. Can be combined with step down care	<ul><li>Ongoing re-enablement following stroke. Nurse led inter-disciplinary care</li></ul>Duration approximately 6–12 weeks

to regain mobility and other abilities. A person who fractures a femur and has successful surgery but develops postoperative complications, such as stroke with associated swallowing, communication and continence problems, will require complex slow stream rehabilitation.

Rehabilitation is the process of enabling a person to regain the highest possibly level of ability after illness or injury. The characteristics of rehabilitation are[6]:

- Is centred around the needs, desires, hopes and aspirations of the individual
- Is interdisciplinary though it may be led by a particular discipline
- Is not limited to therapeutic interventions
- Involves social and environmental interventions
- Has specific objectives within a specific time frame
- Is an ongoing process that is not restricted to the time frame of a formal programme
- Can take place in a range of settings such as hospitals, nursing homes, day centres or the person's own home.

The benefits of rehabilitation

Reorganising our health care system to enable older people to recover following illness and accident is not only humane but also cost effective. Structured rehabilitation programmes could enable at least 20% of people currently cared for in nursing homes to return home[7]. Rehabilitation need not be a threat to nursing homes – it merely involves a change of focus from long-term care to a mixture of long-term, rehabilitation and respite care. The home has three different but complementary types of care provision.

Since the introduction of the community care component of the NHS and Community Care Act in 1993, social services departments have had powerful incentives to admit people with nursing needs to residential homes. Residential homes are less expensive than nursing homes because staffing levels are lower and registered nurses are not employed. Nursing needs are provided by district nursing staff and the costs of district nursing are met by health authorities and not from social services budgets. Many older people who require nursing care are cared for in residential homes[8]. The incentive to place people requiring nursing care in residential homes is now disappearing. In October 2001 government began to fund the costs of registered nursing care of self-funding residents. This scheme will be expanded to cover people funded by social services in April 2003, and the incentive to ignore a person's nursing needs will vanish. If 20% of people admitted to nursing homes could benefit from structured rehabilitation programmes to enable them to return home, an even greater number of people admitted to residential care could also benefit. Rehabilitation services could also be used to rehabilitate people receiving home care. This would enable older people to live more independently and would cut the burgeoning costs of home care.

Rehabilitation services can help ensure that public funds are spent wisely. Efficient use of public funds will enable people to function to capacity. This will reduce the overall costs of care and enable government to introduce systems that provide the right level of care in the right setting with the right resources.

Current rehabilitation policy

The money for rehabilitation services has now come on-stream but there is little evidence of strategic planning. There have been a number of short-lived projects but there is little evidence of a national rehabilitation strategy.

The Victoria Hospital Project in Blackpool was set up in 1998 using winter pressures funding. It was jointly managed by health and social services. Three nursing homes provided care for 26 patients after day surgery. Patients were provided with four days of nursing home care after surgery. Twenty-five of the patients were discharged home after four days; one patient required a further day's nursing home care. When the pilot concluded successfully North West Lancashire Health Authority was unable to find additional funds to continue this work.

The South London total purchasing pilot was set up in 1997. It aimed to prevent unnecessary hospital missions and speed up discharges. A combination of beds in nursing homes, the local geriatric hospital and hospital at home were used to enable early discharge from acute hospital beds. This small project prevented hospital admissions and reduced time spent in acute hospitals.

The East Lancashire fractured neck of femur pilot was launched in 2000. This six-month pilot used six nursing home beds to free up acute beds and provide nursing home-based rehabilitation. Patients were transferred 3–5 days post operatively. The nursing home provided rehabilitative nursing care; physiotherapy and occupational therapy were provided by hospital staff who visited the home. The average stay was two weeks and 90% of patients were discharged home within two weeks. This project delivered effective rehabilitation at half the cost of acute NHS care.

In the absence of a national rehabilitation strategy, projects such as those described above are often unable to secure continuing funding. There is a danger that money provided for rehabilitation will be swallowed up in NHS running costs and older people will not obtain rehabilitation services.

Successful rehabilitation programmes

Successful rehabilitation programmes are well planned and have structures in place to enable the team to succeed. The most important characteristics of successful programmes are that they are patient-centred, involve comprehensive assessment, have clear goals, foster teamwork and interdisciplinary record keeping and have a designated manager. The patient must be at the centre of the rehabilitation programme. It is important to discuss the person's choices and to develop a working partnership with the person.

Assessment, the keystone of community care, is crucial in rehabilitation[9]. Assessment enables professionals to determine an individual's potential for rehabilitation. It enables professionals to determine whether fast or slow stream rehabilitation is most appropriate. At the moment different assessment tools are used in different parts of the UK. The assessment tool used affects the person's access to services. The use of non-standardised assessment tools is unfair[10]. Few assessment tools provide the information required to assess an individual's potential for rehabilitation. We need to develop a standardised assessment tool to determine rehabilitation potential if we are to offer fair access to rehabilitation services. Rehabilitation of people in their eighties and nineties is a new concept and research is required to enable the development of an effective and comprehensive assessment. When comprehensive assessment and goal planning are implemented the risks of an individual requiring hospital treatment or long stay care are reduced[11] and physical and mental function can increase by 35%[12]. Comprehensive assessment enables the rehabilitation team to set clear goals. It is important that goals are patient-centred and agreed with the patient and the team. These goals must be appropriate to the individual and realistic. They should be recorded and regularly re-evaluated to check progress[13]. Many of the rehabilitation schemes currently running do not regularly re-evaluate goals and it is difficult to determine how effective they are.

Joint record keeping is extremely important but relatively rare. If professionals are to offer holistic care they require access to each other's records so that they can all pursue the same goals and offer coherent care. Teamwork is essential when rehabilitation services are being delivered. Rehabilitation requires a wider range of competencies and expertise than any one professional group can provide[14]. It can be difficult for individual therapists who may visit the patient at different times to work together as a team. Successful rehabilitation schemes have a designated manager who manages care and co-ordinates the roles of therapists to ensure that goals are met. Each team member should be able to give a clear explanation of how the team is managed and how individual therapists are contributing to the person's rehabilitation programme.

Purchasing care

Health and social service purchasers are being asked to do something they have never been asked to do before – work in partnership with voluntary and independent sector providers to develop rehabilitation schemes. The money is flowing and the pressure is on to get schemes up and running. In such circumstances there is a temptation to pay insufficient attention to the planning process. This can lead to purchasers buying services they want although those services may not be those that the community they serve needs.

What type of care?

It is important that purchasers work out the needs of the community they serve. Most communities will require a range of rehabilitation services. It is important for purchasers to prioritise and to launch one scheme at a time.

Who are the services for?

If the purchaser does not have clear assessment and eligibility criteria there is a danger that rehabilitation beds can be used as 'dumping grounds' or 'hotel services'. The following is an example of clear assessment and eligibility criteria (based on Sheffield community rehabilitation criteria):

- Over 65 years old and would benefit from rehabilitation
- Willing and able to actively participate in rehabilitation programme
- Has the potential to improve physical function
- Is medically stable
- Does not have severely limited verbal and non-verbal problems comprehending
- Has no severe swallowing problems
- Is not suffering from significant dementia
- Is not suffering from behavioural problems
- Is not suffering from a depressed level of consciousness.

The above criteria exclude some people because their ability to participate is impaired. There is evidence that people with dementia can benefit from specialist rehabilitation facilities tailored to their specific needs.

How many places?

Purchasers need to consider the number of people to whom they aim to offer rehabilitation services. It is tempting to try to treat the maximum number of people by reducing length of stay. This can be counterproductive because older people take longer to recover than younger people so it is important to be realistic about the time people require to regain abilities. It is also important to avoid blocking rehabilitation beds as this can deny people access to rehabilitation services. Purchasers must balance these two issues and determine realistic minimum and maximum lengths of stay. When purchasers have determined the type of services required, eligibility criteria and the likely length of stay, they can examine therapy services.

Therapy services

Some nursing homes provide a total package of care and therapy services. Some provide a full range of nursing and care services but therapists employed by the NHS acute or community trust visit the home to provide therapy services. Purchasers need to be clear about who is to provide therapy services.

What type of contract?

Purchasers need to decide how many beds they need to purchase and on what basis they are purchasing. There are two options: spot and block contracts. Under a spot contract the scheme manager finds a bed in a local nursing home when the person is ready for discharge from acute care. Table 17.2 outlines the costs and benefits of spot contracts.

Table 17.2 Benefits and costs of spot contracts.

Benefits	Costs
Cost effective – the bed is only paid for when it is used	Inability to find beds may lead to discharge delays
Set-up costs minimised	Requires manager to locate bed so ongoing management costs higher
No long-term financial commitment	Homes may not wish to participate and may prefer long-term care residents because of financial uncertainty
	Little influence on quality of service provision
	Difficulty in ensuring quality control because contracting with different providers

If purchasers decide to purchase beds on a spot contract basis they need to be sure that homes in the area have sufficient excess capacity to provide short-term beds at short notice. The nursing home sector is contracting and there are bed shortages in many areas.

Under a 'block contract' the purchaser buys a number of beds for a set period, usually after tendering. The period ranges from one to ten years and beds are paid for regardless of occupancy. Table 17.3 outlines the costs and benefits of block contracts.

Purchasers need to be clear about the standard of facilities they require.

Table 17.3   Benefits and costs of block contracts.

Benefits	Costs
Access to beds is guaranteed	Costs are fixed though demand may vary – purchaser must ensure beds used effectively. Some schemes have 50% occupancy
Possible to develop collaborative partnerships	Purchaser locked into scheme for set period so unable to take advantage of market changes
Provider can afford to invest in staff development	Costs per bed may be higher than if using spot contracts
Purchaser can influence service provision	May be difficult to terminate contract if provider does not deliver

The length of proposed stay influences costs as short stay admissions increase costs by around 25%.

Standards of care

Purchasers need to determine the standards of care and quality required and to identify indicators that the home has the ability to deliver these standards.

A designated unit

National minimum standards require homes offering rehabilitation services to provide a dedicated unit. This standard may deter homes from developing rehabilitation services unless purchasers are unable to purchase ten or more beds on a contract basis. Few homes will be able to afford to set aside a dedicated unit on the off chance that social services will purchase on a spot contract basis.

Medical services

People participating in rehabilitation programmes require a range of medical services. They require medical oversight and may require emergency and out-of-hours medical care. Purchasers need to be clear about who will provide medical services. Sometimes consultants take responsibility for a person's medical rehabilitation but are seldom willing or able to provide out-of-hours and emergency medical cover.

Transport

The person may need to visit hospital-based specialists while in the nursing home. Purchasers need to decide who will provide transport to outpatients' appointments. Will the Trust provide transport or will the home be required to do this? If the home is to provide an escort, can arrangements be made to reduce delays in outpatients? This is important because if the person spends a day in outpatients, a day's therapy may be lost. These issues are particularly important when a person is having fast stream rehabilitation.

Laundry services

People who are participating in rehabilitation programmes dress each day. In hospital-based rehabilitation programmes staff depend on relatives to launder clothing. Purchasers need to be clear about whether they will expect relatives to launder clothes or if they wish the home to provide laundry services.

Dental services

Diseases such as stroke and Parkinson's affect the ability to eat, and inability to eat can impair health. Quality dental services are an important aspect of care[15]. Purchasers need to consider the best way to provide dental services. Will the person be required to use his or her own dentist? This may not be practical if people are being drawn from a wide catchment area. Will the community dentist be able to visit the home? If this is not possible then the purchaser will need to check what arrangements the home has to provide dental services.

Diet

Purchasers need to consider the level of catering services required. Can the home provide nutritious food that meets the dietary needs of the people they will care for? Will the home be able to provide a range of choices and special diets?

Equipment

Nursing homes provide equipment such as hoists and pressure relieving overlays and mattress replacements. If specialist equipment is required this should be specified.

Footwear services

Specialist footwear can enable people to regain mobility and reduce the risk of falls. If the rehabilitation unit caters for people likely to require orthotist services, such as people recovering from stroke, purchasers should check if the orthotist could visit the home on a sessional basis to avoid outpatients' appointments disrupting therapy programmes.

Management

Successful rehabilitation services have a designated manager who integrates the work of therapists and ensures goals are evaluated and holistic care delivered. Managing rehabilitation services is not a task that can be added to a busy manager's job description. Successful rehabilitation schemes need a dedicated manager who has expertise in the care of older people and in rehabilitation. Purchasers need to be clear about who will manage the service. Some purchasers appoint a manager; others ask the home to provide a manager.

Costs

When the purchaser has identified the key elements required to deliver the service and how these are to be provided, the costs of providing the service can be calculated. Quality rehabilitation services are not cheap and it is inappropriate to attempt to deliver them at the same cost as long-term care. In London, at the time of writing, purchasers pay providers £700–£900 a week for quality rehabilitation services. This fee includes physiotherapy, occupational therapy and out-of-hours medical services. In the north-west of England purchasers pay £400 a week for quality care services. NHS staff provide therapy services in the homes.

Contract issues

It is important to decide how long the contract should run. Medium to long contracts encourage commitment but purchasers need to ensure that they retain the ability to terminate contracts if circumstances change. Contracts should be reviewed at least once a year because the purchaser or the provider may wish to change the specifications.

Providing rehabilitation services

At the moment, preparing to offer rehabilitative care requires a leap of faith and an element of risk. Preparing for rehabilitation services demands considerable time and energy. It can also involve capital investment and investment in staff education and training. It is vital to check if there is any demand for rehabilitation services locally before making this investment. There is little point in gearing up for rehabilitation if the major purchaser in your area is about to award a 20 year contract to another home near yours. In such circumstances your home may prefer to concentrate on improving current services or setting up another service that is not provided locally.

Research

If local purchasers are interested in purchasing rehabilitation services you need to find out what type of services they are considering purchasing. If the purchaser wishes to purchase beds to rehabilitate people with dementia, the skills they require from the home's staff will be very different from those required to rehabilitate people following repair of fractured femur.

Managers need to ask themselves if they have expertise with the client group that will require services. If you have expertise in caring for that particular client group, you need to get as much detail about the service specification as possible. What services are purchasers interested in buying, and can you provide those services for the fees offered? It is important to evaluate service specifications and fees offered carefully. Will the fee offered enable you to deliver the specified services? Is the contract being offered on a secure medium to long-term basis? If you decide to offer rehabilitation services, you need to evaluate your ability to deliver.

Structure

The manager needs to evaluate the physical structure of the home and the structure of the organisation. Evaluating the structure of the home is straightforward. It is easy to decide if you can now or in the future offer a designated rehabilitation unit within the home. Deciding if you can provide the facilities that purchasers require is simple. Evaluating the structure of the organisation and the skill levels of staff is more complex. Managers need to examine the organisation dispassionately and work out what skill levels staff possess. In most homes staff will require education and training to enable them to provide rehabilitative care. Introducing annual appraisals (if these are not already in place) will enable you to identify skills gaps. If you have formalised systems of staff supervision these will help you to evaluate staff. It is important though that these evaluations take account of the fact that rehabilitation requires skills, such as the ability to work as part of a multi-disciplinary team, that may not have been considered critical when offering traditional long-stay care. Managers need to work out what further education staff require. You will need to examine ways to deliver that education; options include in-service training and education delivered by university staff in the home[16].

The culture of the home is important. Adopting a rehabilitative focus will turn many homes into very different places. Are staff willing and able to change? Do you have the ability to move the culture of the organisation forward? Most people underestimate the effort required to change an organisation's focus. It is important to create a sense of urgency and a feeling that the status quo is no longer acceptable. Staff need to feel that change is important or they will not make the sacrifices required to change the culture. If you feel that you do have the skills, remember that leaders are made not born. Leadership is 98% work – the rest is talent! Investigate management courses so that you can develop the skills to move the organisation forward.

Process

The term process describes the systems that the organisation has in place. Processes describe how the organisation does a certain thing. The home may have a process that aims to prevent the development of pressure sores. The process may involve risk assessment, using appropriate aids and taking certain actions to prevent pressure sores developing. Managers need to check that the home really has a system to assess, document and evaluate the type of rehabilitative care that will be delivered. The home should have processes such as resident and relative meetings and surveys that enable managers and staff to provide care that is responsive to resident requirements. You may have to develop new processes because the home will be doing new things in new ways. If you aim to offer step down care then it will be important to develop discharge questionnaires to find out what you do well, so that you can continue doing it, and what you do less well so that you can improve it. Remember, expectations of short-stay rehabilitation residents will be different from those for whom your home is their home.

Outcomes

The term outcome describes how effectively the organisation does a certain thing. It measures how effectively the structure and process deliver the desired outcomes. Is the home successfully maximising mobility or are your staff too 'helpful' and offering wheelchairs instead of encouraging walking?

Many homes will be competing for contracts for rehabilitation beds. The homes that will succeed will be those that can demonstrate successful outcomes. It is important that these outcomes are not restricted to professional goals. Outcome measures should also measure residents' perceptions of outcome. Well-planned structures such as staff education levels, equipment and facilities, and processes such as planning assessment and evaluation of care, should enable managers to evaluate outcomes. If the home does not have systems to measure resident perception of functional recovery, the manager may wish to work with purchasers to develop these measures. These measures will probably be as new to most purchasers as they are to managers.

Conclusion

Rehabilitation is a new and exciting area of nursing within nursing homes. For many staff, rehabilitation will involve a change of focus. It focuses on enablement and empowerment of older people so that they can regain abilities and go home again. Rehabilitation can at first appear threatening and overwhelming to staff because it implies that the care we give to long-stay residents is somehow less important. Nothing could be further from the truth; the care we offer to long-stay residents can also enable and empower, even if the person is no longer able to return home. This is explored more fully in Chapter 18.

References

[1] Department of Health (2000) *The NHS Plan: The Government's response to the Royal Commission on Long Term Care.* Presented to Parliament July 2000. CM4818–II. Available from The Stationery Office (Mail, telephone and fax orders only) PO Box 29, Norwich NR3 1GN. General enquiries 0870 600 5522. http://www.nhs.uk/nhsplan

[2] Nazarko, L. (1993) Out of the darkness. *Elderly Care*, **5**(3), 8.

[3] Tierney, A., Worth, A., Jose Closs, S., King, C. & McMillan, M. (1994) Older patient's experiences of discharge from hospital. *Nursing Times*, **90**(21), 36–39.

[4] Holzhausen, Emily (2001) *You can Take him Home now.* Carers National Association, London.

[5] Department of Health (2000) *The NHS Plan: A plan for investment a plan for reform.* Available from The Stationery Office (Mail, telephone and fax orders only) PO Box 29, Norwich NR3 1GN. General enquiries 0870 600 5522. http://www.nhs.uk/nhsplan

[6] Linda Hanford, Lorna Easterbrook, Jan Stevenson (1999) *Rehabilitation for older people: The emerging policy agenda.* Briefing paper 1. The Kings Fund Rehabilitation Programme Rehabilitation Opportunities for Older People, Kings Fund, London.

[7] Nazarko, L. (2001) Quality outcomes in rehabilitation. *Nursing Management*, **8**(2), 22–26.

[8] Schneider, Justine (1997) (ed.) *Quality of Care: Testing Some Measures in Homes for Elderly People.* Report of a study funded though Northern and

Yorkshire NHS Executive under the Department of Health Initiative. Discussion paper 1245. Personal Services Research Unit, University of Kent at Canterbury, Canterbury.

9   Robinson, J. & Turnock, S. (1998) *Investing in Rehabilitation*. King's Fund, London.

10 Stewart, S. (1999) The use of standardised and non standardised assessments in social service settings; implications for practice. *British Journal of Occupational Therapy*, **62**(9), 417–423.

11 Sinclair, A. & Dickinson, E. (1998) *Effective Practice in Rehabilitation: The Evidence of Systematic Reviews*. Kings Fund/Audit Commission, London.

12 Audit Commission (2000) *The Way to Go Home. Rehabilitation and remedial services for older people*. Audit Commission, London.

13 Young, J. (2000) Rehabilitation and older people. *British Medical Journal*, **313**, 677.

14 Hastings, M. (1996) Team working in rehabilitation. In: Squires, A. (ed.) *Rehabilitation of Older People*. A handbook for the multidisciplinary team. Chapman Hall, London.

15 Sheiham, A. & Steele, J. (2001) Does the condition of the mouth and teeth affect the ability to eat certain foods, nutrient and dietary intake and nutritional status amongst older people? *Public Health Nutr.*, **4**(3),797–803.

16 McGinlay, E. & Hawkey, B. (2001) Creating a rehabilitation training programme for nursing home staff. A university and private nursing home partnership. *Presentation at Kings Fund Workshop: Nursing Homes and Intermediate Care*, 8th January 2001. Kings Fund, London.

Chapter 18

Maximising Ability

Introduction

Older people often enter nursing homes at their lowest ebb, following a major life crisis. Illness, accident or the loss of a loved one can cause them to enter nursing home care. They have usually been moved from home to hospital to nursing home. Although efforts have been made to help heal physical damage they have often had little help in coming to terms mentally with a major life event. Older people who enter nursing homes have 'failed' to get better. Many have low expectations of themselves and of the nursing home; most older people would, given a choice, prefer to live at home, and some individuals feel that others have given up on them and transferred them to the nursing home to await death. Life can seem hopeless and worthless to some older people when they enter a nursing home, but many older people admitted to nursing homes have the potential to be rehabilitated and can, with skilled care from a nurse-led multidisciplinary team, enjoy an enhanced quality of life within the nursing home.

This chapter aims to:

- Help you enable residents to regain abilities
- Help you enable residents to retain abilities
- Help you enable residents to function to capacity
- Enable you to enhance your residents' quality of life

The aims of rehabilitation are to enable the older person to recover from the major life event that necessitated their admission to the nursing home. In many cases a full recovery and subsequent discharge is not possible. It is possible, though, to help the older person to make as full a recovery as possible. The individual who regains skills and is able to carry out some aspects of care regains a measure of independence and an enhanced quality of life.

Assessing for rehabilitation

A full assessment should be carried out prior to the older person being admitted to the nursing home; details are given in Chapter 2. On admission this assessment should be reviewed as some time may have elapsed from assessment to admission, or the patient's condition may have changed rapidly. It is helpful if a dependency score is used. The dependency score provides a baseline assessment and it is then possible to determine progress by scoring again at a later date.

It is impossible to plan a rehabilitation programme without the consent and active participation of the patient. An extremely ill older person who has been admitted with a pressure sore may lack the will to begin a rehabilitation programme. It is important to talk to the individual and discover the individual's priorities. Basic needs such as freedom from pain, having sufficient food and fluids and being able to feel safe to express such needs, are normally the older person's first priorities. It is only possible to begin working towards rehabilitation when these basic needs have been met. The nurse, though, must plan ahead. If, for example, an older person has been admitted to the home immobile and suffering from a sacral pressure sore, the nurse must determine short and long-term goals.

The short-term goals would be to ensure that:

- Pain was controlled
- Psychological needs were met
- A diet with sufficient calories, protein and nutrients was offered and consumed
- Pressure relieving devices were used
- An appropriate dressing was used to promote wound healing.

The long term goals may include:

- Ensuring that suitable shoes are provided to correct shortening following surgery
- Organising physiotherapy to build muscle strength
- Ordering a walking frame.

You must work with the person to ensure that, while the most pressing needs are met quickly, work continues to meet long-term goals. In some cases the person and the professional will have differing priorities and goals. An older person with restricted mobility who enjoys reading and has lost her glasses may view her first priority as obtaining new glasses so that she can continue to keep in touch with the world by reading the paper. Your priority may be to take a wound swab and ensure that her pressure sore is not infected. The sensitive and aware nurse will balance nursing and the individual's priorities to ensure the individual's needs are met, and will work in partnership with the person towards common goals. The nurse who delays organising an optician's appointment for an older person may find that the older person becomes depressed and unwilling to eat or work with the nurse towards rehabilitation.

Barriers to rehabilitation

Nursing practice plays an important part in enabling older people to fulfil their full potential, and in preventing premature disablement and unnecessary dependence on nursing staff. Nursing can actively foster disability by discouraging older people from walking, by thoughtlessly placing obstacles in an older person's path, or by leaving walking frames, shoes and aids out of the older person's reach.

Nursing staff may encourage older people to rely on nursing staff pushing them around in wheelchairs 'because it's quicker' or because 'it must be such a struggle for poor Mary'. Some nursing staff move people who are able to transfer independently and insist on dressing people who are able to dress themselves slowly. These actions undermine an older person's abilities and foster a sense of powerlessness and apathy: 'What's the sense of trying; they'll only say I did it wrong'.

If the nurse is working with an older person to enable them to regain skills, it is vital that all nursing staff are aware of the rehabilitation programme and work together to support the older person. Staff must recognise that older people, like all others, have the right to struggle to regain skills if they so wish. The older person should be offered support and help in ways that do not undermine their efforts to regain skills. The older person should not be made to feel slow or clumsy, and effort and achievement should be praised. The manager's attitude is important to rehabilitation. A manager who stresses that beds must be made by a certain time, or baths completed by a certain time, places staff under pressure to speed up and have work completed to a fixed time-scale. Staff normally respond by encouraging older people to 'hurry up', and it is so much quicker to do something for an older person than to enable them to do it for themselves. In the end the needs of prematurely disabled residents will overwhelm staff, but by dressing Mary they get through the morning. Managers who wish to encourage older people to regain or retain self-care skills must be careful to ensure that staff do not feel pressurised to have tasks completed within a set time-scale.

The older person's relatives can actively undermine attempts at rehabilitation. Many relatives feel extremely guilty about their loved one living in a nursing home. Some family members can pressurise one member of the family (often a daughter or daughter-in-law) to take the older person home and provide care. Relatives in this position can feel extremely threatened by an older person regaining skills, as they may feel that staff are planning to discharge the older person to their care.

Some relatives feel that their loved one has entered a nursing home to be looked after. Nurses who encourage the older person to maintain or regain skills are, in the eyes of such relatives, failing to provide care. It is important to obtain the older person's consent and discuss the aims of any rehabilitation plan with relatives. Relatives who are aware of the advantages of rehabilitation and do not feel threatened by the older person's progress can work together with the older person, nurses and other professionals to enhance care and improve skills.

Enlisting the help of other professionals

Nurses do not possess all the skills required to help an older person rehabilitate. Nurses, though, because of the amount of patient contact they have, are in a unique position to assess the needs of an older person and to organise referral to other professionals. The older person benefits from a home where nurses co-ordinate and work with other professionals towards common goals which have been determined by the older person and the nurse.

Physiotherapy

Many older people benefit from physiotherapy, yet the pace of admission and discharge in hospitals today is so great that many have had little physiotherapy treatment during their hospital stay. The physiotherapist can advise older people on exercises that will improve muscle strength and help them regain function, or will prevent deformity following illness.

There are three methods of arranging physiotherapy services for individuals living in nursing homes. The first is to employ a part-time physiotherapist. Some homes employ one by placing an advertisement in the local paper. It is also possible to obtain details of physiotherapists in private practice from the local Yellow Pages. These physiotherapists typically charge, at the time of writing, from £30 to £45 for a 45 minute treatment session.

Most older people who live in homes are state funded and unable to afford to pay either a directly employed or a sessional physiotherapist. Some older people who have sufficient funds to meet their own fees may be able to afford private physiotherapy. Community physiotherapy is available from the NHS. Nurses are unable to request physiotherapy but can ask the individual's doctor to request it. Many community trusts have a standard physiotherapy referral form that the doctor must complete. You can obtain a supply of these from the local community physiotherapist and they can be kept at the home so that they are available to the individual's doctor when a referral is required. Taking a photocopy of the form and filing it in the older person's notes ensures that the nurse can readily supply a copy of the referral if the original gets lost in the post or at the community physiotherapy offices. You should make sure the referral is obtained and posted off as quickly as possible. There is normally a waiting list that varies nationally from three weeks to three months for an initial assessment.

The physiotherapist normally visits and makes an initial assessment and then decides how often the individual can have treatment. Unfortunately, while the numbers of older people living in nursing homes have increased greatly in recent years and the demands on the time of community physiotherapists have increased, there has not been a corresponding rise in the numbers of NHS community physiotherapists. You must ensure that the older person, all nursing staff and relatives if they wish to be involved, encourage and assist the older person with the physiotherapy programme. This involvement is crucial if any benefit is to be obtained from the extremely limited amount of NHS physiotherapy currently available to nursing home patients.

The limitations of nursing home-based physiotherapy

At the home where I am director of nursing we have a fully equipped physiotherapy department and employ two physiotherapists and one physiotherapy aid. Most nursing homes are small units; the average size is currently 39 beds. Average size nursing homes normally do not have the facilities that some older people require if they are to make an optimal recovery. Some of the larger corporate and voluntary sector homes have fully equipped physiotherapy facilities and equipment such as parallel bars.

Some older people find that their potential to regain skills is limited because equipment and resources are not available within the nursing home. It is possible in such circumstances to ask the community physiotherapist or the individual's doctor to refer to the hospital physiotherapy department. Some hospital physiotherapy departments are unenthusiastic about treating older people from nursing homes and the nurse needs to act as the older person's advocate, adopting a firm but polite stance. If the person is falling frequently you should find out if there is a falls prevention clinic in your area. The National Service Framework for Older People identifies falls as an area for action and recommends setting up fall clinics. Physiotherapy is one of the therapies available at falls clinics.

Useful addresses and telephone numbers

Local community physiotherapist

Private physiotherapist (if used)

Hospital physiotherapy department

Falls clinic

Communication problems

Many older people who are admitted to nursing homes have communication problems. These are a common feature of neurological disease and are commonly seen after strokes if the speech centre in the brain has been affected by the stroke. They can cause different types of problems and full details are provided in Chapter 12.

Speech and language therapists

Speech therapists are now known as speech and language therapists (SALTS). This change of name more accurately reflects their role, which is to work with people who have problems not only with speaking but also with understanding speech and interpreting written work. The nurse can refer individuals directly to the SALT in most areas of the UK, though it is wise to check local policy. SALTS have long fought to retain a policy of open access to their services. This policy ensures that individuals, parents (in the case of children), carers and professionals can readily obtain the services of SALTS. It means that the nurse can refer either by speaking to the SALT, leaving a message on an answerphone or writing a note.

While some community trusts employ SALTS, the majority are still based in hospital but cover a specific area of the community. The therapist normally makes an initial assessment visit, identifies the individual's problems, and plans care. SALTS can be asked if they wish to make notes in the individual's care plan. Most are keen to do so, and documenting the work of all professionals involved in an older person's care helps ensure continuity of care. The SALT works with the individual and the nursing staff involved in caring for the individual, to ensure that everyone is using the same methods to communicate, and working towards the same ends.

If primary nursing is used at the nursing home, the primary nurse should if possible be on duty when the initial assessment takes place. The therapist may give the individual details of exercises to be carried out to improve fine muscle control to the mouth and lips; a communication card may be supplied so that the individual can point to everyday items. You can begin a scrapbook that has one picture, such as a bath, on each page, with the word 'bath' written clearly and in large letters underneath. This can be used to increase the range of needs an individual can communicate.

SALTS normally decide how often they will visit after the initial assessment visit; it is usually once or twice weekly. Therapists emphasise that nursing staff have an important role to play in helping individuals with language problems to communicate, and they suggest that nurses ensure that all staff and relatives encourage the person to use language.

Obtaining aids

Many older people require aids to enable them to carry out the activities of daily living. A walking frame can enable an older person to walk safely around a home, and will reduce the risk of falling. Older people who are unable to grip walking frames, perhaps because of arthritis, can benefit from a gutter frame. Some older people lack the physical strength required to lift a frame, and benefit from a walking frame with wheels. Individuals who have suffered from strokes and who have a residual hemiplegia, or marked weakness of one arm, are seldom able to manage a walking frame. A tripod often helps such individuals to walk.

Individuals who suffer from arthritis, or other conditions which make it difficult for them to bend, can find a Helping Hand aid invaluable. This is a long, thin, flat, stainless steel aid that has two claw like pincers at the end. It can be used to pull up stockings, pick up items which are out of reach and even, with practice, change television channels.

The policy on obtaining aids varies from region to region. In some areas physiotherapists are responsible for ordering aids while in others this is the responsibility of the occupational therapist. It is important that individuals are assessed and the correct aid to help is selected. People come in all shapes and sizes and it is important that the walking frame supplied is the right height for the individual. Too high a frame on a small person encourages tip toe walking and poor balance, and can lead to falls. Too small a frame for a tall person leads to the individual hunching over the frame; this leads to poor posture and the individual tends to hang their head. This often means that the individual cannot see ahead clearly and can easily fall or collide with others. A walking frame with wheels is a boon to a weak arthritic individual but can be a hazard when supplied to an older person who tends to move fast. The individual can easily fall or collide with others. Some tripods have the facility for the handle to be turned around so that they can be used either right or left handed; others do not. The individual who has a hemiplegia should have a tripod supplied that is of a suitable height and is designed for the appropriate hand.

You should check who is responsible for supplying aids in your area and how these are obtained. In some areas you may be required to fill out a form and in others you may simply telephone or write a note asking for an assessment for the individual with a view to supplying a certain aid. It is important that older people are supplied with aids that are appropriate to their needs, but these can easily become mixed up in a home. Two individuals can sit down to lunch with their frames placed side by side; after lunch they could both pick up the wrong frame. The easiest way to ensure that individuals retain their own aids is to name each aid. This can appear very institutional so the nurse may prefer to label the underside of an aid. Some older people, though, prefer a large, clearly written or printed label to be visible on their aid, enabling them to identify it readily. Some older people prefer to personalise their aids in a variety of ways; some have stickers while others might prefer to have a ribbon or an artificial flower tied to the aid.

Useful address and telephone number

Person and department responsible for supplying aids

Obtaining repairs

Most community health trusts have a community supplies department (known in some areas as medical loans). This is often situated at the central offices of the community trust. The community supplies department normally keeps records of the names and addresses of individuals, and details of the aids supplied to them. The rubber ends which are attached to walking frames and tripods are called ferrules. These often wear down and the metal from the frame is in direct contact with the floor. Worn down ferrules destabilise frames and can predispose an individual to falls. All equipment can be returned to the community supplier department for repair. Unfortunately repairs can take some time; delays normally vary from three days to three weeks and are dependent on staffing levels and current workload. Community supplies departments will make every effort to supply replacement aids if repairs cannot be carried out quickly. If ferrules are worn down you can contact community supplies and give the individual's name, address and the aid; the supplies department can identify the type of aid and post ferrules to the home where these can be quickly replaced by the home's maintenance staff. It is not usually possible to remove ferrules from unused aids as there are several different sizes and fitting the wrong size can lead to accidents.

Useful address and telephone number

Community supplies department responsible for supplying and repairing aids

Wheelchairs

Some individuals bring their own wheelchairs to the home. Normally the community supplies department keeps a register of all individuals who have been issued with wheelchairs. You should inform community supplies, preferably in writing (and retain a copy of the letter), of the individual's change of address. This is important as contractors asked to repair wheelchairs are supplied with a list by community supplies and will only repair chairs if details of the individual match their records. Individuals who are admitted from out of the local area must have their chairs registered with the local community supplies department for the same reason.

In most areas the individual's doctor must complete a wheelchair request form before a wheelchair is supplied. The procedure varies from area to area. In some areas this form is sent to the physiotherapist who assesses and measures the individual and orders the appropriate wheelchair. In other areas the form is sent direct to community supplies who employ contractors to assess the individual, measure them and supply the appropriate wheelchair. Your local community supplies department or physiotherapist can advise you of local procedure.

Each home is supplied with a list of individuals and the type and serial number of each wheelchair. This list should be kept in a safe place. Each wheelchair should be identified with the individual's name. Some older people may wish to use stickers to personalise their wheelchairs. This often enables them to identify them more quickly.

It is important that the nurse ensures that wheelchairs are kept in a state of good repair. Flat tyres can make it difficult for individuals or nursing staff to propel the chairs. Tyres should have a reasonable amount of tread and will need replacing from time to time. Flat or badly worn tyres can affect the brakes and can mean that a chair can move despite the brakes being on. This can lead to falls and injury. Footplates should move easily and sides should slip off easily to enable older people to transfer easily. Chairs should fold without difficulty. Ensuring that wheelchairs are well maintained makes it easier for older people who are wheelchair dependent to move freely around the home. Relatives are also more willing to take an older person on trips and outings when they are not forced to struggle with a wheelchair which is difficult to push because of flat tyres, or is difficult to fold and place in the boot of the car.

The home's maintenance staff can ensure that tyres are pumped up and that moving parts are oiled. The policy for having repairs carried out varies from area to area. In some areas community health trust staff visit the home and carry out repairs or take the chair away for major repairs or replacement. In other areas the community trust has appointed contractors to carry out such repairs. The nurse should check what the arrangements are in the local area. When repairs are required you should contact the appropriate repair staff. Details of the individual's name and the wheelchair identification code are required. If you are unable to supply the serial number or identification code which has been supplied, repairs are delayed.

Useful address and telephone number

Local trust/contractor responsible for repairing wheelchairs

Exercise sessions

There has been a revolution in the provision of recreational facilities for residents in nursing homes over the last seven years. Now recreation is a high priority in homes, but exercise is not always considered to be recreation. Sometimes older people and their families think that people in nursing homes are too old or too frail to benefit from exercise.

Exercise is important at all ages and many older people benefit from regular exercise. Extend (Exercise Training for the Elderly and Disabled) is a registered charity which trains exercise teachers. EXTEND teachers specialise in working with older people. All older people, including those individuals who are wheelchair bound or extremely frail, can take part in

EXTEND classes. Music is an important part of the classes, which have a carefully graded programme of exercises tailored to the differing abilities of individuals within the class. The programme comprises a number of exercise sequences, each one exercising a different part of the body and all designed to mobilise muscles and joints. EXTEND teachers usually work on a sessional basis. You can obtain details about local EXTEND teachers from: EXTEND, 1a North Street, Sheringham, Norfolk NR26 8LJ. Tel. 01263 822479. A stamped addressed envelope is appreciated if requesting information.

Recreational activities

Recreational activities are important if the nursing home is to feel like home and not an institution. Older people who live in nursing homes come from many different backgrounds and have different interests. Recreational activities should reflect this. If possible the home should employ an activities co-ordinator to work with older people and nursing staff to organise a variety of activities. The activities co-ordinator can be a part-time appointment. If it is not possible to employ an activities co-ordinator it may be possible to find a volunteer or a number of volunteers who would be willing to co-ordinate activities within the home. Homes who employ an activities co-ordinator should also supplement this with volunteers and members of the local community. The local Citizens Advice Bureau (CAB) can give details of organisations that keep registers of volunteers willing to offer their time and skills. Local churches and organisations such as the Rotary Club are often keen to become involved in voluntary activities within the home.

Local clubs and societies may be willing to come to the home and give a talk or show slides. A local representative of the Royal Society for the Protection of Birds may be able to give a talk to the elderly bird-watcher. The older person who enjoys chess but cannot find anyone in the home to play may find a partner from the local chess club who will come in and play. Volunteers come from all walks of life, newly retired people, people who are studying for professional qualifications part-time, mothers of school age children and unemployed people all offer a wealth of skills. One volunteer may be able to offer painting lessons, another flower arranging, another may be able to play the piano (if the home has one) or an electronic organ, and offer sing-songs. Volunteers can also befriend individuals who do not have a family and can visit for a chat. An older person who has a particular interest and who is visited by a member of, for example, the local amateur photographer's association may become involved in the social activities of the group. Activities and involvement with local groups can enrich an older person's life, and a life that has seemed empty and worthless can become full and enjoyable.

Government have emphasised the importance of volunteers in all walks of life and have designated 2002 as the year of the volunteer. You are now required under national minimum standards to provide volunteers with induction and support and to check references because they have access to vulnerable adults.

Many people when they consider recreational activities think of group activities. Individual activities and activities involving small groups are also important. Many older people find it difficult to take part in activities because of disabilities. It is possible to get games which have been modified to enable people with poor vision or poor muscle control to take part, for example, Scrabble is available with large tiles, and larger than normal playing cards are available.

Reading

Many older people enjoy reading. Library books and a range of daily newspapers should be available in the home. Local councils provide a special service to nursing homes. Normally the home registers with the local library service, and the librarian visits and explains about the range of books available. There are thousands of titles available in large print, and most of the books delivered can be large print. Normally the library offers a selection of books such as crime, adventure, romance, historical, etc. The nurse can ask older people what type of books they like and who their favourite authors are. The library service will include these books in the selection sent to the home. Library books are normally changed every three months but the service can visit more frequently if required.

Useful address and telephone number

Local library service

Books and newspapers for the blind

Many older people who are no longer able to read can still enjoy books and newspapers. Many books are available on tape and cassette and are provided by the Talking Book Service. Individuals must be registered as blind or partially sighted to qualify for this service. The local council is required to keep a register of such individuals. Nurses who wish to obtain Talking Book services on behalf of individuals should contact the local council who can supply details.

A local member of the Royal National Institute for the Blind normally visits the individual and notes the reading/listening preferences; these are used to choose suitable books. Tapes are posted to the individual in a padded plastic pouch; when the tape is to be returned the label is reversed (the sender's address is printed on the back) and the package returned post free.

The Royal National Institute for the Blind (RNIB) can provide details of the local Talking Books group and can offer help and advice on recreational activities for blind and partially sighted individuals. Contact RNIB, 224 Great Portland Street, London W1N 6AA. Tel. 020 7388 1266.

Useful address and telephone number

Talking Books service

Films and television programmes

Many older people visited the cinema frequently in their youth. They often enjoy watching films from the 1930s, 1940s and 1950s. Many films that interest older people are shown either mid afternoon or very late at night. In the afternoon the home can be busy or visitors can interrupt an enjoyable film. If the home has a video recorder, staff (and relatives) should be encouraged to find out what type of films the older people enjoy and to record these films. Video hire shops often stock older type films that can be hired inexpensively. Showing films in the evening can encourage older people to sit up, chat and enjoy an evening's entertainment.

Music

Music has a powerful effect on mood and many people enjoy listening to their favourite music. Older people can be encouraged to bring their favourite records and tapes and these can be played in the lounge, the dining area or in the individual's room. Many older people enjoy hearing music played quietly in the dining room at meal times.

Outings

Everyone enjoys going out and older people are no exception. It need not involve a great deal of planning. You should encourage individuals living in the home to get out and about. Many nursing home residents are unable to go out alone. Nursing staff and relatives should be encouraged to take the older person out of the home. A trip to the local coffee shop, a visit to a shop to choose toiletries, or popping into the pub for a pint, can be enjoyable trips out. Relatives would often like to have their loved one home for tea or a meal at weekends, but hesitate to suggest this to nursing staff. Nursing staff who work with relatives can suggest that the family might wish to take the individual on outings. Local churches, charities and other organisations often arrange special trips for older people living in nursing homes. You should encourage such invitations; staff, relatives and volunteers can help at such events if required.

Working with residents

Establishing regular meetings with residents enables nurses to ensure that all services within the home, including recreational services, meet the needs of individuals living in the home.

Celebrations and special occasions

It is important that individuals are able to continue celebrating special occasions such as Christmas, Easter and birthdays when they live in nursing homes. Older people and their families should be involved in planning such events. Providing a cake and cards and singing Happy Birthday can make an older person who entered the nursing home fearful and apprehensive, finally feel that they are 'at home' and among friends.

Conclusion

Many older people who enter nursing homes benefit from rehabilitation, which can improve quality of life. The older person and nurse can work together to determine the aims and priorities of the older person. The nurse can co-ordinate and continue the work of other professionals to enable older people to fulfil their potential. Rehabilitation and activities can transform an older person's life and enable the individual to lead a full life within the home. The nurse's role is essential to this process.

Chapter 19

The Way Forward

What does the future hold for nursing homes?

Nursing homes are entering a period of great uncertainty. The number of homes is falling and there are bed shortages in some areas.

Impact of political and legislative changes

Many of the changes predicted in the first edition of this book are now being introduced. The Care Standards Act (see Chapter 1) will change the way homes are inspected. Homes will now work to new standards and there are fears that some of these standards will drive homes to close. Some of the new standards will require a lot of investment but homes are poorly funded and may not be able to borrow money to upgrade.

The growth of large homes

The amount that social services departments pay for care has fallen in real terms in recent years but the impact of the shortage of registered nurses and the impact of the minimum wage have raised the costs of delivering care. These changes mean that many small homes are no longer economically viable. Already some homes have closed and bed shortages are developing in some areas. Some larger providers from both the independent and voluntary sector are closing their small homes and building larger homes because they can benefit from economies of scale.

When homes become larger there are fewer of them and relatives, especially in rural areas may have to travel some distance to the home. The larger a home, the more difficult it becomes to offer personal care. Inspectors and health authorities no longer seek to limit the size of homes because they realise that the drive to meet new standards is forcing homes to become larger merely to survive.

The challenge now is for providers to ensure that new homes are built in ways that enable nurses to care for people well. This means that homes should be built so that they are subdivided into smaller units. Some providers are meeting this challenge by providing homes that are divided into separate floors, wings or units so that the home does not begin to resemble the large geriatric hospitals that we left behind.

When homes become large, the role of the manager changes; it is much more difficult to be 'hands on' and work with staff when you have responsibility for 80, 100 or 300 people. The challenge for managers is to ensure that they remain accessible to staff and residents and develop the talents of staff to enable them to nurse well. Managers need to develop systems that enable staff to operate on a human scale and provide individualised care even in larger homes.

Inspection

The merging of social services and health authority inspection units to create an independent inspection unit will mean that homes that were formerly 'dual registered', caring for people in residential and nursing beds, will have a single inspection. Inspectors will have training and education to enable them to carry out their role and inspection will no longer be seen as a 'job for life' but merely a step on a career path. Inspectors will in future concentrate on the same standards as those outlined in national minimum standards. There is a danger that the nursing voice will be lost in the newly merged inspectorate and that non-nurses will inspect and comment on nursing care.

Changes in medical care

Government are pushing forward huge changes in primary care. Primary care groups have been created and primary care trusts are now beginning to emerge. The National Service Frameworks for Older People, Diabetes, Coronary Heart Disease and Chronic Obstructive Airways Disease have set GPs targets in health promotion and disease management. Older people will benefit from more proactive medical care but GPs may find their workload much heavier. The scene is set for the introduction of gerontological nurse specialists and nurse practitioners to begin working with homes via Primary Care Groups (PCGs) and Trusts (PCTs) and the newer Care Trusts. When PCG/Ts and Care Trusts begin to pool budgets they may realise the importance of using consultant geriatricians to support GPs and improve the health of older people living in homes. This would avoid unnecessary hospital admissions.

Changes in the education of registered nurses

The National Boards that were responsible for validating nurse education courses, such as the ENB 941 in Care of the Older Person, have now gone. Nurse education is no longer constrained by the National Boards and it is possible for universities to develop educational modules and pathways that lead to degree and master's level qualifications. South Bank University is now developing a degree and master's degree in gerontology concentrating on the nursing home sector[1].

Role of staff with National Vocational Qualifications (NVQs)

National minimum standards require homes to ensure that 50% of care assistants have an NVQ level 2 qualification by 2004. The NVQ level 2 qualification enables care assistants to care. The NVQ level 3 qualification is a more in-depth qualification and closely mirrors the old two-year enrolled nurse qualification, though there are gaps. Now NVQ level 3 qualifications are becoming more valued. People with NVQ qualifications have the entry qualifications for nurse education. At the moment some universities are offering people with NVQ level 3 qualifications accelerated nurse education programmes. The person with an NVQ level 3 enters the common foundation programme halfway through. These are pilot projects and will be evaluated within the next few years.

We are facing the worst shortages of registered nurses in living memory and some inspectors are suggesting that managers use NVQ level 3 staff to provide additional support to registered nurses. In some areas inspectors are saying you must have three registered nurses on an early shift or two registered nurses and one NVQ level 3. The suggestion is not that the NVQ level 3 is equivalent to a registered nurse, but that the contribution made by an experienced level 3 who knows the residents is preferable to using an agency nurse who does not know residents.

The 2002 NHS pay award recognised the contribution of NVQ qualified staff for the first time by paying a premium of £400 a year to NVQ qualified staff. Some homes already pay a premium to NVQ qualified staff; others will follow because NVQ staff increasingly expect a differential over non-NVQ qualified care assistants.

It is important to work with care assistant colleagues and to remember that they are an aid not a substitute for the registered nurse.

Growing inequalities

Devolution is leading to growing inequalities in care for older people. In Scotland older people who have savings and property above income support levels receive a large percentage of the costs of care. In Wales registered nursing care is paid at a flat rate. In England there is assessment and banding. We have one unified tax system but three funding systems. The English system has been condemned as unfair and it may well be unsustainable.

Future growth?

Government statistics suggest that by 2011 over a million people will be aged over 85 and we will need a 65% increase in home capacity in order to care for them. If diseases such as Alzheimer's are not conquered and if older people continue to have a period of disability in their final years, there will be a huge shortage of places. Government may have to encourage the growth of homes to provide care.

The future is uncertain but what we do know is that the registered nurse makes a huge difference to the quality of life of older people and will continue to do so. The challenge now is to have the government and professionals recognise the unique contribution that the registered nurse makes to an older person's quality of life.

Reference

[1] For details contact Allan Hicks. Tel. 020 7815 4785. email hicksa@sbu.ac.uk

Index